DISCOVER THE CARDIAC CARE PLAN THAT HAS HELPED THOUSANDS OF HEART-DISEASE SUFFERERS!

Let Dr. Julian Whitaker show you how to reverse heart disease by:

- Following a heart-healthy diet that is low in fat and high in fiber
- Taking nutritional supplements, such as Vitamins E and C and Niacin
- Exercising regularly to condition the heart and improve brain function
- Getting a handle on negative emotions to ease stress and depression
- Using natural hormone therapy to fight heart disease in men and women
- Harnessing intense therapies such as EECP for advanced disease

DR. JULIAN WHITAKER'S

REVERSING HEART DISEASE

"Well-documented and understandable . . . used in concert with regular visits to a physician, Whitaker's book may set the ailing heart patient on the road to recovery."
—*Booklist*

"Brimming with recipes, yes, but much, much more . . . could help extend the life of heart patients *without surgery.*"
—*Philadelphia Daily News*

"A [illegible] le changes that may limit and eve[illegible] . . worthwhile."
—*Kirkus Reviews*

Also by Julian Whitaker, M.D., and Warner Books

Reversing Hypertension
Reversing Diabetes

REVERSING HEART DISEASE

A VITAL NEW PROGRAM TO HELP PREVENT, TREAT, AND ELIMINATE CARDIAC PROBLEMS *WITHOUT SURGERY*

JULIAN WHITAKER, M.D.

WARNER BOOKS

An AOL Time Warner Company

NOTE: Dr. Julian Whitaker is a medical doctor with extensive experience in the fields of preventive medicine and natural healing. Although recommendations in this book have met stringent criteria for safety and effectiveness, they have not been reviewed by the U.S. Food and Drug Administration. Dr. Whitaker's recommendations are not intended to replace the advice of your physician, and you are encouraged to seek advice from a competent medical professional for your personal health needs.

Warner Books, Inc., 1271 Avenue of the Americas, New York, NY 10020

Visit our Web site at www.twbookmark.com.

 An AOL Time Warner Company

Printed in the United States of America

First Printing: March 2002

10 9 8 7 6 5 4 3 2

Library of Congress Cataloging-in-Publication Data
Whitaker, Julian M.
Reversing heart disease / Julian Whitaker.—Rev. ed.
p. cm.
Includes bibliographical references.
ISBN 0-446-67657-8 (alk. paper)
1. Coronary heart disease—Treatment. 2. Coronary heart disease—Prevention. 3. Coronary heart disease—Diet therapy. 4. Coronary heart disease—Exercise therapy. I. Title

RC685.C6 W473 2002
616.1'23—dc21 2001053614

I would like to dedicate this book to any and all individuals who read it, use it, and in any way, shape or form benefit from that experience

Contents

Part III: The Whitaker Wellness Institute Program for Reversing Heart Disease

Part IV: The Dietary Program for Reversing Heart Disease

Part V: The Program in Action

Acknowledgments

This book could not have been written without the enormous contribution of the hundreds of scientists who have published thousands of pages of research on heart disease. It is unfortunate that much of this important research has failed to have an impact on clinical medicine—simply because it runs counter to prevailing beliefs and practices. It would be impossible for me to cite each of these individuals, but they have my utmost respect and admiration for their contributions.

Closer to home, I want to thank Peggy Dace for her help in updating this book. I would also like to acknowledge Kelly Griffin for her research and editing, Tammy Faridi and Stacey Murray for their fact-checking, Elena Granofsky for typing portions of the manuscript, and Diane Lara, who compiled the recipes and menus that make up an important part of this book. My editors at Warner Books (Diana Baroni for the second edition and Bernie Shir-Cliff and Marge Schwartz for the first edition) were extremely patient, tolerant, and helpful through multiple revisions. And a special thanks is due to Dr. Henry McIntosh for his invaluable editorial input in the hardcover edition.

Last but not least, I owe a firm debt of gratitude to everyone who has completed the program for reversing heart disease—my patients at the Whitaker Wellness Institute and the people who read the first edition of this book, put the program into action, and shared their successes with me. These people have validated the principles outlined in this book by dramatically improving their health and enhancing the quality of their lives. The credit is theirs, and their experiences and inspiring stories are what motivated me to write this book.

Foreword to Revised Edition

The one constant in life is change, and this is certainly evident as I look back on everything that has happened in medicine and particularly in the area of heart disease since I wrote the first edition of *Reversing Heart Disease*. The scientific literature on the understanding and treatment of heart disease has exploded, and so has our access to it. When I was writing the first edition of this book, I spent hours and hours in the medical library, poring over musty volumes of scientific studies and scribbling notes on yellow legal pads. Today I have instant access to ten million studies through the National Library of Medicine's Web site.

In the mid-1980s, we were just beginning to understand how arterial blockages developed. In the intervening years, dozens of biochemical interactions involved in this complex process have been identified. Back then, elevated cholesterol was felt to be the sole cause of heart disease. Today we know it is only one of a number of factors that contribute to this multifaceted condition. In the past seventeen years new screening tests have been developed, scores of new drugs have been introduced, and new surgical techniques have been perfected for the treatment of heart disease.

Yet the more things change, the more they stay the same. Although thousands of studies demonstrating the powerful therapeutic effects of nutrition and exercise have been published since

I wrote the first edition of this book, most physicians pay them little heed. Cardiologists still have the same inclination to prescribe lifelong drug regimens. And despite the well-documented proof that bypass surgery and angioplasty do not save lives, prevent heart attacks, or improve quality of life for the vast majority of patients undergoing these procedures, they are being performed in record numbers.

One positive trend I have observed has been a dramatic increase in patient interest in diet, nutritional supplementation, and other safe, noninvasive therapies. Patients are no longer content to meekly follow their doctors' orders. They are much better educated than they used to be, and far more proactive. Fewer Americans are smoking, we're eating less fat, and our average cholesterol level has dropped considerably. Although heart disease remains our number one killer, rates of death from heart disease have declined significantly during the past seventeen years, and the credit goes not to doctors, drugs, or surgeries but to the people who have made these positive changes in their lives.

When I first wrote *Reversing Heart Disease* and described the lifestyle program I was using to treat patients with serious diseases, the Whitaker Wellness Institute was only six years old. Just a few years before, I had been in the middle of a residency in orthopedic surgery, when doubts about my chosen profession assailed me. I wasn't sure how satisfied I could be as a surgeon. I preferred patient interaction to the drama of surgery, and I was disturbed by the inside politicking aimed at getting hospital privileges and patient referrals. I decided to take a year or two off from my residency—with the full intention of returning and completing my surgical training.

Cut loose from specialty training, I was free to use the most valuable skill to be acquired in a medical education: the ability to use the medical library. And what I learned as I delved into the research on nutrition and exercise—which I had not been told about in medical school—radically altered the way I practice medicine. I never did return to the confines of conventional medicine, and I've never looked back.

The Whitaker Wellness Institute is now twenty-three years old, and more than 30,000 patients have come to the clinic for medical evaluation and treatment, education, and help in implementing lifestyle changes. I continue to use exercise, diet, and nutritional supplements as my primary therapies, and this treatment program continues to be unbelievably effective. By adhering to these simple, inexpensive therapies, blood pressure routinely plummets, risk factors for heart disease improve, blood sugar normalizes, and aches and pains disappear. Time and time again patients are able to get off prescription drugs and even opt out of surgery.

This book is a product not only of my experience in treating all these patients, but also of thirty years of continued research into the latest data on nutrition, exercise, and other nonconventional therapies. My work with heart patients has been exciting and fascinating because it has been new territory. I could never have acquired the special knowledge or developed the treatment program we use at the Whitaker Wellness Institute if I had not struck out in my own direction.

As a physician, I take pleasure in watching people undertake a diet, exercise, and supplement program and begin to understand what true health and optimal well-being are all about. Interest in these modalities has increased dramatically over the years, and some of what was considered alternative when I wrote this book seventeen years ago is now mainstream. My approach to heart disease will not put established medicine out of business, nor would I want it to. Improvements will continue to be made in diagnostic tools, surgical techniques, and drugs—marvelous developments when used appropriately. But we must remember that these high-tech modalities are aimed at the treatment of symptoms, not the causes of illness.

I have revised this book for the same reasons I wrote it in the first place. In order to prevent or reverse heart disease you must have a basic understanding of what causes it and how various treatments work—for you are in charge of the treatment yourself. Hurling yourself into a nutrition and exercise program without guidance and information may do more harm than good. This book is designed for use with your own physician. It provides you with a step-by-step program designed to produce the maximum results that can be reasonably expected from lifestyle changes. This book is not intended to challenge your physician's role in your treatment; rather, it is designed to help your doctor help you. Many cardiologists are very supportive of the principles in this book, but their practices and responsibilities make it difficult for them to help their patients understand and implement them. *Reversing Heart Disease* simply provides both you and your physician with the proper tools to improve your health.

An extremely complex and costly technology for the management of coronary heart disease has evolved, involving specialized ambulances and hospital units, all kinds of electronic gadgetry and whole platoons of new professional personnel to deal with the end results of coronary thrombosis. Almost everything offered today for the treatment of heart disease is at this level of technology, with the transplanted and artificial hearts as ultimate examples. When enough has been learned for us to know what really goes wrong in heart disease, we ought to be in a position to figure out ways to prevent or reverse the process; and when this happens, the current elaborate technology will be set to one side.[1]

—Dr. Lewis Thomas

Unless the doctors of today become the dieticians of tomorrow, the dieticians of today will become the doctors of tomorrow.[2]

—Alexis Carrel

The doctor of the future will give no medicine, but will interest his patient in the care of the human frame, in diet, and in the cause and prevention of disease.[3]

—Thomas A. Edison

It appears to me necessary for every physician to be skilled in nature and to strive to know, if he would wish to perform his duties, what man is in relation to the articles of food and drink and to his other occupations, and what are the effects of each of them on everyone. Whoever does not know what effects these things produce upon man cannot know the consequences which result from them. Whoever pays no attention to these things, or paying attention to them does not comprehend them, how can he understand the diseases which befall man? For by every one of these things a man is affected and changed this way and that, and the whole of his life is subjected to them—whether in health, convalescence, or disease. Nothing else, then, can be more important and necessary than to know these things.[4]

—Hippocrates

PART I

Heart Disease: Causes and Controversies

CHAPTER 1

The American Way to Die

HEART DISEASE IS NOT A TRENDY DISEASE. PEOPLE DON'T WEAR brightly colored ribbons on their lapels to announce their support of the fight against this disease. Few celebrities lend their names to the cause, and there are no highly publicized, star-studded fund-raisers to underwrite research in this field. Unlike those with cancer or other newsworthy diseases, people who die of heart disease are rarely touted as courageous fighters or unfortunate victims. If there is a big story about heart disease, it's because someone famous has died of a heart attack or there is some "breakthrough" new heart drug or surgical procedure. Heart disease per se is simply not newsworthy.

Yet more Americans die of heart disease than any other cause. More than twelve million Americans have been diagnosed with heart disease, and half a million succumb to this condition annually.[5] While such deaths have declined rather dramatically in the past thirty-five years, heart disease is and will continue to be a major cause of death and disability, not only in the United States and other developed nations but throughout the world, as developing countries adopt a Western diet and lifestyle habits.

It's time we move heart disease into the spotlight—where our number one killer surely belongs. It is important for you to realize that this disease is not just a malady of the elderly. It isn't the merciful release at the end of a long life. Heart disease is killing people in the prime of life. It is the fatal tragedy you read about daily in the obituary section of your newspaper; it kills without warning. And when it doesn't kill it often disables, burdening its victims with chest pain, shortness of breath, and fears of an impending heart attack.

But common as death from heart disease is, it is no more natural than death by gunshot or car accident. The high rate of heart disease in this country is a distinctly unnatural phenomenon. I'm always taken aback when I hear that a person in his or her fifties or sixties has died of "natural causes" (which almost always translates into heart disease). There is nothing natural about dying of heart disease at this age.

WHAT IS HEART DISEASE?

Before we go further, let's define what heart disease is. It is, of course, a type of cardiovascular disease, a very broad category that encompasses dozens of diseases of the heart and blood vessels. Hypertension, or elevated blood pressure, for example, is a very prevalent and significant cardiovascular disease, but it isn't the focus of this book—although we will touch on it repeatedly, for it is a very significant risk factor for heart disease. Congestive heart failure, an inability of the heart to adequately circulate blood caused by a weakening of the heart muscle, is likewise an often-coexisting condition, but it isn't what we commonly refer to as heart disease. Nor is atrial fibrillation or other heart rhythm disturbances.

When we talk about heart disease, we are generally referring to the following:

Atherosclerosis: Buildup of arterial plaque (deposits of fat cholesterol, white blood cells, smooth muscle cells, and fibrous tissue) in the arteries, which damages and narrows them.

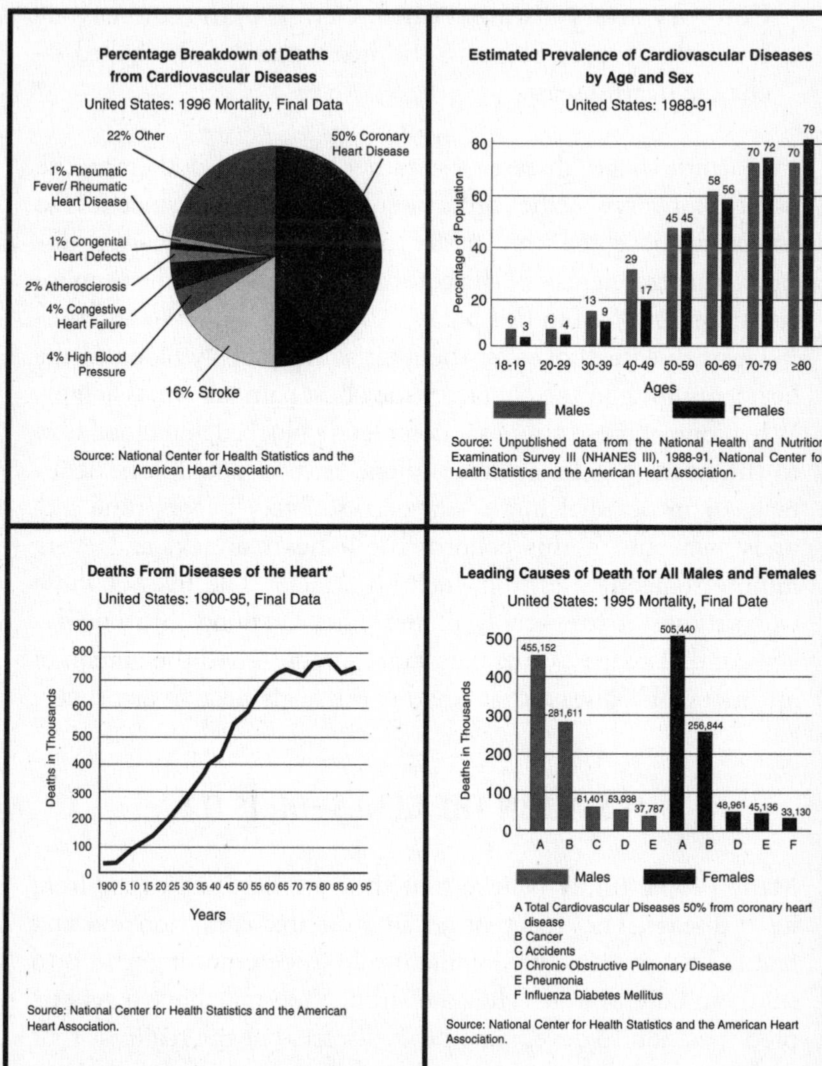

1998 Heart and Stroke Statistics Update, American Heart Association.

FIGURE 1: Heart Disease Is Our #1 Killer.

Coronary artery disease: Atherosclerosis of the coronary arteries that supply blood to the heart muscle; also called ischemic heart disease.

In truth, heart disease is a rather simplistic and imprecise name for a very specific cardiovascular disorder, but since it is so commonly accepted—and easier to say than coronary artery disease or atherosclerosis of the coronary arteries—it is the term we will use most often in this book.

Heart disease chokes off the arteries that supply blood to the heart, resulting in the characteristic chest pain known as angina. When one of these arteries is completely blocked and blood flow to the heart muscle, or myocardium, is interrupted, a heart attack, or myocardial infarction, occurs. Every twenty-nine seconds someone in this country has a heart attack, and every minute someone dies from such an attack.[6] The lives of those who survive are irrevocably altered. They are flung onto a merry-go-round of surgery, drugs, and more surgery—and the burden of an "incurable" disease that could rear its ugly head at any time.

IT'S ALL IN THE GENES—OR IS IT?

Many people firmly believe that they are destined to die from heart disease. They feel that it is an inherited condition and that family history plays the dominant role in determining who is to suffer and die from it. They are wrong. You may have a genetic predisposition to developing heart disease, but the reality is that for the overwhelming majority, heart disease is a lifestyle disease, and family history plays only a secondary role.

Yet it is easy to see why this disease is thought to be inherited. Since heart disease is our leading cause of death, it is hard to find a family that has escaped its clutches. If your father, uncle, grandmother, and brother all die from a heart attack, concerns about your own fate are understandable. However, just because heart disease strikes many families does not mean that genes are the only factor at work. A perfect example of this is heart disease risk among Japanese immigrants to the United States. In Japan, the incidence of heart disease is much lower than in this country. However, when Japanese move to the United States and adopt our diet and lifestyle, within one generation their rate of heart disease dramatically escalates, approaching that of Americans. If heart disease were primarily an inherited disease, the protection afforded the native Japanese would come with them to this country.

True, there is an inherited tendency in a small group of individuals for extremely high cholesterol levels, which is a risk factor for heart disease. Such individuals generally have cholesterol levels above 300, and many of them do indeed die prematurely from heart disease. However, while one in five Americans die from heart disease, this genetic trait occurs in only about one of every 500, so it is obviously not a significant factor for the overwhelming majority with heart disease.

Even more important, people who have inherited a tendency toward elevated cholesterol have not inherited atherosclerosis. Plaques must develop in their arteries, just as they develop in the rest of us. And unlike hemophilia or other truly inherited diseases that can be traced to a single defective gene, heart disease isn't just about high cholesterol levels. It is multifactorial, as we will discuss in the next chapter, and you can control most of the risk factors associated with it. For some of you, the task may be more challenging than for others, but for no one is death from heart disease a foregone conclusion.

RISK FACTORS YOU CAN'T CONTROL

Although genetics is only a secondary determinant in whether you'll die of heart disease, it is one of several factors beyond your control that do to some degree place you at increased risk of heart disease. Here are some others.

Age

Not surprisingly, advancing age increases your risk of heart disease. The wear and tear on the heart and arteries caused by normal metabolic processes accumulates with age. Just as your skin wrinkles and your hair turns gray, these age-associated changes are inevitable. However, there are things you can do to slow down the aging of the cardiovascular system, and we will discuss them in this book.

One thing you need to realize is that even though heart disease is more likely to manifest as a heart attack later in life, the process of atherosclerosis begins at a tender age. This was first made clear in 1953 in a landmark study published in the *Journal of the American Medical Association.* Researchers examined the coronary arteries of healthy soldiers averaging age twenty-two, who had been killed in combat during the Korean War, and reported the presence of advanced atherosclerotic lesions in the coronary arteries of a majority of these young men.[7] Subsequent studies found fatty streaks (beginning stages of plaque) in the arteries of children during their first decade of life, indicative of early atherosclerosis.[8]

Sex

The sterotypical heart attack victim is a hardworking, driven, middle-aged male—and the reality isn't too far from this popular image. By the age of sixty, one in five American men will have had some type of coronary event, compared to only one in seventeen women of similar age. After this age, however, the gap closes. Both men and women over age sixty have a one-in-four chance of dying from heart disease.[9]

The reduced risk of heart disease among younger women has long been attributed to the protective effects of estrogen.

Men and Women: Different at Heart

For years the research on heart disease primarily involved male study subjects. It was just assumed that what's good for the gander was good for the goose. Now that more studies include both genders (and some, such as the ongoing Nurses' Health Study, are limited strictly to women), we know that—surprise!—men and women are not the same. Here are some of the more significant gender differences regarding heart disease:

- Only one in seventeen women under the age of sixty will have a heart attack, compared to one in five men. After age sixty, one in four men and women die of heart disease.[10]
- Heart attacks are more lethal in women than in men. Thirty-eight percent of women who have a heart attack die within a year, compared to 25 percent of men.[11]
- An elevated level of triglycerides is one of the most significant predictors of heart disease in women—but not in men.[12]
- Diabetes is an even stronger risk factor for heart disease in women than in men.
- Although elevated LDL cholesterol is a risk factor for women, it is not as significant as it is for men. A low HDL level, on the other hand, is directly related to risk of heart disease in women, and even small rises in HDL confer protection.
- The symptoms of a heart attack in women are sometimes different from those in men, often less severe and more likely to be felt as something other than chest pain. Women also tend to take longer to get to a hospital after first experiencing symptoms.

(In Chapter 17 we will examine the latest research on this.) Interestingly, although the death rate from heart disease has fallen off rather dramatically in the past three decades, declines among men have outpaced those of women. One likely explanation is smoking—women just aren't quitting at the rate men are. Another reason is rising rates of obesity, which climbed by 38 percent from 1980 to 1990, with women leading the pack.[13]

Race

There are racial differences in rates of death from heart disease. For African American males the mortality rate is 20 percent higher than for Caucasian males, and deaths among African American females outstrip Caucasian females by 31 percent—until the age of sixty-five, when the Caucasians' likelihood of having a heart attack surpasses the African Americans'. Much of this is due to the fact that African Americans are twice as likely to have high blood pressure as Caucasians, and 20 to 30 percent of them die from complications of hypertension. Native Americans and Latinos are also at increased risk of heart attack, as are people of South Asian descent. Chinese- and Japanese-Americans, on the other hand, have lower rates of cardiovascular disease than those of European extraction.

The reasons for these differences will likely be uncovered as advances continue to be made in unlocking the human genome. However, I have no doubt that other factors are instrumental here as well. Poverty, stress, cultural food preferences, and other differences must also be considered. All told, the role of race in the etiology of heart disease is far less important than lifestyle factors.

If your family tree is riddled with heart disease, if you are in a high-risk ethnic group, if you are male, or if you are over age sixty, don't despair. Let this knowledge motivate you to implement the lifestyle changes outlined in this book. The bottom line is that of the top ten factors identified as increasing the risk of heart disease, only three are outside the sphere of your influence. You hold the reins of the others. You can prevent and reverse heart disease, and I'll show you how.

OUR UNPRECEDENTED LIFESTYLE

If heart disease is not inherited or caused strictly by race, age, or gender, why do so many of us have it? In a word, lifestyle. The way we live is unprecedented in human history. Unlike our prehistoric ancestors, we are no longer required to engage in strenuous physical activity merely to survive. We don't spend the better part of our days hunting or foraging for food—we drive to the grocery store. Yet the human body needs exercise. Without it our muscles atrophy, our hearts weaken, and our overall health suffers.

Our diets have also changed dramatically. Our earliest ancestors ate indigenous plants and, when times were good, wild game (which is extremely low in fat compared to today's feedlot animals). About 10,000 years ago agrarian societies emerged, and humans added to their diet cultivated grains and produce, along with milk and meat from domesticated livestock. There were few concentrated sources of sugar or fat, and foods were eaten in their natural state.

Skip to the twenty-first century. Americans consume on the average 34 percent of their calories as fat and eat 152 pounds of sugar a year. We eat bacon and eggs or sugary cereals for breakfast, hamburgers for lunch, and hearty dinners centered around a slab of meat—downed with sodas and topped off with sugar-laden desserts. We are conditioned to the tastes and consistency of the foods we have eaten since childhood. A thick, juicy steak not only tastes good but is a not-so-subtle statement that "all is well." And the reward for good behavior or a clean plate? Cookies, cake, and ice cream.

Other lifestyle factors are at play in the etiology of heart disease, including smoking, excess weight, immoderate use of alcohol, and psychological issues such as unmanaged stress, anger, and depression. So are diseases like high blood pressure, high cholesterol and triglyceride levels, syndrome X, and diabetes, which are themselves largely attributable to poor diet and lack of exercise. Of course, there are some factors that are beyond your control, as we discussed above. But for the most part, the things you do—or don't do—every day are the primary contributors to heart disease and other chronic illnesses that plague modern America.

LIFESTYLE CHANGES: STRONG MEDICINE

Dismal as the current statistics on heart disease are, I don't want to paint too dark a picture. Strides have been made in reducing the incidence of heart disease in the past thirty-five years. Deaths from heart attack peaked in 1968 and, except for a few bumps in the road, have been on a downward curve ever since.

The medical community has been quick to take responsibility for this decline, pointing to high-tech diagnostics, more drugs, and improved surgical techniques. Yet regardless of how loudly conventional medicine toots its own horn, the truth is that the downward trend in heart disease stems primarily from changes in lifestyle.

In the mid-1980s, the World Health Organization mounted an international study to determine the factors responsible for the dropping rates of heart disease. Called the Multinational Monitoring of Trends and Determinants in Cardiovascular Disease (MONICA), this large, long-term research endeavor involved the efforts of hundreds of researchers from twenty-one countries around the world. In a 1999 analysis of this study, researchers concluded that although improvements had been made in the medical treatment of patients who had had a heart attack, two-thirds of the decline in the death rate were attributable to reductions in coronary events such as heart attacks.[14] In other words, although some lives were saved by medical management, the primary reason behind the drop in deaths from heart disease was that fewer people were having heart attacks in the first place.

In another arm of the MONICA project, researchers set out to determine exactly what was responsible for this reduction in the incidence of heart attacks. What factors really made the difference? The answers were clear: a decline in smoking and improvements in blood pressure and cholesterol levels.[15] Each and every one of these factors is related to lifestyle choices, illustrating that lifestyle changes are very powerful medicine indeed.

HEART DISEASE IS NOT INEVITABLE

While these trends are encouraging, heart disease remains our number one cause of death. However, as I hope I have made clear, it is far from inevitable. Its causes are reasonably well understood, and steps to prevent its onset are universally acknowledged. Even more encouraging, scientific research proves that if you already have heart disease, it is possible to reverse its progress and restore your cardiovascular system to a healthier state.

How? Well, here is where I part company with conventional medicine, with its emphasis on drugs and surgery. I have been practicing medicine for almost thirty years, and for most of that time I have specialized in the treatment of heart disease, hypertension, and diabetes. Long ago I came to the realization that heart disease and other degenerative diseases can be treated successfully with safe, noninvasive, natural therapies.

As a young physician I undertook an intensive study of the medical literature and unearthed research that changed the way I practice medicine. I discovered that the negative effects of many of the drugs prescribed to patients with heart disease outweighed their benefits. I learned that the effectiveness of bypass surgery and angioplasty was questionable when compared to a more conservative treatment course. And I found that millions of patients were being frightened into having these unnecessary and potentially harmful invasive procedures.

Most important, I discovered the power of low-tech, inexpensive lifestyle changes in the prevention and treatment of heart disease. As I began to put these therapies to work with my own patients and observed how well they responded, I became convinced that conventional medicine's approach to heart disease was just plain wrong—and their resistance to utilizing these inexpensive, safe, and highly effective therapies unconscionable. Thirty years and thousands of patients later, my convictions are stronger than ever. The following story of a typical patient at the Whitaker Wellness Institute may help you understand why I am so confident and passionate about the approach to heart disease outlined in this book.

Lester's Story

When Lester M. was sixty-four, he had a stroke that affected his left arm and leg. Four years later, after a frightening episode of angina, his doctor ordered an angiogram to determine the extent of his heart disease. It was serious—four blocked arteries—and he was recommended to have quadruple coronary artery bypass surgery. However, because of his history of stroke, Lester was considered a poor operative risk, so he was prescribed medications instead. Over the next few months, more drugs were added to his regimen. He wasn't doing much better, but his doctor told him that nothing could be done except to continue on his growing list of medications.

Discouraged but determined, Lester and his wife began searching for alternatives. They learned about the Whitaker Wellness Institute from their daughter, who had heard me on a radio interview, and enrolled in our program. After a complete physical exam and extensive testing, Lester was started on a nutritional supplement regimen with vitamins and minerals that target the cardiovascular system. I took a hard look at all the drugs he was taking, eliminated some of them, reduced the dosages of others, and monitored him closely during his stay at the clinic.

Lester and his wife joined a small group of patients to learn the principles of the low-fat, high-fiber diet and exercise program that is an integral part of our therapeutic approach. More important, they were shown how to put these principles into practice. They were led in an exercise regimen and taught how to shop for and prepare heart-healthy food. They left the clinic with a true understanding of their treatment options and were encouraged and inspired to continue on the program at home.

Within four months Lester reported dramatic improvements in his cholesterol and triglyceride levels. His exercise tolerance improved, he had no more episodes of angina, he lost ten pounds, and he looked and felt better than he had in years. Most important, he had regained a sense of hope and the empowering knowledge that he was actively improving his health.

WHAT THIS BOOK IS ALL ABOUT

The program that Lester followed, which is outlined in this book, is based on lifestyle changes. If you respond appropriately to the seemingly trifling choices you are faced with every day (what foods you select, how much you exercise, whether or not you smoke or take nutritional supplements, how you manage stress), you will likely never be faced with monumental decisions such as whether to undergo angioplasty or bypass, or to take one drug versus another. These little things you do every day largely determine the health of your cardiovascular system.

That is the gist of this book. In the next three chapters, I want to make sure you understand what heart disease is all about. We will take a close look at the anatomy of the heart and vascular system, how heart disease gets started, and why it progresses. We will go beyond the old paradigm that a high cholesterol level is the sole cause of heart attacks and explore the latest research into the causes of heart disease. We will also examine the ways in which other medical problems such as hypertension, diabetes, insulin resistance, and obesity, affect the heart and arteries, and why it is so important to get these conditions under control.

In Part II I will give you my views on the industry that has been created around the treatment of heart disease. I want you to know the truth about the relationship between our current system of medical education and the multibillion-dollar pharmaceutical industry. I'll show you how bypass surgery and the other invasive procedures that form the backbone of modern cardiology came into being and cite research that will truly astound you—and make you think twice, should your physician recommend surgery. This is an important section, for you are unlikely to get this information anywhere else, and especially not from your cardiologist.

Finally, in Parts III, IV, and V, I will share with you the details of the Whitaker Wellness Institute program for reversing heart disease. I will teach you everything we teach the patients who spend a week with us at my clinic in Newport Beach, California. I will provide you with the same dietary guidelines and recipes for gourmet, heart-healthy meals our professional chef prepares for our patients. You will get the same step-by-step instructions in setting up an exercise program that we give our patients. I will help you create a nutritional supplementation program like that used at the clinic for our patients with heart disease, and I will walk you through the stress reduction exercises we teach our patients.

I will also tell you about the specialized, cutting-edge therapies for heart disease that we offer our patients at the institute. Although these treatment modalities are exceptionally effective and are supported by solid scientific research and years of clinical experience, you are not likely to hear about them from a conventional physician.

Heart disease *can* be reversed. You are to be congratulated on your initiative in taking the first step toward gaining control of your health. Let's get started.

CHAPTER 2

Atherosclerosis: The "Heart" of Heart Disease

A man is as old as his arteries.

THE IDEAL PATIENT-PHYSICIAN RELATIONSHIP IS A PARTNERSHIP OF honesty and trust. First, the physician lays out the options and explains the pros and cons of various treatments. The patient digests this information, asks questions, does independent research, and perhaps even seeks a second opinion. Then with the help of the physician, the patient determines his or her own course. All this takes time and effort on the part of both, but for me it is the only way to practice medicine.

For patients with heart disease, this requires a basic understanding of the cardiovascular system and why problems develop in the heart and arteries. Therefore, I want to begin this chapter by giving you an overview of your body's elegant and efficient cardiovascular system.

THE CARDIOVASCULAR SYSTEM

In its simplest terms, your cardiovascular system is basically a pump-pipe system. Your heart is the pump, your blood vessels the

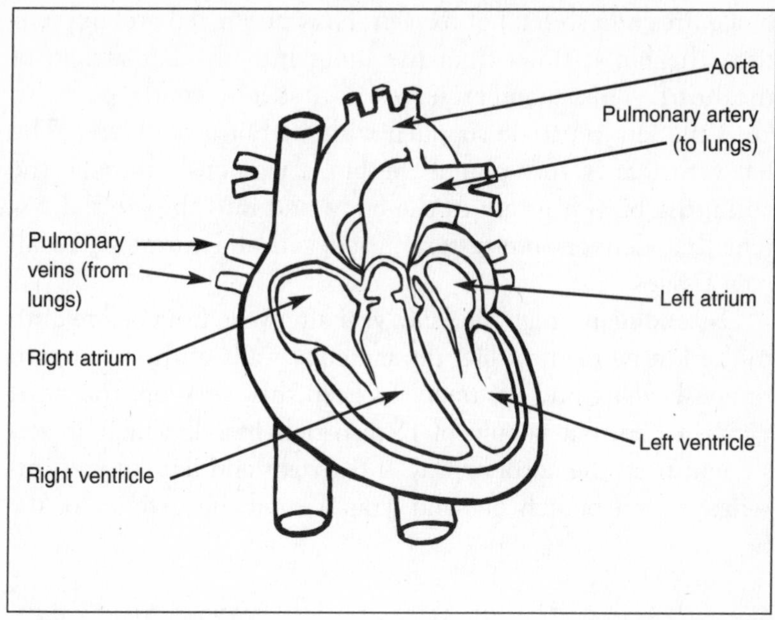

FIGURE 2: The Heart

pipes, and your blood the fluid that carries oxygen, nutrients, hormones, and other vital constituents to every cell in your body. The blood's round-trip journey begins as it leaves the heart and flows into the large arteries, which branch into smaller arterioles, then into tiny, thin-walled capillaries, where life-sustaining oxygen and nutrients are handed off to the cells and the waste products of metabolism are picked up. The blood then begins its trek back toward the heart and lungs through small venules and into larger veins that empty into the heart, where it is readied for another round of deliveries.

The heart is the engine that drives the blood through the body. The bluish deoxygenated blood transported by the veins flows into a chamber of the heart called the right atrium. (See the diagram above.) From there it enters the right ventricle, which contracts and pumps this blood through the lungs, where it acquires a fresh load of oxygen. Now bright red and oxygen-rich, the blood flows from the lungs into the left atrium of the heart. This chamber serves as a steady, gentle pump to keep the left ventricle supplied with fresh arterial blood. The left ventricle in turn pumps the blood vigorously through the aorta, the biggest artery in the body, and into the arterial system that delivers life-sustaining oxygen and nutrients to all your tissues.

Day and night, night and day, year after year, from before birth to the last moment of life, the muscular walls of the heart continuously relax and contract. To keep this work up, the heart needs a constant supply of oxygen-rich blood, which it gets straight from the aorta by way of the right and left coronary arteries, which branch out and wrap around the exterior of the heart.

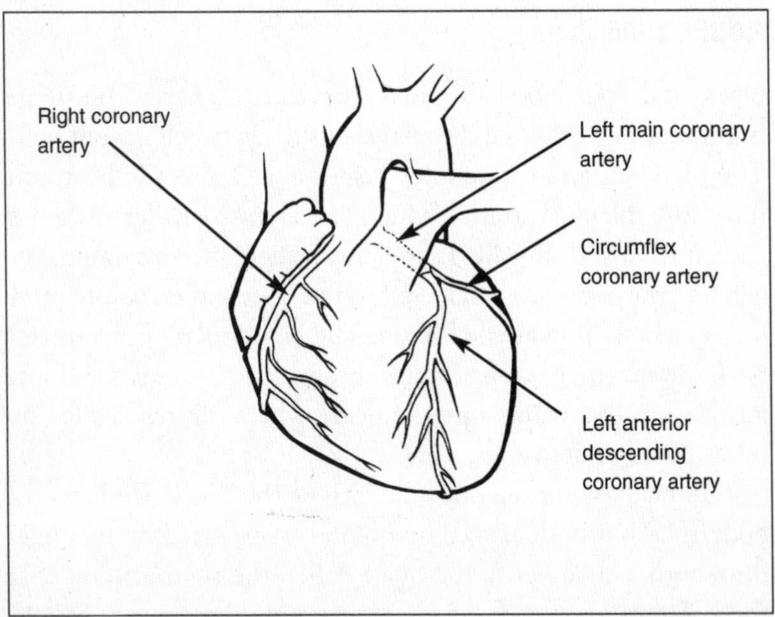

FIGURE 3: The Coronary Arteries

WHY THINGS GO WRONG

When you consider how hard the heart muscle and the coronary arteries work (the heart beats an average of 100,000 times and the arteries get an incredible amount of action as a result), you may be amazed that things go right as often as they do. The human body is an awesome masterpiece of art and engineering. However, glitches do occur. Arteries clog, the heart muscle fails, and disease sets in. A number of things can go wrong.

Sometimes the problem is with the blood itself. The vascular system of arteries and veins, as I mentioned above, is a network of progressively smaller vessels, ending in tiny capillaries where the actual exchange of oxygen and nutrients take place. Some of these capillaries are so small that the red blood cells must pass through single file—and sometimes these individual cells are actually required to bend and flex in order to pass through! The system obviously works best when the blood is thin and fluid. However, when you throw excess fat into the diet, some of it ends up in the blood, making it thicker and stickier. Clotting factors may also get out of balance, causing red blood cells to clump together and resulting in more viscous blood. Circulation becomes impaired, and the heart is required to work harder to pump blood through the small arterioles and capillaries.

The fault can also lie in the heart muscle, which may be enlarged or weakened by disease or subject to rhythmic disturbances. The left ventricle, the chamber that pumps blood into the arteries, is of particular concern in heart disease. Poor left ventricular function, which is often caused by uncontrolled hypertension, worsens the prognosis of patients with heart disease. However, problems with the heart muscle (such as cardiomyopathy and congestive heart failure) and rhythm (like atrial fibrillation) are not synonymous with coronary artery disease, and they are beyond the scope of this book.

As its name implies, coronary artery disease is primarily a disease of the arteries. Damage to the coronary arteries narrows these important passageways, restricting blood flow to the hungry heart muscle. It is caused by atherosclerosis or buildup of plaque in the arteries, and it is responsible for the vast majority of heart disease in this country. This same process occurring in other arteries may bring on strokes, poor circulation in the legs, gangrene, and even erectile dysfunction: All these conditions involve impaired circulation caused by deterioration of the arteries.

The word *arteriosclerosis* is sometimes used interchangeably with atherosclerosis, so I want to differentiate between the two. Arteriosclerosis describes the general process of damage and subsequent hardening and thickening of the major arteries. (*Arterio* means artery and *sclerosis* hardening or scarring). It is associated with any process that damages the arteries, including relatively rare forms related to syphilis, lupus, or polyarteritis nodosa. Atherosclerosis, the most common form of arteriosclerosis, is the specific process of thickening and hardening of the arterial walls by depositions of plaque.

And atherosclerosis of the coronary arteries is what heart disease is all about. It is hardly surprising that these arteries are prone to problems—just think about the workout they get. Not only are they continuously contracting and relaxing in response to the pulsation of blood flow from the aorta, they are also constantly in motion due to the vigorous movements of the heart muscle that they supply. Heart attack, massive coronary, coronary infarction, myocardial infarction . . . these are all names for the same thing: a severe blockage in one or more of the coronary arteries, making it unable to deliver fresh blood and oxygen to the throbbing heart muscle.

OUR PRECIOUS ARTERIES

The arteries are the passageways for blood flowing from the heart throughout the body. However, they are far from the passive conduits you might envision. Instead, these thick muscular tubes are extremely active participants in the goings-on of the cardiovascular system. Highly responsive to changes in pressure caused by the rhythmic pumping of the heart, they are able to contract or dilate in response to a number of physiological stimuli. For example, when you exercise, the arteries of your active limbs expand to allow for the increased oxygen and nutrient requirements of muscles at work. When you get up from a reclining position, they quickly divert blood to your brain, so you won't feel lightheaded.

The arteries are composed of three layers: 1) the sturdy, dense outer *adventitia*, made of connective tissue and anchored with a network of nerves and blood vessels; 2) the layers of smooth muscle tissue in the middle called the *media*; and 3) the inner layer, or *intima*, which is lined with specialized cells called *endothelial cells*, or the *endothelium*. The endothelium gives the artery a slick surface ideal for blood flow through the lumen, or opening inside the artery, and serves as a barrier between the blood and the muscle cells of the artery wall.

This single layer of cells lining the arteries is much more dynamic than anyone imagined only a few years ago, and it is key to the development of atherosclerosis. The endothelium contains sensors that gauge blood pressure and blood flow by picking up signals from hormones and other blood-borne chemicals. It produces a number of specialized substances, including compounds that affect cell growth—an important function, since the arteries, like most tissues in the body, are in a constant state of remodeling, and cellular growth is a prerequisite.

Endothelial cells also produce chemical messengers that govern the muscle tone of the arteries, instructing them to constrict or relax in order to direct the blood where it is needed most. One of these is angiotensin-converting enzyme (ACE), which converts an inactive blood component into angiotensin II (A II). A II is a powerful and useful constrictor of the arteries. However, when there is an excess of A II, the vessels constrict too much, raising blood pressure and increasing the risk of heart attack.[1]

At the other end of the spectrum, with actions directly counter to those of A II, is another important compound released by the endothelium, nitric oxygen (NO). NO has emerged as a very important determinant in atherosclerosis. It used to be called endothelial-derived relaxing factor, an appropriate name because that's exactly what NO is: the most potent vasodilator, or relaxer of blood vessels, yet discovered. Because it controls tension in the arteries, NO is a primary regulator of blood pressure. It also guards against atherosclerosis, for it prevents platelets and white blood cells from adhering to artery walls. In addition, it discourages the aggregation or clumping together of platelets, thus preventing the formation of potentially dangerous blood clots. Finally, NO also keeps the underlying muscle cells from multiplying and thickening, yet another factor in atherosclerosis.[2]

THE PROCESS OF ATHEROSCLEROSIS

Progressive atherosclerosis is the essence of heart disease. It develops quietly. Because there are no nerve endings inside the arteries, you don't feel pain as your arteries are injured and fill with plaque. Damage is well under way before you realize anything is wrong. Never forget that the first symptom of heart disease for many people is death from a heart attack.

What exactly causes atherosclerosis? The most widely accepted explanation is the response-to-injury hypothesis. Atherosclerosis is triggered by some sort of injury or insult to the endothelial cells. It may be physical trauma. A sudden spasm in an artery, propelled by a stress-related surge in hormones that causes the arteries to constrict, may cause a minute tear in the endothelium. It could be hypertension. High blood pressure in-

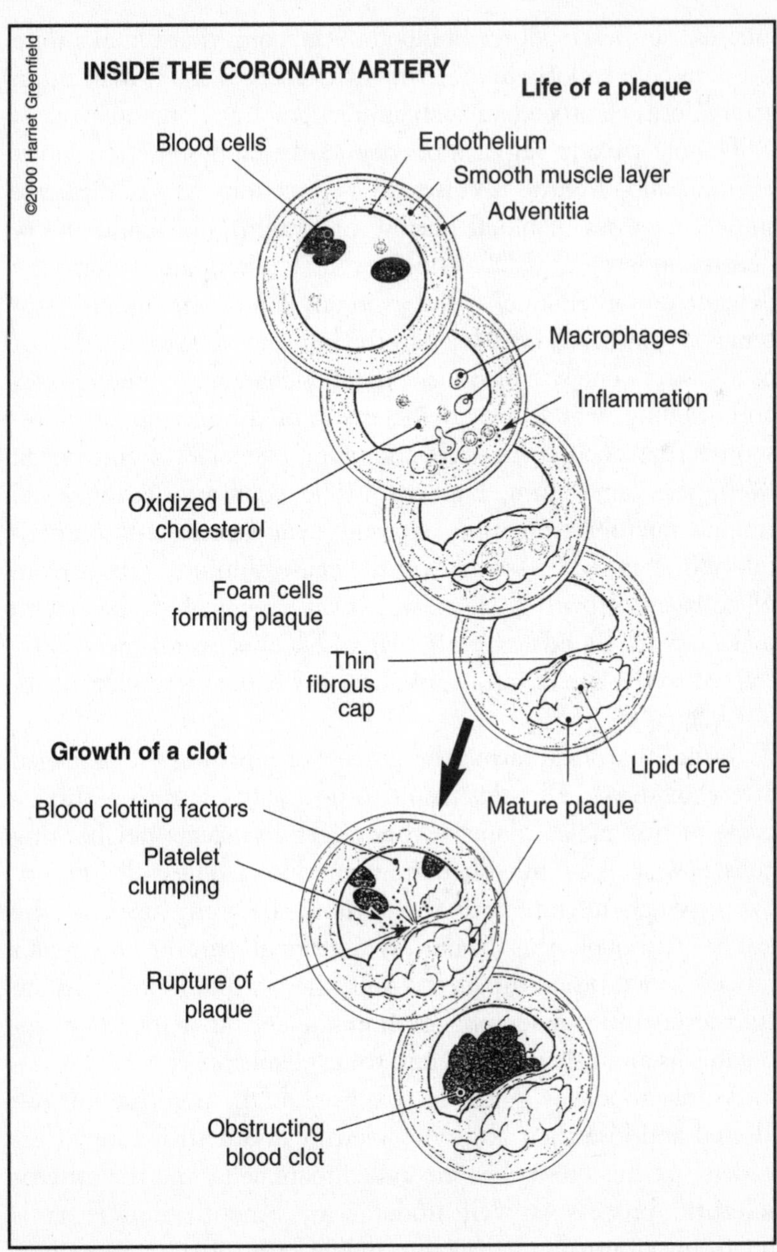

FIGURE 4: The Process of Atherosclerosis

creases the shearing force of blood to the point that it may injure the sensitive endothelium. It might even be a small nick in an artery during a procedure such as angiography or angioplasty.

The most likely perpetrators of endothelial dysfunction, however, are blood-borne toxins such as infectious agents, cigarette smoke, excesses of blood glucose or insulin, and oxidized low density lipoprotein (LDL) cholesterol.[3] These toxins damage the delicate endothelial cells, and as in any injury, the immune system goes to work. Think back to the last time you sustained a cut or abrasion. The site of injury probably developed some redness and swelling, which are characteristic of the inflammatory response that occurs when your immune system kicks into gear. Well, the same thing happens inside your arteries. Physical trauma, microbial infection, exposure to metabolic, environmental, or dietary toxins—whatever the cause of injury, a fix-it team of collagen, growth factors, and other chemicals rushes in to make repairs. Blood fats, particularly LDL cholesterol, are also attracted to the site of injury, and here is where atherosclerosis really begins.

Rather than facilitating the process of repairing the damaged artery, oxidized LDL adds insult to injury. It sets into motion a cycle of free radical damage that adversely affects neighboring cells as well. Also unleashed are white blood cells called monocytes, which migrate into the intima, the inner layer of the artery. Although this begins as a normal part of the repair process, once inside the artery wall, these white blood cells are transformed into macrophages, immune cells that ingest microorganisms and other foreign and toxic elements.

As macrophages gorge on oxidized LDL, they are further altered and lose their ability to identify and destroy foreign invaders. At this point they are called foam cells, and the atherosclerotic process is well under way. Smooth muscle cells migrating from the media (the middle layer of the artery) join the foam cells, multiply, and more cholesterol is taken up. This is known as the *fatty streak* stage. As atherosclerosis progresses, the smooth muscle cells lay down collagen and elastin fibers that thicken the intima, forming plaques filled with a thick gruel of dead and dying foam cells, LDL cholesterol and other fats, and additional white blood cells.

There are various types of plaques. Some are large, hard, and fibrous. They protrude into the lumen, narrowing its diameter by as much as 80 percent. The popular view of what happens in a heart attack is that a blood clot becomes lodged in one of these narrowed arteries and cuts off blood flow to the heart. Indeed, a multibillion-dollar-a-year industry is dedicated to an intensive search-and-destroy mission to eradicate these large plaques. These are the plaques picked up on angiography and the type that drive many patients into bypass surgery. However, hot-off-the-press research makes it clear that these large, stable plaques are not the primary culprit in heart disease.

THE VULNERABLE PLAQUE

Research conducted over the past few years suggests that the most important determinant in whether or not an arterial plaque will precipitate a heart attack is not its size but its composition. We now know the vast majority of heart attacks are caused not by the large plaques observed on angiography but by far smaller, yet much more deadly lesions. Known as *vulnerable*, or *unstable, plaques*, these small lesions have a soft, lipid-rich core topped with a thin, fibrous cap. The reason they are so troublesome lies, as their name suggests, in their susceptibility to rupture.[4]

Mechanical forces such as a sudden increase in blood pressure, pulse rate, or force of heartbeat (triggered by stress-related hormonal surges) may cause these lesions to open. Biochemical factors within the plaque, such as bleeding and an increase in inflammatory activity, can also weaken the cap of the lesion, making it more prone to bursting open. Once ruptured, its contents are spilled into the artery, attracting clotting factors and inflammatory chemicals in the blood to form a thrombus, or blood clot.[5] If the blood clot blocks a coronary artery, you have a heart attack.

Long-standing myths about heart disease and atherosclerosis have been shattered in recent years, and the fiction that has fallen the hardest concerns large, stable plaques. With each passing year the research supporting the importance of vulnerable plaques in the etiology of heart disease grows. Yet, as we will discuss in Part II, conventional cardiology continues to treat large, stable plaques as public enemy number one, attacking them by the hundreds of thousands every year with angioplasties and bypass surgeries. Yes, such procedures may reduce chest pain as blood flow and oxygen delivery are restored to the heart. However, they do little to prevent heart attacks or slow the progression of heart disease.

SIGNS AND SYMPTOMS OF HEART DISEASE

Atherosclerosis is silent and stealthy. As I mentioned in the first chapter, it begins in childhood. By the time most Americans reach their twenties, they have measurable blockages in their coronary arteries. Yet relatively few have chest pain or other signs or symptoms of heart disease. Only after atherosclerosis has progressed to the point that oxygen delivery is severely restricted do symptoms appear.

You may first notice it when you climb a flight of stairs or when you're exercising. It may come on when you are emotionally distressed or even when you're exposed to extremely hot or cold weather. Most people describe it as a feeling of tightness or constriction in the center or left side of the chest. Others experience it as compression-like pain of varying severity in the same area. Still others report the radiation of tightness or pain to the left arm, neck, jaw, back, or even the teeth. It is *angina pectoris* and it is the predominant symptom of heart disease.

Caused by insufficient blood supply to the heart, angina is appropriately named: It comes from the Greek word meaning "strangulation." The coronary arteries, narrowed by plaque and unresponsive to signals to dilate and allow more blood through, simply cannot deliver enough oxygen-rich blood to the heart, and it cries out in pain. There are two types of angina. *Stable angina*, the most common kind, generally comes on when there is an increased need for oxygen by the heart, during physical activity or periods of emotional extremes, stress, or excessive heat or cold, when hormonal surges constrict the arteries. Stable angina is not a heart attack. It generally lasts no more than a minute, and once it passes, things go back to normal—until the next time.

A second type of angina, *unstable angina*, is considered to be far more serious. It may occur at rest, and it tends to be progressive in frequency, severity, and duration. Unlike stable angina, which occurs in a predictable fashion, unstable angina is precipitated by an abrupt coronary event: a spasm in an artery, the rupture of a plaque, or the formation of a blood clot in an artery. Although this type of angina isn't a heart attack either, there may be a fine line between the two. In fact, unstable angina is sometimes called "intermediate coronary syndrome" or "preinfarction angina."

I want to mention one more manifestation of heart disease: *silent ischemia*. Even though it is caused by the same mechanism as angina—temporary deprivation of adequate oxygen to the heart—it isn't felt at all. In fact, people with silent ischemia don't even know they have it. It shows up only on an electrocardiogram (EKG) or other diagnostic test. We don't know why some patients with heart disease have anginal pain and some

Do You Know the Signs of a Heart Attack?

Everybody is familiar with the signs of a heart attack and the importance of getting immediate medical attention—or are they? Two recent studies suggest that many patients and even medical personnel lack information about how to recognize and respond to a heart attack. In one study, records of 400,000 patients treated for heart attacks at hospitals across the United States revealed that one-third of them did not have the classic symptoms of chest pain when they arrived at the hospital. These patients were less likely to be diagnosed with a heart attack on arrival in the emergency room and twice as likely to die in the hospital as patients who had chest pain.[6] The other study discovered that the average delay between the onset of symptoms of heart attack and arrival at a hospital was 140 minutes—well over two hours![7]

Get familiar with all the symptoms of a heart attack—this knowledge may save your life. The most common symptoms are pressure, fullness, squeezing or pain in the center of the chest, or pain that radiates to the shoulders, neck, or arms. Less common warning signs that should be taken seriously include unusual chest pain, stomach or abdominal pain, dizziness or nausea with or without chest pain, shortness of breath and difficulty breathing, intense sweating, palpitations, and general weakness. If you notice one or more of these signs in yourself or another person, call 911 immediately, for time is of the essence. In addition, chew and swallow a full-strength (325 mg) aspirin at once. (We will talk more about aspirin in Chapter 9.) This can substantially reduce the chances of death from heart attack.

don't. Nevertheless, silent ischemia is as significant a sign of heart disease as painful angina.

Of course, the worst thing that can happen in patients with heart disease is a heart attack, or myocardial infarction. When the heart muscle is deprived of oxygen by obstruction of a coronary artery, white blood cells called lymphocytes and other inflammatory cells rush to the area. They prompt the production of massive amounts of free radicals, which damage the heart tissue, or myocardium. Often an insult of this magnitude interrupts the rhythm of the heart, resulting in fibrillation, or chaotic beating, that cannot properly circulate blood. When this happens and medical intervention is not immediate, the usual result is sudden cardiac death. If damage to the myocardium is not too great, patients survive. However, according to American Heart Association statistics, only one-third of them make a full and complete recovery.[8]

Don's Story

Don Williams, a patient of mine, relates the story of his heart attack in his book, *Dead by Now*. Don was an insurance agent. At his company he was known as the "shock troops," for he was the guy who was sent in to close difficult clients or salvage sales on the verge of collapse. He was obviously under a lot of pressure to appease and persuade clients and produce results. Don was very good at his job, but it required long hours and frequent travel.

One day, after finally closing a difficult sale, he celebrated with a late-night steak dinner. He got back to his motel room around eleven, turned on the evening news, and settled onto his bed. Suddenly he felt a crushing sensation in his chest, radiating into his arm. The pain was unbearable—it felt as if "a big boot had stepped on my chest." Don lay on the bed, scared to death but hoping he was suffering a bad case of indigestion, and he eventually dozed off. When he awoke the next morning, he was covered in sweat and ached all over, but the crushing pain was gone.

Believe it or not, Don kept his appointments that day, but as soon as he got home he went to the emergency room, where an EKG revealed that he had had a heart attack.

The next few days passed in a blur. In a chain of events that Don later described as "medical terrorism," he was told he would have to have bypass surgery. Because it was close to Christmas, the procedure was delayed—which gave Don enough time to evaluate his options. He read everything he could get his hands on about bypass, as well as numerous books on the therapeutic benefits of exercise and diet. He decided to forego bypass surgery even though he was told that without it he would be dead within two years. Instead, Don made dramatic changes in his lifestyle. For more than twenty-five years after Don's heart attack, he was periodically threatened and bullied by his cardiologists (one actually told him he had only minutes to live), but he never did have that bypass.[9]

Don's story is typical in many ways—the crushing pain, even the irrational belief that he was suffering from bad indigestion. Yet it is dramatically different from that of the millions of patients who get caught in the net of conventional cardiology. Let Don's experience serve as testimony that you too can tackle heart disease on a more fundamental level. Like Don, you can actually improve the health of your heart and arteries and essentially reverse heart disease.

I hope this chapter has given you a basic understanding of the cardiovascular system and the complex, multifaceted process of atherosclerosis. In the next chapter, we will approach heart disease from a slightly different angle by exploring the factors that have been positively identified as causing or contributing to the progression of the disease.

CHAPTER 3

The Culprits in Cardiovascular Disease

NOT LONG AGO SCIENTISTS BELIEVED THAT A HIGH CHOLESTEROL level was the sole cause of heart disease. The accepted explanation of atherosclerosis was that consumption of a high-fat, high-cholesterol diet led to the buildup of cholesterol deposits in the artery walls, setting the stage for a heart attack. Then came the discovery that the cholesterol issue wasn't quite as simple as previously thought. Researchers discovered that while some types of cholesterol, particularly LDL cholesterol that had been altered by free radicals, were indeed harmful, one type actually had a protective effect on the arteries.

Things got more complicated when homocysteine, a by-product of amino acid metabolism, entered the picture and was found to be a primary instigator of the endothelial damage that precipitates atherosclerosis. Then the research on inflammation started rolling in, and it was revealed to be among the most significant risk factors of all. Add to this new information on clotting factors in the blood, triglycerides, and insulin resistance, plus decades-old research on how diabetes, hypertension, and smoking compound the risk of heart disease, and we end with a whole lineup of suspects.

Yet to this day, most physicians point the finger at cholesterol and cholesterol alone. This is absurd. Half of all Americans who suffer a heart attack have cholesterol levels within the normal range! There are obviously other processes at work—and ways to identify and address them. The good news is that by following the program outlined in this book, you can rein in each and every one of these risk factors. Let's look at exactly how and why each of these factors figures into heart disease.

THE CHOLESTEROL CONNECTION

By now everyone knows that a high cholesterol level is a major risk factor for cardiovascular disease. But did you know that this waxy lipid (fat) is also essential to life? It is required in the production of steroid hormones, which include the sex hormones (estrogen and testosterone) and other adrenal hormones. Cholesterol is also a component of our cellular membranes, giving them needed stability. In addition, it is necessary for the synthesis of vitamin D, the myelin sheaths that surround nerve cells, and bile, an important factor in digestion.

Much of the research on the relationship between cholesterol and heart disease has come out of the Framingham Study. Begun in the early 1950s, this study, which is funded by the National Heart, Lung and Blood Institute (NHLBI), is one of the longest-running studies ever conducted. In fact, it continues to this day and now includes offspring of the initial participants. It has followed thousands of residents of Framingham, Massachusetts, for more than fifty years now and has been a gold mine of data on lifestyle and heart disease.

One of Framingham's most significant findings appeared in a landmark paper authored by Framingham Study director William Castelli, M.D., and colleagues. They reported that the cholesterol levels of patients who had suffered a heart attack over the twenty-five-year study period ranged from 220 to 260, with an average of 244. They also found that the incidence of heart attack in study participants with very low levels of cholesterol was almost nil. This was the first study to definitively link an elevated blood cholesterol level to increased risk of heart disease.[1]

A flurry of research followed, and the dangerous and unequivocal relationship between high cholesterol levels and heart disease has been upheld in hundreds of worldwide studies. It was also discovered that when cholesterol levels can be brought down, risk of heart attack drops. This was most strikingly demonstrated in the Lipid Research Clinic Coronary Primary Prevention Trial, which followed 3,806 men with elevated cholesterol at various medical centers for seven and a half years. These men were treated with lifestyle interventions such as diet as well as cholesterol-lowering drugs in an effort to bring down their cholesterol levels. The results of this study showed that every 1 percent drop in cholesterol was accompanied by a 2 to 3 percent drop in the frequency of coronary artery disease events.[2]

LDL VERSUS HDL

You know the old saying "Oil and water don't mix." This is as true of the lipids in your bloodstream as it is of an oil slick on the ocean. Fat is light, and it floats on top of fluids rather than dissolving in them. In order for cholesterol to be transported through the bloodstream, it must attach itself to various water-soluble protein complexes. These are known as lipoproteins, and this piggyback arrangement allows cholesterol, as well as other fats called triglycerides, to be delivered wherever they are needed in the body.

There are three major types of cholesterol, each named according to the protein complex that transports it:

- **HDL cholesterol** is attached to a relatively heavy carrier made up of more protein and less fat called high-density lipoprotein. It is often referred to as "good" cholesterol, for it mobilizes excessive cholesterol out of the cells and artery walls. People with high levels of HDL cholesterol are less prone to having heart attacks.

- **LDL cholesterol** rides on low-density lipoprotein, a lighter particle made mostly of fat that transports cholesterol to the tissues. LDL cholesterol that has been oxidized, or damaged by free radicals, is deposited into artery walls and contributes to atherosclerosis and its associated misery. Therefore, elevated levels of LDL cholesterol are undesirable.
- **VLDL cholesterol** is the lightest transporter, containing even more fat than LDL. It is primarily a carrier of triglycerides. Because an elevated level of triglycerides is another risk factor for heart disease, and because some VLDL cholesterol is converted into LDL cholesterol, a high level of this type of cholesterol is also bad news.

As we discussed in the previous chapter, the harm done by excess cholesterol—more specifically oxidized LDL cholesterol—results from its interaction with injured or dysfunctional endothelial cells. It is attracted to the site of arterial injury, where it further irritates the endothelium by setting off a chain reaction of free radical damage. Oxidized LDL cholesterol also enters the artery wall and is incorporated into the fatty streaks and foam cells that are the essence of atherosclerosis. Chronically elevated levels of LDL cholesterol fuel the process of plaque formation.

HDL, on the other hand, puts the brakes on atherosclerosis. It removes excess cholesterol from the bloodstream and blood vessels and returns it to the liver, where it is escorted into the gastrointestinal tract and out of the body. This fraction of cholesterol also inhibits the oxidation of LDL cholesterol.[3] HDL cholesterol is so protective that a low level is considered to be an independent risk factor for heart disease. According to the Framingham Study, each 4 mg/dl decrease in HDL is accompanied by a 10 percent increase in risk.[4] Suboptimal HDL levels are also associated with more severe coronary artery disease and increased

Classification of LDL, Total, and HDL Cholesterol (mg/dl)

Executive Summary of the Third Report of the National Cholesterol Education Program (NCEP) Expert Panel on Detection, Evaluation, and Treatment of High Blood Cholesterol in Adults (Adult Treatment Panel III), 2001.[5]

LDL Cholesterol	
less than 100	optimal
100–129	near or above optimal
130–159	borderline high
160–189	high
greater than or equal to 190	very high
Total Cholesterol	
less than 200	desirable
200–239	borderline high
greater than or equal to 240	high
HDL Cholesterol	
less than 40	low
greater than or equal to 60	high

likelihood of restenosis, or return of blockages, following angioplasty. (More on angioplasty in Part II.)[6] The flip side of this is that a high HDL cholesterol level is considered to be a "negative" risk factor: It actually lowers the risk of heart disease.

So it's easy to see that total cholesterol readings tell only part of the story. Proportions of LDL and HDL cholesterol are much more predictive of heart disease risk, a fact that has been underscored by the latest guidelines from the National Heart, Lung and Blood Institute. In May 2001, an NHLBI expert panel unveiled the National Cholesterol Education Program's updated recommendations for cholesterol testing and management, and the focus is on LDL cholesterol. The guidelines also include ranges for HDL and total cholesterol and figure in other risk factors for heart disease, such as smoking, hypertension, diabetes, and age. However, the program's primary target is getting LDL cholesterol into the normal range.

Let's look at an example of two men. Each has a total cholesterol level of 220, but one's LDL cholesterol is 165 and his HDL 35 (the remaining 20 is VLDL). The other man has an LDL cholesterol of 135, with an HDL of 65. Although their total cholesterol levels are the same, the first man is at significantly higher risk of having a heart attack than the second because of his higher LDL and lower HDL cholesterol.

An easy way to quantify this risk is to calculate what is commonly called the risk ratio: the ratio of total cholesterol to HDL cholesterol. For instance, the first man's total cholesterol of 220 and HDL of 35 give him a risk ratio of 6.3 (220 ÷ 35 = 6.3). The second man's risk ratio is considerably lower at 3.4 (220 ÷ 65 = 3.4). This is a fairly accurate predictor of heart disease. A ratio of less than 3.1 is desirable—the higher it is, the greater your risk. If your total cholesterol level happens to be very low, 160, say, the ratio is irrelevant because your harmful LDL cholesterol is so low that it will rarely promote atherosclerosis.

The best news about cholesterol levels is that they are very responsive to lifestyle changes. Eat a diet high in saturated fat, sit back in your easy chair, and watch your cholesterol soar. Follow a prudent diet, exercise regularly, and take the targeted nutritional supplements that are part of this program for reversing heart disease, and the majority of you will be able to bring your level into the acceptable range—without resorting to drugs.

VLDL: A MARKER OF TRIGLYCERIDES

You likely know your cholesterol level, and perhaps even your HDL or total cholesterol/HDL ratio. But what about your VLDL? For years, this third type of cholesterol was viewed as inconsequential—it was just too large to enter the artery walls like LDL cholesterol does. Although Yale University researchers suggested decades ago that a high triglyceride level might be even more predictive of heart attack than high cholesterol, the cholesterol theory of heart disease had such a firm grip on medicine that this research was ignored. However, in recent years triglycerides have emerged as an independent risk factor for heart disease, and VLDL, the major carrier of triglycerides in the blood, is being given more consideration.

What exactly are triglycerides? Grab ahold of your love handles, and you've got a handful of triglycerides. Eat a steak or an avocado, and you've got a mouthful of them. Simply put, triglycerides are the primary form in which fat is found in nature. Triglycerides are shuttled around the body on two types of lipoproteins: chylomicrons and VLDL. Chylomicrons, which are formed in the small intestines, pick up triglycerides that are absorbed into the bloodstream after you eat. VLDL, on the other hand, is produced by the liver and mobilizes stored triglycerides.

The more VLDL your liver churns out, the higher your triglyceride level. This means that more fat is circulating in your blood. This is not a good thing. It makes the blood sluggish and lowers its oxygen-carrying capacity. A high level of VLDL also goes hand in hand with a low level of protective HDL cholesterol. Furthermore, some VLDL is converted into harmful LDL cholesterol—and it's a smaller, denser, more easily oxidized type of LDL. Excessive triglycerides damage the arteries in yet another way. Partially degraded VLDL and chylomicrons, called remnant lipoproteins, which remain in the bloodstream after they've unloaded their cargo of triglycerides, are highly destructive to arterial walls and play a role in atherosclerosis.[7]

Elevated triglycerides are particularly harmful for women. In fact, a high level of triglycerides is among the best predictors of heart disease in females. A 1999 review of seventeen studies examining the link between triglyceride levels and cardiovascular disease revealed that each 86-point rise in triglycerides was accompanied by a 31 percent increase in risk in men—and a 76 percent increase in risk in women![8]

Keeping your triglycerides in check is a significant step in reversing your risk of heart disease. (NCEP guidelines define normal as less than or equal to 135 mg/dl.)

According to Gerald Reaven, M.D., of Stanford University, insulin resistance, which we will discuss in detail in the next chaper, is a primary cause of elevated triglycerides. High insulin levels prompt the liver to make more VLDL, which results in higher triglyceride levels. Fortunately, triglycerides are very responsive to exercise and dietary modifications, as well as one of the nutritional supplements we will discuss in part III.[9]

LIPOPROTEIN(a) AND ATHEROSCLEROSIS

Lipoprotein(a) (Lp[a]) is a low-density lipoprotein-protein combination that is recognized as another important risk factor for heart disease. According to a British review of twenty-seven studies published in *Circulation* in September 2000, patients with elevated levels of Lp(a) had a 70 percent increased risk of heart disease.[10] Although there is general accord that Lp(a) contributes to atherosclerosis, there is less consensus regarding how it does so.

Some researchers speculate that Lp(a) is taken up by foam cells and incorporated into the plaque in arterial walls. Others suggest that it promotes the growth of the smooth muscle cells of the arteries, thickening the arteries and making them less responsive. Still others believe that Lp(a) is involved in the inflammatory aspect of atherosclerosis. One of the most interesting theories about Lp(a) was put forth by the late Nobel Prize–winning scientist Linus Pauling, Ph.D., and Matthias Rath, M.D., in 1990.[11]

These innovative scientists described Lp(a) as an LDL molecule surrounded by a sticky band of protein that easily adhered to areas of endothelial damage within the arteries. Noting that Lp(a) goes up when vitamin C levels in the blood are low, they suggested that the presence of ample vitamin C and other antioxidants in the blood might keep Lp(a) in check and protect the vascular walls. This theory represented a radical shift in focus from cholesterol and other factors that damage the arteries to the health of the arteries themselves and their ability to resist injury and infiltration.

As you might expect, this theory was not well received by the medical establishment. However, as with virtually everything that the brilliant Dr. Pauling championed in his lifetime, this idea has more than a kernel of truth. Lp(a) and risk of heart disease can be lowered with high doses of supplemental vitamin C, as well as other antioxidants.

HOMOCYSTEINE: A METABOLIC TOXIN

In 1969 Kilmer S. McCully, M.D., made a discovery so revolutionary that it should have shaken the very foundations of cardiology. Instead, Dr. McCully, a Harvard pathologist at the time, was shunned and ridiculed by a scientific community committed to the cholesterol theory of heart disease. In fact, he was eventually asked to leave Harvard because of his renegade research. However, in recent years the theory first put forth by this innovative physician—that elevated homocysteine is a highly predictable risk factor for heart disease—has been validated, and Dr. McCully has been vindicated. In fact, according to a 1997 study, "An increased plasma total homocysteine level confers an independent risk of vascular disease similar to that of smoking or hyperlipidemia."[12]

Homocysteine is produced during the normal metabolism of methionine, an amino acid found in protein. Although the body utilizes small amounts of homocysteine, it becomes toxic when levels are elevated (above 8 mmol/l). Fortunately, your body has an efficient means of detoxifying and eliminating excesses of homocysteine as well as other cellular toxins: a process called methylation. Methylation is one of your body's housecleaning services—it is as important to a healthy body as cleaning is to the maintenance of your home. If you never washed the dishes, vacuumed the carpets, or dusted, your home would deteriorate beyond repair. In a similar fashion, without adequate methylation in your body, homocysteine and other metabolic by-products build up, initiating and accelerating not only atherosclerosis but also Alzheimer's disease, cancer, and other maladies.

Homocysteine is extremely damaging to the arteries. It decreases the production of nitric oxide, which, as we discussed in Chapter 2, protects the endothelium by preventing the adhesion of substances that initiate atherosclerosis. Homocysteine also irritates the muscle cells of the arteries, and it makes the platelets stickier, increasing the likelihood of blood clots that may cause heart attacks.[13] Fortunately, keeping the methylation process in tiptop shape is fairly easy. All it requires is adequate amounts of folic acid and vitamin B12. Although vitamin B6 does not directly facilitate methylation, it also lowers homocysteine levels by converting homocysteine to cysteine, a harmless amino acid. We will discuss these vitamins further in Chapter 14.

OVERZEALOUS CLOTTING FACTORS

The coup de grâce in most heart attacks is a blood clot, which cuts off blood supply to a coronary artery and starves an area of the heart muscle of vital oxygen. Yet blood clots serve an invaluable function—without them we would bleed to death from the smallest of nicks. Whenever there is a break in a blood vessel, platelets, rallied by a chemical messenger called thromboxane A2, rush to the injured area and form a temporary plug. A number of coagulation factors in the blood are activated to transform the blood at the injury site from a liquid to a gel-like clot to stop blood loss. One of these is fibrinogen, which forms a net of proteins called fibrin that holds platelets tightly together and seals the hole. After healing begins, fibrin is broken down in a process called fibrinolysis (*lysis* means dissolution or decomposition). A chief player in fibrinolysis is plasminogen, which produces a clot-busting enzyme that eats up fibrin and removes the now-useless clot.

Sometimes this elegant system goes awry and a clot develops spontaneously or is triggered by the rupture of a vulnerable plaque within a blood vessel. This is called a thrombus, and if it forms within a coronary artery, it may trigger a heart attack. A thrombus may also break off, travel in the bloodstream, and lodge in a small vessel in the lungs, causing a pulmonary embolism, or in the brain, precipitating a stroke.[14]

It is easy to see how elevated blood levels of certain clotting factors could exacerbate the formation of thrombi and risk of heart attack. Excesses of thromboxane A2 lead to excessive clumping of platelets, and high levels of fibrinogen may stimulate the formation of unnecessary clots. Plasminogen activator inhibitor-1 (PAI-1), which inhibits the breakup of blood clots, is yet another factor.[15] There are powerful drugs that modulate coagulation. But there are also natural therapies, which we will discuss in Part III, that safely and effectively address these clotting factors.

LOW ANTIOXIDANT STATUS AND ATHEROSCLEROSIS

Free radicals are natural by-products of normal metabolism. Any chemical reaction that involves oxygen (oxidation), such as the production of energy in the cells, creates free radicals. Because free radicals are missing an electron, they are very unstable and highly reactive. In an attempt to stabilize themselves, they steal electrons from other molecules, which, in turn, destabilizes those molecules and sets them into motion. The activity of free radicals reminds me of Super Balls, those small, hard rubber balls you or your kids might have played with. If you bounce a super ball hard enough in a small room, it will wreak havoc, ricocheting against walls, ceiling, and floor, knocking over vases, lamps, pictures, and whatever else is in its path.

Nature's answer to free radicals is antioxidants. Antioxidants intervene in the chain of free-radical destruction by giving up electrons to stabilize these free-wheeling, highly reactive molecules. Thus they work on several fronts to reduce the risk of atherosclerosis. Antioxidants nurture the endothelial cells lining the arteries and protect them from injury. They stop the transformation of LDL cholesterol into its harmful, oxidized form. Certain antioxidants also help boost HDL cholesterol and strengthen the capillary walls. Low blood levels of antioxidants are a decided and independent risk factor for atherosclerosis. In a study conducted by the World Health Organization, low blood levels of vitamin E were much more predictive of heart attacks than better-recognized risk factors such as elevated cholesterol and high blood pressure.[16]

Blood tests are available to determine antioxidant levels. However, we don't routinely order them at the Whitaker Wellness Institute. The tests are expensive, the results are variable, and, in my opinion, they are not all that helpful. Instead, we recommend that *all* our patients increase their antioxidant levels through diet and supplementation. Plant foods are our best dietary sources of these important nutrients. By following the dietary program described in Part IV, you will dramatically increase your antioxidant intake. However, the best way to be sure you're getting protective levels of antioxidants is to take nutritional supplements as recommended in Chapters 13 and 14.

INFLAMMATION: AN EMERGING MARKER

The once-heretical concept that atherosclerosis is an inflammatory disease has been almost universally accepted over the past few years. It hinges on the fact that every injury in the body, whether it is an abrasion on your skin or damage to the endothelial cells lining your arteries, alerts the immune system to mount an inflammatory response. As I explained in the previous chapter, inflammation facilitates healing of an injured area—it is a normal part of the immune response. Unfortunately, the same white blood cells and inflammatory chemicals that are involved in the healing process may also burrow into the artery walls and contribute to atherosclerosis.

It is likely that minor injuries to artery walls heal without consequence. However, decades of injury and irritation to the endothelium result in arteries littered with large, stable plaques and smaller, vulnerable plaques filled with inflammatory compounds. The overburdened immune system may turn from friend to foe and trigger changes in these vulnerable plaques that lead to plaque eruption and thrombus formation, and possibly to a heart attack. Chronic inflammation is thus a cause—and a consequence—of heart disease.

Levels of inflammatory compounds are reliable determinants of heart disease risk. One of the best markers of inflammation is C-reactive protein, which is manufactured in the liver in response to inflammation anywhere in the body—including the arteries. In a study published in the *New England Journal of Medicine* in 1997, Harvard researchers used as their database 22,071 men in the ongoing Physicians' Health Study. When these men enrolled in the study in 1982, they were run through a battery of tests, and blood samples were taken and frozen for future analysis. They were all healthy at the time with no history of heart disease. Eight years later, 543 of the men had had a heart attack, stroke, or a blood clot in a major vessel. The frozen blood samples of these men were analyzed and compared to samples from 543 men who were free of cardiovascular disease. They found that the men with the highest level of C-reactive protein were twice as likely to have had a stroke and three times as likely to have suffered a heart attack. And elevated C-reactive protein levels were present in the blood six to eight years before the cardiovascular event took place![17]

Paul M. Ridker, M.D., a cardiologist and researcher at the Brigham and Women's Hospital and Harvard Medical School in Boston, has spearheaded several studies demonstrating that C-reactive protein is a very strong predictor of future heart attack or other coronary events—even stronger than cholesterol. In one study, women with the highest levels were at 4.4 times the risk as women with the lowest levels.[18] In another study Dr. Ridker rated the various risk factors in an attempt to see which best predicted future risk of heart attack. He found that the most accurate of all was a combination of C-reactive protein and the ratio of total cholesterol to HDL.[19]

Of all the risk factors for heart disease discussed in this chapter, inflammation may be the most difficult to curb. However, a growing body of research suggests that dietary measures coupled with small doses of aspirin and natural anti-inflammatory agents may dampen inflammation and be one of your best defenses against heart disease.

IS INFECTION AT THE HEART OF ATHEROSCLEROSIS?

Because inflammation is so closely associated with infection, the possibility of a microbial component in atherosclerosis has logically come up, and certain chronic, low-grade bacterial and viral infections have been linked with increased risk of heart disease. It has been theorized that these microorganisms migrate to the arteries, possibly on white blood cells, set up residence, damage the endothelium, and initiate atherosclerosis.

One proposed culprit is the common herpes simplex virus type 1 (HSV-1), which causes cold sores on the mouth. A 2000 study of more than 600 individuals revealed that people who had antibodies to HSV-1 were twice as likely to have suffered or died from a heart attack as those who had not been exposed to the herpes virus.[20] Another suspect is cytomegalovirus (CMV). This virus is found in as many as half of all Americans over the age of forty, but it causes no symptoms in most. Researchers from the Washington Hospital Center in Washington, D.C., found that infection with CMV was an independent risk factor for coronary artery disease in women.[21]

Chlamydia pneumoniae, a microorganism that is most significantly associated with infections in the lungs, has also been studied, as have bacteria associated with gum disease. Researchers at the Ann Arbor Veterans Administration Hospital in Michigan discovered that men with severe periodontal disease were four and a half times more likely to have heart disease than men with healthy gums. These same individuals may also be at increased risk of stroke. According to researchers at Columbia University College of Physicians and Surgeons, the buildup of plaque in the carotid arteries (a major risk factor for stroke) was 50 percent greater in individuals with diseased gums than in those with healthy gums.[22]

The newest and most intriguing microbial suspect in atherosclerosis is *Nanobacterium sanguineum*. Nanobacteria, which are 1/10,000 the size of regular bacteria, are commonly found in the blood of animals and humans. Researchers at the Academy of Nanoscience have amassed data suggesting that nanobacteria are implicated in atherosclerosis, kidney stones, and other disorders involving calcification. Nanobacteria are pleomorphic, meaning that they have several different forms during their life cycle, and one form is characterized by a unique cell membrance that secretes a "gooey slime" film. This film, which protects the nanobacterium and links it with others, is foreign and toxic to the human body, so the immune system mounts an inflammatory response. Clusters of nanobacteria are walled off, and the film calcifies and hardens, leaving areas of calcified plaque in the coronary arteries and elsewhere in the body.

There is still a lot of controversy surrounding the infection–heart disease theory. Although direct relationships between these microorganisms and heart disease are not definitive, the research is compelling. Even if microorganisms do not actually infect or damage the arteries, the presence of these foreign organisms elsewhere in the body causes the immune system to be constantly on guard, releasing white blood cells and inflammatory chemicals that are most definitely involved in atherosclerosis. This was recently supported by a study involving 10,000 adults, in which subjects with gum disease were found to have higher levels of fibrinogen and C-reactive protein.[23] Not only are elevated levels of these two compounds indicative of infection, each is independently associated with increased risk of heart disease.

As I said at the beginning of this chapter, heart disease is a lot more complicated than most people think. Yet for each and every one of the culprits in cardiovascular disease that we have discussed, there is a safe and natural therapy. The program for reversing heart disease is actually much simpler than the process of developing heart disease in the first place. All it requires is that you pay attention to what you eat, exercise regularly, and take a few targeted nutritional supplements.

Before we get into the particulars of the treatment of heart disease, I want to make sure you're aware of a few medical conditions that dramatically increase your risk of atherosclerosis.

CHAPTER 4

Partners in Disease

HEART DISEASE DOES NOT EXIST IN A VACUUM. DON'T BELIEVE IT when you hear about a "perfectly healthy" person who has dropped dead of a heart attack. The human body is much too finely engineered to self-destruct like that. That's not to say that health problems are always evident. They are not, and heart disease is particularly sneaky. A high cholesterol or triglyceride level doesn't make you feel ill. Elevated homocysteine or C-reactive protein won't send you running to the doctor for a pain pill. Atherosclerosis begins at a very early age, usually in childhood, yet gives no inkling of its presence until it is quite advanced. Unless you educate yourself on the underlying causes of heart disease and proactively take stock of your risk factors, you too could breeze along, never knowing you had any hint of heart disease. As I mentioned earlier in this book, sudden death from heart attack is the first sign of heart disease in far too many people.

It is vital that you become familiar with the factors that put your cardiovascular system in jeopardy. These include not only the subtle events going on at the cellular level, which we covered in the previous chapter, but also better known, more obvious conditions that are blatant warning signs of heart disease. If you have hypertension, odds are that you also have heart disease—it is the number one risk factor for heart attack. Diabetes, insulin resistance, obesity: All these conditions are "partners" in heart disease, and a diagnosis of any of these disorders means that you are at dramatically increased risk.

HYPERTENSION: THE NUMBER ONE RISK FACTOR FOR HEART DISEASE

High blood pressure is intimately related to heart disease because it promotes atherosclerosis. The relentless stress on blood vessel walls due to hypertension damages the endothelium and causes the heart and arteries to age before their time. Hypertension triples the risk of dying of a heart attack, quadruples the risk of heart failure, and increases the risk of stroke sevenfold!

When your blood pressure is taken, you will get a reading of two numbers, which indicate how much force is being exerted by the blood on the vessels. The top number, or systolic blood pressure, is the higher of the two, and it measures the pressure just after the heart contracts and pushes blood into the arteries. The bottom number is the diastolic reading, and it denotes pressure when the heart is at rest.

As in any pump-pipes system, blood pressure is affected by three things: pumping intensity of the heart, volume of blood, and resistance on the vessels. Blood pressure can vary significantly throughout the day. For example, it rises during exercise as the heart beats harder and faster to meet the muscles' demand for blood and oxygen. It is increased by stress, which tirggers the release of chemicals that signal the arteries to constrict. It is not unusual for a patient's blood pressure to be elevated in a doctor's office—just being there is stressful to many—while it is normal at home, a condition known as white-coat hypertension. However, chronically elevated blood pressure signifies a problem.

According to the Joint National Committee on the Prevention, Detection, Evaluation, and Treatment of High Blood

Pressure, optimal blood pressure is less than 120/80, and normal is under 130/85. High normal is considered to be 130–139/85–89, and anything above that falls into the classification of hypertension. (140–159/90–99 is stage 1, or mild, hypertension, 160–179/100–109 is stage 2, or moderate, and 180+/110+ is stage 3, or severe.)[1]

Fifty million Americans have hypertension, yet a third of them are unaware of it. Those who have been diagnosed with elevated blood pressure are often saddled with ever-expanding drug regimens rather than being instructed in much safer, less expensive lifestyle therapies. Ironically, some of the drugs commonly used to lower blood pressure may actually increase the risk of death from heart attack. Nevertheless, good blood pressure control, whether by the diet and other lifestyle modalities which we will discuss in Part III, or by drug therapy, reduces the risk of heart attack and other cardiovascular diseases.

DIABETICS BEWARE

Diabetes and heart disease go together hand in glove. It may surprise you that 75 percent of diabetics die from heart attacks. A 2001 study in the *British Medical Journal* suggests that elevated blood sugar is in and of itself a powerful predictor of heart disease.[2] Excess glucose in the blood damages the blood vessels, in part by increasing free-radical damage. It makes the blood thicker, more concentrated, and less able to deliver oxygen and other nutrients. Circulation is impaired, and blood flow to important organs, including the heart, is restricted.

The diabetic condition also accelerates another biochemical process in the body that is a well-known contributor to overall degeneration and aging. Glycation occurs when glucose binds to and chemically alters proteins, fats, and other molecules. These damaged molecules, called advanced glycation end products

(AGEs), accumulate in the cells and hamper their normal functioning. AGEs are involved in diabetic complications of the eyes and kidneys. Recent research suggests that they also are party to the heart disease so common in diabetics.

When AGEs link to collagen in the arteries, these blood vessels lose their elasticity and responsiveness. Accumulations of AGEs also attract platelets that encourage the formation of blood clots. They bind to LDL cholesterol, making it more susceptible to oxidation, and interfere with its clearance, thus contributing to elevated levels of this harmful type of cholesterol.[3] Furthermore, some researchers have suggested that when AGEs are incorporated into artery walls, they promote chronic low-grade inflammation, which is a hallmark of atherosclerosis.[4]

Diabetes, which is diagnosed when fasting blood sugar is higher than 126 mg/dl, is increasing in epidemic proportions. Worldwide its incidence has tripled in the past thirty-five years and is expected to double in the next twenty-five. Once a condition largely confined to older people, diabetes has wormed its way into all segments of our society, including our children. This is yet another unfortunate consequence of our sedentary lifestyle, appetite for unhealthy food, and growing problems with obesity.

INSULIN RESISTANCE MEANS INCREASED RISK

Even more prevalent than diabetes is insulin resistance, which affects an estimated 25 to 30 percent of the American population and is the underlying cause of type 2 diabetes (the kind that affects 90 to 95 percent of all diabetics). Insulin resistance is not caused by a failure of the pancreas to produce insulin (the essence of type 1 diabetes). Rather, it is caused by an inability of the cells to allow insulin to usher in glucose, resulting in excessive levels of both glucose and insulin in the blood.

Yet insulin resistance encompasses much more than type 2

diabetes. Abnormalities in blood lipids, hypertension, abdominal obesity, and increased risk of heart disease are its common companions. Stanford University School of Medicine researcher Gerald Reaven, M.D., who has been studying insulin resistance for thirty years, has given the cluster of conditions that stem from insulin resistance a name: syndrome X. (It is also called Reaven's syndrome, the "deadly quartet," metabolic syndrome, and insulin resistance syndrome.) Dr. Reaven believes that insulin resistance may be involved in half of all heart attacks and that it may be as accurate a predictor of heart disease as elevated LDL cholesterol.[5]

Insulin resistance is characterized by hyperinsulinemia (high levels of insulin in the blood). This bodes poorly for the arteries because it upsets the normal metabolism of fats. It cues the liver to make more very-low-density lipoprotein (VLDL), the primary carrier of triglycerides in the blood. As we discussed in the previous chapter, an elevated triglyceride level is a risk factor for atherosclerosis, and VLDL has been discovered to have damaging effects of its own. When levels of insulin remain high, protective HDL cholesterol falls, and small, dense, and very harmful LDL cholesterol particles are created.

In addition to its effects on lipids, hyperinsulinemia is linked to inflammation. It raises levels of fibrinogen and plasminogen activator inhibitor-1, which are involved in the formation of blood clots, as well as C-reactive protein. Individuals with insulin resistance are often overweight as well, and Dr. Reaven reports that approximately 50 percent of all patients with high blood pressure also have insulin resistance.

All these add up to one thing: increased risk of heart disease. If you are more than fifteen pounds overweight and carry that weight in your abdominal area, or if you have hypertension, high triglycerides, or low HDL cholesterol, you might consider having a fasting blood glucose test and perhaps a glucose tolerance test. If your fasting glucose is greater than or equal to 110 mg/dl and your glucose tolerance test higher than 140 mg/dl (these are lower than the diabetic ranges), you likely have insulin resistance and all its accompanying risks.

Fortunately, insulin resistance and its many manifestations respond well to the same nutritional and exercise measures (plus a few additional nutritional supplements) that comprise my program for reversing heart disease.

OBESITY: A WEIGHTY RISK FACTOR

In the past fifteen years the number of overweight Americans has grown by leaps and bounds. Today almost 55 percent of us are above normal weight and 22 percent are classified as clinically obese.[6] This is bad news for the cardiovascular system: Being 20 percent above your ideal weight more than doubles your risk of heart disease.

One explanation for this is the increased risk of hypertension and diabetes that goes with a forty-inch waistline. The common ground here is insulin resistance. Scientists are not certain if extra weight increases the risk of insulin resistance or if insulin resistance causes the body to store more fat and gain weight. Regardless of the exact nature of their relationship, the two are so closely intertwined that weight loss almost always improves insulin resistance and in many cases "cures" the conditions associated with syndrome X.

Obesity also triggers chronic inflammation. Researchers at the Free University in Amsterdam and the National Institute on Aging in Bethesda, Maryland, analyzed data on 16,000 men and women and found that obese men were five times as likely to have high levels of C-reactive protein, an inflammatory marker of heart disease risk, as lean men. Obese women were even more prone toward inflammation. They were thirteen times more likely to have elevated levels than thin women.[7]

Where you carry that weight is also important in heart disease.

Love handles and a big belly are typical of abdominal or "apple-shaped" obesity, which places you at increased risk. You may not like your extra pounds any more if they're on your hips and thighs, but that is definitely a healthier place to carry them. In fact, Harvard studies have reported that waist circumference and waist-hip ratio are independent risk factors for heart disease in women,[8] and that an apple shape is a strong predictor of death from cardiovascular disease in older men.[9] Abdominal fat is more metabolically active. It breaks down more easily into fatty acids that enter the bloodstream and raise triglyceride levels.

If you aren't sure if you are apple-shaped or the healthier pear shape, take a tape measure and measure the circumference of your waist at its narrowest point, just above the hipbones. Measure your hips at their widest, and then divide your waist measurement by your hip measurement. For example, if your hips are 37 inches and your waist is 28 inches, you have a hip/waist ratio

Height	Weight																					
	100	105	110	115	120	125	130	135	140	145	150	155	160	165	170	175	180	185	190	195	200	205
5'0"	20	21	21	22	23	24	25	26	27	28	29	30	31	32	33	34	35	36	37	38	39	40
5'1"	19	20	21	22	23	24	25	26	26	27	28	29	30	31	32	33	34	35	36	37	38	39
5'2"	18	19	20	21	22	23	24	25	26	27	27	28	29	30	31	32	33	34	35	36	37	37
5'3"	18	19	19	20	21	22	23	24	25	26	27	27	28	29	30	31	32	33	34	35	35	36
5'4"	17	18	19	20	21	21	22	23	24	25	26	27	27	28	29	30	31	32	33	33	34	35
5'5"	17	17	18	19	20	21	22	22	23	24	25	26	27	27	28	29	30	31	32	32	33	34
5'6"	16	17	18	19	19	20	21	22	23	23	24	25	26	27	27	28	29	30	31	31	32	33
5'7"	16	16	17	18	19	20	20	21	22	23	23	24	25	26	27	27	28	29	30	31	31	32
5'8"	15	16	17	17	18	19	20	21	21	22	23	24	24	25	26	27	27	28	29	30	30	31
5'9"	15	16	16	17	18	18	19	20	21	21	22	23	24	24	25	26	27	27	28	29	30	30
5'10"	14	15	16	17	17	18	19	19	20	21	22	22	23	24	24	25	26	27	27	28	29	29
5'11"	14	15	15	16	17	17	18	19	20	20	21	22	22	23	24	24	25	26	26	27	28	29
6'0"	14	14	15	16	16	17	18	18	19	20	20	21	22	22	23	24	24	25	26	26	27	28
6'1"	13	14	15	15	16	16	17	18	18	19	20	20	21	22	22	23	24	24	25	26	26	27
6'2"	13	13	14	15	15	16	17	17	18	19	19	20	21	21	22	22	23	24	24	25	26	26
6'3"	12	13	14	14	15	16	16	17	17	18	19	19	20	21	21	22	22	23	24	24	25	26
6'4"	12	13	13	14	15	15	16	16	17	18	18	19	19	20	21	21	22	23	23	24	24	25

FIGURE 5: What Is Your Body Mass Index?

of 0.75, which is within the normal range. If, however, your hips are 36 inches and your waist is 37 inches, your ratio is a much less desirable 1.03. A healthy hip/waist ratio for women is less than 0.8; for men it is less than 0.95.

Another common measurement of obesity and overweight is the body mass index (BMI). Use the chart on page 55 to figure out your BMI. Aim for a BMI in the healthy range of 19 to 25; 26 or higher places you at increased risk.

Americans spend $33 billion per year on weight-loss aids like diet books and prescription and over-the-counter diet pills, looking for the magic trick that will override the dozens of genes, hormones, and brain chemicals that influence appetite and metabolism. What we really need to do is improve our diets (we spend $110 billion per year on fast food[10]) and lift ourselves out of our easy chairs and get active. There's simply no escaping the first law of thermodynamics. If you eat more calories than you burn, you'll gain weight. More on this in Part III.

A COMPREHENSIVE APPROACH

Anyone concerned with heart disease needs to pay special attention to the conditions we have covered in this chapter, for if you ignore them, you're playing with fire. But let me reassure you that the treatment program for reversing heart disease, which is the basis of this book, is in reality a program for engendering health. Many of the biochemical processes involved in heart disease that we've discussed in these opening four chapters have nothing personal against your cardiovascular system. Disease is systemic. When you take measures to improve the health of your heart and arteries, you are benefiting your entire body. The focus of this book is reversing heart disease, but the beautiful part of the Whitaker Wellness Institute program is the improvements you'll see in many aspects of your health.

My program for reversing heart disease is pretty simple—so simple that you may be skeptical that it could possibly work. All it requires is that you pay attention to what you eat, exercise regularly, learn to manage stress, and take a few targeted nutritional supplements. Do not be deceived by its simplicity. Here are some of the things you might expect by following the program described in this book.

- All of the known risk factors for heart disease will be lowered or eliminated. Your total cholesterol, LDL, and triglyceride levels will fall. Your HDL will rise, and your homocysteine and other markers of heart disease risk will normalize.
- You likely will reduce or eliminate your medications for heart disease. In some cases, this reduction will occur within a few weeks.
- Your blood pressure almost certainly will fall, and you may be able to get off medication for hypertension.
- Chest pain likely will diminish or stop entirely as the oxygen-carrying capacity of your blood increases.
- You will probably lose weight. The average weight loss with this program is four to seven pounds a month, until your weight stabilizes near your ideal.
- Your physical endurance will improve, as will your muscular strength.
- Your cells will become more sensitive to insulin, which in turn will reduce your risk of developing insulin resistance and diabetes. If you have type 2 diabetes along with heart disease (a very common combo), your need for diabetic drugs likely will be reduced or eliminated.
- Your gastrointestinal system will receive a tune-up. If constipation has been a problem, it likely will disappear.
- As your heart health improves, you will probably notice changes for the better in all aspects of your health. You'll

feel better, have more energy, and notice improvements in your mood, memory, and sexuality.

I have found that these improvements take place to some extent in virtually every patient who undertakes this program, and in many the changes are striking. If the benefits of this program could be provided in a pill, it would be heralded as a miracle cure for heart disease. But of course there is no such pill, only a program of lifestyle changes that you must learn about, understand, and persevere in following.

Part II

The Conventional Approach to Heart Disease

CHAPTER 5

Heart Disease and Modern Medicine

WHEN PRESIDENT DWIGHT EISENHOWER HAD A HEART ATTACK IN 1955, he was rushed to the hospital, where he remained for almost two months, confined to bedrest. Before 1962, when the first coronary care units opened, there was little to offer patients who had suffered a heart attack other than rest, watchful concern, and hope that the injured heart muscle would heal.[1] Without question there have been enormous advances in the tools available for the treatment of patients with heart disease.

Today patients are placed in high-tech coronary wards, hooked up to machines that constantly monitor heart rhythm and other functions. Their hearts are looked at from every angle conceivable with high-resolution X rays, ultrasound, and other sophisticated scanning devices. They are even examined from the inside, with catheters snaking up through the body into the coronary arteries.

Whereas physicians in President Eisenhower's day had at their disposal a handful of drugs to manage heart disease, today there are more than a dozen major classes of pharmaceuticals and scores of individual drugs aimed at ailments of the heart. There are drugs that regulate the rhythm of the heart, slow it down, or speed it up. Others reduce the amount of oxygen required by the heart muscle or improve oxygen efficiency. Lower blood pressure, dilate the arteries, improve cholesterol and triglyceride levels: you name it and there's a drug that "fixes" it.

Even more astounding advances have been made in the operating room. We now have the technology to stop the heart completely while doctors perform elaborate surgery on the heart's blood vessels, a procedure undreamed of in the 1950s. We can ream out, prop open, or even bypass blockages in the arteries altogether. Lasers and robotics have entered the picture—chest pain can be relieved by drilling tiny holes in the heart with lasers, and surgeons can control tiny instruments in minimally invasive procedures.

These advancements are believed by physicians and patients alike to save the lives of hundreds of thousands of patients with heart disease every year. But do they? Where is the proof?

IS SURGERY SCIENTIFIC?

The introduction of surgical procedures follows quite a different path than the more familiar road of drug development and approval. You probably know that before a drug comes to market, it must undergo a series of clearly defined steps to gain approval by the Food and Drug Administration (FDA). It is first subjected to extensive animal testing to determine its safety and effectiveness, followed by carefully controlled human trials in which the drug is slowly and painstakingly studied for both its efficacy and adverse effects. Only after it meets all these requirements is a drug approved for routine use. And despite all this testing, some of the drugs that gain approval turn out, as I will show you, to be more dangerous than suspected and are ultimately banned from use.

Surgical procedures have no such approval process. Animal research, when it is done at all, is performed primarily to perfect the surgical technique, rather than to assess the procedure's dangers or ultimate usefulness. Many, if not all, new surgical procedures are developed on the *assumption* that they might help; then they are tried on human beings to see if they *do* work. In other words, they are performed, often for years, without any proof of efficacy. Sometimes a surgical procedure—such as tonsillectomy, a childhood rite of passage when I was growing up in the 1950s—is eventually abandoned or sharply curtailed after scientific studies show lack of benefit. Meanwhile, millions of patients serve as guinea pigs for untested procedures.

I personally believe that all surgical procedures should be subjected to the same type of controls that are required for new drug approvals. A new operation should first be done on animal models of the disease to determine its effectiveness and safety. If these animal experiments demonstrate a significant benefit, then carefully controlled studies in human volunteers would follow. Half of the volunteers would have the operation while the other half would be treated more conservatively. Both groups would be followed for a period of five years to determine if the procedure does indeed alter the natural course of the disease or have significant benefits, and to monitor its short- and long-term adverse effects. If the surgery's benefits outweighed its risks, then and only then would the surgical community be allowed to include it in their repertoire, and surgeons would be required to receive training in the new technique prior to utilizing it.

Do not interpret this discussion as a blanket criticism of surgery or of surgeons. I feel that many of our surgeons are among the most caring, competent, and concerned physicians in the country. Nevertheless, their craft includes so much risk that simply allowing procedure after procedure to be haphazardly developed, then abandoned and replaced by other untested procedures, doesn't make much sense.

OUR DRUG CULTURE

Like surgery, drugs are so embedded in the conventional practice of medicine that we can hardly imagine them as anything but lifesaving, health-enhancing wonders. The current system of medicine and medical education is tightly intertwined with the pharmaceutical industry. One lesson every medical school graduate walks away with is that drugs are the primary therapy for virtually all conditions. Links with drug companies become even stronger after medical school. Ongoing education for most physicians comes from medical journals (most of which are filled with pharmaceutical advertisements), from drug company sales representatives, and from pharmaceutical industry–sponsored conferences and events, where physicians are "educated" on the use of specific drugs.

Drug companies defend costs by reporting that they spend billions per year on research, but they neglect to mention expenditures on marketing and promotion—including billions of dollars on advertisements directed at consumers.[2] And their marketing efforts are paying off. Our health-care system is being bankrupted by more and more prescriptions and costlier drugs.

If drugs were safe, that would be one thing. But they aren't. Drugs are unnatural agents (You can't patent anything found in nature). They alter biological systems to bring about a desired effect. However, because they are foreign to the human body, they also have side effects and adverse reactions that are often completely unanticipated. More than 2.2 million adverse reactions to prescription drugs are reported in this country every year, and 106,000 deaths are caused by drugs used exactly as prescribed.[3] Believe it or not, prescription drugs kill more people in any given year than stroke, diabetes, pulmonary disease, AIDS, accidents, murder, or illegal drugs!

PREVENTION VERSUS TREATMENT

More than 100 billion dollars are spent each year in this country on the treatment of cardiovascular disease, yet it remains our leading killer.[4] This is not to say we've made no progress against heart disease. After sharp increases in the 1950s and early 1960s, a dramatic decrease in the death rate from coronary heart disease began. According to Dr. Robert I. Levy, former director of the National Heart, Lung, and Blood Institute, from 1968 to 1978 heart deaths decreased by 29 percent.[5] During the 1980s, the decline continued at a yearly rate of 3.5 percent.[6] And in the last decade of the century it fell again by half.

The medical establishment doesn't hesitate to take credit for falling mortality rates associated with heart disease, pointing to advances in surgical techniques, medical devices, and drugs. But newer isn't necessarily better, and these high-tech gadgets and powerful medications aren't all they're cracked up to be. Consider bypass and angioplasty, the big guns of cardiology. In Chapters 7 and 8 I will provide you with clear and perhaps startling evidence that these invasive procedures have made little to no significant contribution to the decline in the death rate from heart disease. Despite the popularity of these procedures—more than a million are performed every year in the United States alone—there is well-documented evidence that these interventions do not prolong life for the vast majority of patients who undergo them.

Then there are drugs. Pharmaceutical companies point to the development of life-saving drugs as a major factor in the declining death rate from heart disease. Some drugs are beneficial. However, to suggest that drugs play the dominant role in the reduction in deaths from heart disease that began in the late 1960s is disingenuous. These drugs were not widely used until the mid-seventies, a time when the fall in the death rate was already well under way. According to a 2000 World Health Organization study, "When the decline began in the USA, the revolution in coronary care had not started and the current powerful drugs were not available. Countries with rising or stable rates were using and adopting new treatments at the same time as the USA.

If new drugs and treatments are the main contributor to the decline in coronary-event rates between the mid-1980s and mid-1990s, this finding cannot be extrapolated back to the 1960s and 1970s or, necessarily, into the future. . . ."[7]

One area that has had some impact on declining deaths from heart disease is the medical care of patients immediately after a heart attack. In President Eisenhower's day, only two out of every three patients who made it to a hospital after suffering a heart attack left the hospital alive, compared to 90 percent today. The accessibility and frequent use of thrombolytic therapy (clot-busting drugs), aspirin, and anticoagulants administered after a heart attack appear to be responsible for much of the improvements in survival after heart attack.[8] Other in-hospital interventions also may contribute to some of the positive changes in mortality statistics.

However, most who die from heart attacks die *before* they reach the hospital. Therefore, even though medical treatment of the acute heart attack victim has improved, it is not and cannot be the explanation for the dramatic drop in deaths from heart disease over the last forty years.

If treatment isn't driving down our rates of heart deaths, what is? As I explained in the opening chapter of this book, it is prevention. A large international study funded by the World Health Organization and published in 1999 concluded that although improvements in the acute treatment of heart attack patients could indeed lay some small claim to declining death rates from heart disease, the real reason was that *fewer people were having heart attacks*.[9] The true heroes are not surgeons or drug manufacturers or hospitals but the people who are getting a handle on their risk factors by stopping smoking, eating better, and exercising more.

I recognize that there will be continued advancements in the treatment of heart disease, and some (though certainly not all) of them will benefit patients. However, very few of the tools used by today's physicians are geared toward eliminating the underlying causes of atherosclerosis or, for that matter, slowing down its progression. More than a million Americans submit to the cardiologist's knife or catheter every year, convinced that their lives are being saved. Tens of millions dutifully take drugs that they've been told are keeping them alive. These presumptions simply are not true, and in the next few chapters I'll tell you why.

CHAPTER 6

The Slippery Slope of Diagnostics

CHARLIE PICKED UP A FLIER IN A DRUGSTORE ADVERTISING A health fair at his community hospital. Several physicians would be speaking on health-related topics, and free screenings for vision, blood pressure, blood sugar, and cholesterol were offered. It sounded interesting, so Charlie and his wife showed up and made the rounds of the various lectures, exhibits, and screenings. A couple of weeks later Charlie got a phone call from a physician's office informing him that his cholesterol test had just come back, and his level was high. Since his blood pressure had also been recorded as somewhat elevated, he was advised to set up an appointment to come in and discuss these findings. Although Charlie felt great and had no significant health problems, this news worried him a little, so he scheduled an appointment.

Although he was unaware of it at the time, Charlie had stepped onto the slippery slope of the heart disease industry, and unfortunately for him, he took a plunge. First, he was told that he needed to have an exercise stress test. A slight abnormality on this test led him to the angiography lab, where blockages were discovered in two of his coronary arteries, and from there he was pushed into the surgical suite for coronary artery bypass surgery. All this in a patient who had never had a single sign or symptom of heart disease!

I wish Charlie's story were a fluke, but it is not. During my near thirty years as a practicing physician I have seen this scenario played out hundreds of times, and each and every time it fuels my drive to educate people about the inner workings of the heart surgery industry. In this chapter I want to tell you about the most common diagnostic and screening tests for heart disease and how they can be a gateway to unnecessary and injurious invasive procedures. For the uninformed patient, like Charlie, a simple, seemingly harmless diagnostic test is all that is needed for yet another unnecessary bypass operation.

ANGIOGRAPHY: THE TARNISHED GOLD STANDARD

Most of the medical establishment holds that the gold standard in cardiology diagnostics is angiography, or cardiac catheterization. Angiography is an invasive X-ray procedure that provides a close look at the anatomy of the coronary arteries. A patient checks into a cath lab in a hospital and is prepped and given a local anesthetic and mild sedative. A hole is punctured in the femoral artery in the groin and a long, thin catheter is inserted. It is snaked up the artery and directed into one or more of the arteries in the heart. Once there, a dye is injected through the catheter, and X-ray pictures are taken. The catheter is then removed, and pressure is placed on the femoral artery to stop bleeding. After a few hours of bedrest, the patient is released. By reading these pictures, a radiologist or cardiologist determines the location and severity of blockages in the coronary arteries.

This test is widely assumed by both patients and physicians to be a very accurate method of assessing the degree of blockage in the heart arteries. In truth, angiograms are far from accurate. Technical problems can undermine the accuracy of this test. When the dye is injected into the artery, the pressure of the injection can distend an arterial segment and give false readings. And as with any X-ray procedure, positioning of the X-ray beam can distort, magnify, or completely miss alterations in the flow of dye in the artery.

Technical errors aside, there are inherent inaccuracies in angiography. The dye that illuminates the arteries detects blockages as a series of lumps or bumps that are interpreted as prime offenders in heart disease. However, as we discussed in detail in Chapter 2, atherosclerosis is generally diffuse, with smooth and symmetrical layers of buildup as well as random projections into the lumen, or opening of the artery. Since an angiogram shows only pronounced intrusions into the lumen and misses the smaller, smoother buildup, it routinely misinterprets the degree of blockage in the artery.

According to Steven E. Nissen, M.D., director of cardiology at the Cleveland Clinic Foundation in Ohio, it also misses the smaller, vulnerable plaques, which are much more susceptible to rupturing and instigating a heart attack than the large plaques that are picked up.[1] In a 2001 presentation, Dr. Nissen presented evidence that angiography fails to pick up an astounding 95 to 99 percent of all atherosclerotic plaques.[2] Angiography scouts out the war against heart disease on one front—seeking out large plaques—while ignoring the far more serious battles going on elsewhere.

To see exactly how inaccurate angiography is, Ernest N. Arnett, M.D., from the National Heart, Lung and Blood Institute and the Department of Medicine of the National Naval Academy in Bethesda, Maryland, performed autopsies on patients who died shortly after having a coronary angiogram. He examined in detail sixty-one coronary arteries from these patients and found that angiography routinely underestimated the severity of the disease and in some cases missed severe blockages altogether. Most of the arteries examined showed 25 to 60 percent diffuse plaque obstruction throughout.[3]

ANGIOGRAMS JUST AREN'T VERY ACCURATE

Yet another serious drawback of angiography is what is known as interobserver variability. Angiograms are read by radiologists or cardiologists, who estimate the degree of blockage. However, studies have shown that there are marked inconsistencies in interpretation—from 7.5 to as much as 50 percent—from one physician to another.[4] Leonard M. Zir, M.D., of the Department of Radiology at Massachusetts General Hospital, compared the readings of four experienced angiographers interpreting twenty consecutive coronary angiograms. These doctors had been working together for years reading angiograms as a group. However, when asked to read the angiograms individually, Dr. Zir found wide variations in interpretation, and he concluded that this posed a considerable problem. "Interobserver variability in the interpretation of lesions in the coronary vessels might be similarly translated into different decisions about the necessity for coronary artery bypass surgery or, if coronary bypass is to be performed, which vessels are bypassable. Interobserver variability is a significant limitation of coronary angiography and clearly requires further study."[5]

A group of researchers from the University of Iowa delivered what in my opinion should have been the knockout punch to the assumed accuracy of angiography. Carl W. White, M.D., and colleagues measured the blood flow through the coronary arteries of patients undergoing bypass surgery and compared these blood flow measurements to angiograms on the same arteries. They discovered that the angiographic findings had no correlation at all to the actual blood flow measured during surgery! For instance, there was no significant difference in blood flow through the arteries that had appeared on angiogram to have a 60 percent blockage, compared to arteries pegged with 90 or even 95 percent blockages. In fact, some of the arteries with a 95 percent blockage according to angiography had greater blood flow than arteries read as having only a 40 percent blockage.

These researchers rightly concluded: "The results of these studies should be profoundly disturbing to all physicians who have relied on coronary angiograms to provide accurate information regarding the physiologic consequences of individual coronary stenosis."[6] Disturbing to physicians, but what about the patients?

BEFORE GETTING AN ANGIOGRAM, GET A SECOND OPINION

Thomas B. Graboys, M.D., a cardiologist at Harvard Medical School, is an astute physician and researcher. Although he functions in a conservative bastion of medicine, he has always refused to accept standard cardiology practices on faith alone. His push for thorough and unbiased validation of current medical practices has resulted in several breakthrough studies, including one that challenges the "let's catheterize" attitude of his colleagues.

In this study, 168 patients with angina who had been recommended to have an angiogram came in of their own accord for a second opinion. Using information obtained from noninvasive tests, such as the exercise stress test and echocardiogram, Dr. Graboys and his colleagues determined that *only six* of the 168 actually needed to have an angiogram. Another 28 patients were recommended to defer angiography pending further studies. The remaining patients—80 percent—did not require it at all.

The group then followed these patients for an average of four years to see how they fared *without* the angiogram that would likely have steered them toward bypass surgery. Over that four-year period, these patients experienced a 1.1 percent annual death rate from heart disease—less than the death rate for patients undergoing bypass surgery at that time. The Graboys team concluded that angiography, which they described as a "conduit" to bypass and angioplasty, is unnecessary for a majority of the patients who are urged to undergo it. Furthermore, this study clearly demonstrated that most patients, even those with severe blockages, can be treated safely with conservative measures.[7]

The lesson here is simple: If your doc tells you to have an angiogram, consider it carefully. And if he or she tells you that you cannot be treated unless an angiogram has been obtained, don't buy it. Treatment decisions should be based on your clinical condition: how much pain you are having and what brings it on, your exercise tolerance, and the results of your exercise stress test, echocardiogram, and blood tests—all of which can be obtained by efficient, advanced, noninvasive testing.

Before submitting to angiography, you had best get a second opinion—a true second opinion and not just a nod of agreement from a physician cut from the same cloth. Take the list of references from this chapter pertaining to angiography to your local medical library and obtain copies of these key articles. Read them carefully, and present them to the physician who renders your second opinion.

The profile of the patient described by Dr. Graboys in the study mentioned above who did not need immediate angiography (the vast majority of the patients who had been referred for the test) was simple. The patient had predictable symptoms—angina with exercise but not while resting or during the night. He or she had adequate heart function as determined by ejection fraction and an exercise stress test free of exercise hypotension (low blood pressure). The presence of ST-segment depression (an irregularity on exercise stress testing that often drives patients toward immediate angiography) was a nonissue in this study. If noninvasive screening tools demonstrate evidence of significant impairment of the heart during exercise or severe chest pain or shortness of breath that cannot be controlled by medication and the lifestyle changes we will discuss in Part III, then angiography could reveal a condition that would warrant invasive therapy.

To recap, although angiography is often billed as simply a diagnostic or screening test, it is more often a prelude to invasive heart procedures—the final and deciding step on the slippery slope of bypass surgery and angioplasty. Therefore, it should be used only as a last resort.

DON'T BET ON THE ULTRAFAST CT SCAN

There is another screening test that is funneling people into unnecessary heart procedures. You may have heard a commercial on your local radio station or seen ads in your paper touting a painless, noninvasive test to predict your risk of heart disease. These very provocative ads often end with the testimonial of a grateful patient who, thanks to this test, was "fortunate" enough to have had an angiogram and an angioplasty—leaving him and many listeners convinced that the test saved his life.

The test is electron beam computed tomography (EBCT), commonly called ultrafast or rapid CT scan. It uses a specialized X-ray machine that takes extremely fast, stop-action pictures of the heart. Like other CT scans, it visualizes cross sections of an organ. Unlike traditional CT, its speed allows it to take pictures of moving organs, such as a beating heart. The ultrafast CT scan identifies calcium in the arteries of the heart. Because calcium is incorporated into arterial plaque, proponents tout it as an excellent screening tool for atherosclerosis and risk of heart attack. Patients are given a calcium score of minimal, slight, moderate, or marked, which they are told correlates with their degree of heart disease.

This whole presumption, in my opinion, is unsound. First, calcium deposits in the arteries do not in and of themselves predict heart attack or death from heart disease. Several studies have demonstrated that the death rate of patients with one blocked artery was no lower than that of patients with two and sometimes with three obstructed arteries. If calcium-containing arterial blockages—as determined by angiography, ultrafast CT scan, or any other screening tool—were predictive of death or heart attack, then patients with multivessel disease would inevitably have had higher heart attack and death rates than those with single-vessel disease. This just wasn't the case.[8]

Furthermore, the absence of calcium deposits in the arteries does not preclude the risk of atherosclerosis. It has been well documented that some patients who have had heart attacks have little or no calcium in their coronary arteries. Calcium tends to be present in large, stable, calcified plaques but less prevalent in the smaller, softer but more deadly vulnerable plaques involved in most heart attacks.

One of the most complete studies of the ultrafast CT scan's power to predict heart attack was published in 1999. The 1,196 subjects recruited for this study averaged sixty-six years of age, and although they were at high risk for heart disease, they had no outright symptoms. They were screened with ultrafast CT scan, as well as with tests of common, established heart disease risk factors (elevated cholesterol, low HDL cholesterol, high blood pressure, and elevated body mass index). Sixty-eight percent of the study participants had detectable coronary calcium on ultrafast CT. However, at the end of this three-year study, the calcium score proved to be no better than the conventional risk factors at predicting heart attacks. Since the ultrafast CT scan added no significant information to the conventional risk factors, the authors concluded that its use in clinical screening was not justified.[9]

One of the problems that plagues angiography is also endemic in the ultrafast CT scan: accuracy. According to Robert C. Detrano, M.D., professor of medicine at UCLA, reproducibility of findings varies widely among investigators, even in same-day repeat testing in the same patient. He cited a Mayo Clinic study that showed a 49 percent variability![10] Such inconsistency is bound to result in a rash of false positives, tests interpreted as showing problems when, in fact, no problems exist.

I am more than a little worried about this test because it is being so heavily advertised directly to the public. Three out of four patients undergoing ultrafast CT scanning at major medical centers come in of their own accord. These people, many of them without any signs of heart disease whatsoever, plunk down their $400 to $500 for the test and, when told of their elevated calcium score, join the swelling ranks of the "worried well."[11] Such individuals, dealing with the fear of lurking disaster, may hastily

Diagnostic Testing the Whitaker Wellness Way

What is the best way to assess your risk of heart disease? At the Whitaker Wellness Institute we rely heavily on a patient's medical history and examination. It is amazing how much a physician can learn during an office visit. By asking the right questions, drawing the patient out, and really listening and observing, a physician can uncover more information than you might imagine possible. In fact, it is not unusual for the patient, directly or indirectly, to make the diagnosis.

Of course, we also do a thorough physical exam, and we obtain invaluable information from the blood tests discussed in Chapter 3, such as blood fats, homocysteine, high-sensitive C-reactive protein, and blood sugar. In addition, we utilize two noninvasive tests that do a superb job of screening for cardiovascular disease: the exercise stress test, which shows how well the heart functions during exercise, and the echocardiogram, which monitors the heart's anatomy. Used appropriately, these screening tests are valuable tools in assessing the health of the heart and structuring reasonable and effective programs for the overwhelming majority of patients with heart disease.

agree to unwarranted interventions. Avoid the ultrafast CT scan. It is yet another gateway to invasive heart procedures.

THE VENERABLE EXERCISE STRESS TEST

The exercise stress test has been around for a long time. In 1908 Willem Einthoven first identified changes in the electrocardiogram (EKG) with exercise, and in 1932 exercise EKG was first used to diagnose angina. Although many physicians prefer newer, more high-tech tests on the assumption that they are superior, I've remained loyal to the exercise stress test. Its predictive value for heart disease is unsurpassed. It is an excellent screening tool for healthy people with no signs of heart disease (I recommend it to anyone over the age of forty before beginning a vigorous exercise program) and for people with diagnosed or suspected heart disease to determine degree of severity.

As its name implies, this test is simply an EKG taken during exercise to evaluate the function of the heart under stress. As with any EKG, electrodes that detect electrical impulses generated by the heart are attached to the arms, legs, and chest. The patient then walks on a treadmill or rides a stationary bike at gradually increasing speeds and degrees of difficulty (the treadmill is elevated and the resistance on the bike is increased). During the average ten-minute test, blood pressure, heart rate and rhythm, and symptoms such as chest pain, shortness of breath, and fatigue are constantly monitored. All the while, the electrodes send impulses to a machine, where they are recorded as a series of waves representing each beat of the heart.

We can learn a lot from an exercise stress test. For example, failure of the systolic pressure (the top number in the blood pressure equation) to rise during exercise usually indicates problems with the heart's pumping efficiency. Heart rate, arrhythmias, blood pressure changes during exercise, how quickly your heart rate returns to normal after exercise—all these things are factored in. Among the most highly predictive findings on a stress test are how long you can exercise and how you feel. If you can keep up with the expected duration and intensity for your age without having chest pain or shortness of breath, that is an excellent sign of good heart health.

Like any test, the exercise stress test isn't perfect, nor is it always analyzed accurately. Several studies have shown that the stress test is less accurate in women, who tend to have a higher rate of false positives. In addition, false negatives (a normal test when heart disease is present) are not uncommon in young men. Furthermore, it has been my experience that some physicians overemphasize minor abnormalities and tell patients they have heart problems when in reality nothing of significance is present.

Exercise stress testing is safe, although it can, like any form of exercise, induce angina in patients with severe heart disease, and a few heart attacks during testing have been reported. Overall, however, the exercise stress test meets the criteria for safety and accuracy to be considered one of our best screening tests for heart disease. According to a 2000 article published in *The Lancet*, ". . . the simple exercise stress test can in most cases outperform the newer tests. . . . Brief, inexpensive, and done in most cases without the presence of a cardiologist, the exercise test offers the highest value for predictive accuracy of any of the noninvasive tests for coronary artery disease."[12]

ECHOCARDIOGRAPHY GIVES AN INSIDE VIEW

Echocardiography is a procedure that allows us to visualize the anatomy and function of the heart. It utilizes an ultrasound, a machine that transmits sound waves, which bounce off organs with varying intensity, then captures them and translates them into pictures. Ultrasound has all kinds of diagnostic purposes and is so safe that it has been utilized for decades to monitor pregnancy. Its use in cardiology goes back even further, and numerous variations have evolved, such as color-flow Doppler (which visualizes blood flow), transesophageal echocardiography (a probe is inserted so the heart can be visualized from behind), and stress echocardiography (in which the patient exercises by pedaling a bicycle-like contraption while lying on the table, or drugs are administered to increase the heart rate).

The standard echocardiogram is completely noninvasive. The patient lies on a table and a technician positions a probe directly on the skin over the heart. Guided by an image of the heart on a screen, he moves the probe around to examine various aspects of the heart and prints pictures of important areas. Echocardiography provides a wealth of information about the heart. It clearly reveals heart valve abnormalities, abnormalities in the pericardium (the thin membrane covering the heart), blood clots within the heart, and even unusual heart rhythms. It also shows the size of the heart: enlargement indicative of heart failure and thickening of certain areas common in uncontrolled hypertension. Of particular importance is the size and function of the left ventricle, the chamber that ejects blood into the aorta.

One of the most significant pieces of information that echocardiography provides is the ejection fraction. The ejection fraction is the percentage of blood ejected from the left ventricle with each beat, and it is a crucial indicator of heart function. If the heart is filled to a capacity of 100 cc of blood and the next stroke pumps out 70 cc, the ejection fraction is 70 percent. If it pumps out only 35 cc, the ejection fraction is 35 percent. The healthier the heart—the stronger and more efficient—the higher the ejection fraction. A normal ejection fraction is considered to be in the 50 to 75 percent range.

The ejection fraction and thus the function of the left ventricle is a pretty reliable indicator of heart disease risk. According to the Coronary Artery Surgery Study (CASS) (a landmark study of the merits of bypass surgery that we will discuss in detail in the next chapter), patients with an ejection fraction of 50 percent or greater had a very low risk of heart attack or death from heart disease. Even if such a patient had blockages in one, two, or even three coronary arteries, if the heart was pumping efficiently the chances of having a major coronary event were about one in 100—without invasive treatment. Patients with a poor ejection fraction, less than 50 percent, had a less optimistic prognosis.

OTHER DIAGNOSTIC AND SCREENING TOOLS FOR CARDIOVASCULAR DISEASE

There are other screening and diagnostic tools for heart disease that I want to review briefly. Nuclear imaging using radioactive isotopes is one of the most high-tech types of heart imaging techniques. The most popular nuclear imaging tool is the thallium scan. Thallium is injected into the bloodstream during maximum exercise. Because it is rapidly taken up by healthy heart tissue but not by damaged areas of the heart, it delineates the extent of damage to the heart muscle. Single-photon emission computed tomography (SPECT), positron emission tomography (PET), and radionuclide ventriculography are other imaging techniques that provide high-resolution pictures of the heart.

Magnetic resonance imaging (MRI) uses the magnetic properties of subatomic protons to provide three-dimensional pictures of the heart and vessels. The patient is placed in a chamber and subjected to a strong magnetic field that lines protons up. The protons are then disturbed with radio-frequency energy pulses, which cause them to resonate at specific frequencies that can be transmitted to a monitor as a picture.[13] When MRI was introduced, it was limited to tissues such as the brain and joints—a beating heart was hard to visualize. New techniques permit improved visualization. There are high hopes for this tool, for it may be able to identify the smaller vulnerable plaques that are most often involved in heart attacks.[14]

These tests are, for the time being anyway, quite pricey and their use is limited primarily to patients whose coronary status cannot be determined by the screening and diagnostic tools discussed earlier.

Testing aside, there's an even better way to stay ahead of heart disease: *Presume* that you have atherosclerosis and act accordingly. Begin a regular exercise program. Eat a heart-healthy diet. Take a potent multivitamin and mineral supplement with high doses of antioxidants and B-complex vitamins. Even if you don't have heart disease, this program will improve your overall health and dramatically lower your risk of ever having a heart attack.

CHAPTER 7

Bypass Surgery: Pros and Cons, Risks and Benefits

HERE IS A SCENARIO PLAYED OUT MORE THAN HALF A MILLION times a year in this country. The dedicated heart surgeon enters the surgical suite. Armed for battle and supported by his loyal entourage, he approaches the prepped patient, and the action begins. Hours pass. He finally emerges with good news for the awaiting family: He has saved the life of the patient. Sometimes the outcome is different, and he must be the bearer of bad news. "I'm sorry. I did all I could to save the patient, but his heart disease was just too far advanced."

If you haven't experienced this yourself or known someone who has, then you've seen it enacted on TV, where the heart surgeon as hero is a familiar character. Fiction aside, coronary artery bypass surgery, angioplasty, and the supporting industry they have spawned are firmly entrenched in modern medicine. These invasive procedures are recommended with such confidence and enthusiasm by so many cardiologists that there appears to be almost no question as to their need or value. Heart surgery is viewed as the last chance for unfortunate patients suffering with heart disease. The lucky ones who get to have surgery are almost assured of a longer, better life, while the unfortunates who for one reason or another cannot go under the knife are likely on their way out.

I have one goal in the next two chapters, and that is to dismantle this preconceived notion. The common perception that surgery is the best or only option for patients with heart disease and that it consistently saves lives and improves quality of life is simply wrong. Of course, some patients do benefit from invasive procedures to open their coronary arteries, but only a small subset of patients falls into this category. There is a plethora of scientific data clearly demonstrating that for the vast majority of patients, heart surgery is expensive, dangerous, and unnecessary.

I am not alone in my opinion. Peter Libby, M.D., chief of cardiovascular medicine at Brigham and Women's Hospital and professor of medicine at Harvard Medical School, has stated that the real problem is not large, stable plaques but the smaller, vulnerable plaques we discussed in Chapter 2. "We have a new therapeutic goal—the stabilization of lesions rather than extirpating them by surgery or angioplasty. We have also come to recognize that none of our high-technology therapies for treating ischemia, including surgery and angioplasty, actually reduces the incidence of MI [myocardial infarction, or heart attack] or prolongs life, except in selected subgroups of patients."[1]

In this chapter we will dismantle the myths about coronary artery bypass grafting, the king of the heart surgery industry, and in the next chapter we will tackle angioplasty, the crown prince.

WHAT IS CORONARY ARTERY BYPASS GRAFT SURGERY?

Before we enter the fray of the controversy surrounding coronary artery bypass surgery, I want to review what this surgery actually involves. Let's take the case of my patient John. When he was sixty-three years old, John was rushed to the hospital with severe chest pain, in the throes of a heart attack. He was told that in order to prevent another, likely fatal heart attack, he needed immediate bypass surgery. Scared out of his wits, John agreed.

He was prepped and taken to the surgical suite, and the medical team got to work. After John was anesthetized, an electric saw cut through his breastbone and split his chest down the center. A device, appropriately called a rib spreader, separated his rib cage to expose his heart and lungs. The heart surgeon cut and peeled away the pericardial sac that covers the heart to reveal the heart muscle. Meanwhile, another surgeon was making an incision on John's leg and removing the saphenous vein, a nonessential blood vessel that runs the length of the leg, from thigh to ankle, to be used as a graft to bypass the blocked arteries.

Next, John was placed on the heart-lung machine. Tubes were inserted into the veins that normally deliver blood to the heart, and into the aorta, the main artery exiting the heart that carries blood to the arterial system. His blood was diverted from the heart and through this machine, which took over the pumping and oxygenating functions of the heart and lungs. His heart was then stopped with an injection, and the actual bypass surgery then began.

The heart surgeon first attached a portion of the vein harvested from John's leg to the aorta and then sewed it onto the diseased artery downstream of the blockage. He repeated this procedure on another blocked coronary artery and attached the left internal mammary artery to yet another blocked artery. These grafts allowed blood to flow to the heart muscle through new blood vessel segments that "bypassed" the blockage, hence the name. Once the grafts were in place, his heart was restarted, he was taken off the heart-lung machine, the rib spreader was removed, and his breastbone was closed with stainless steel wire. His incisions were sewn up, and he was wheeled into the intensive care unit, where he would be closely monitored for several days. John would eventually leave the hospital in good spirits, convinced and grateful that his life had been spared.

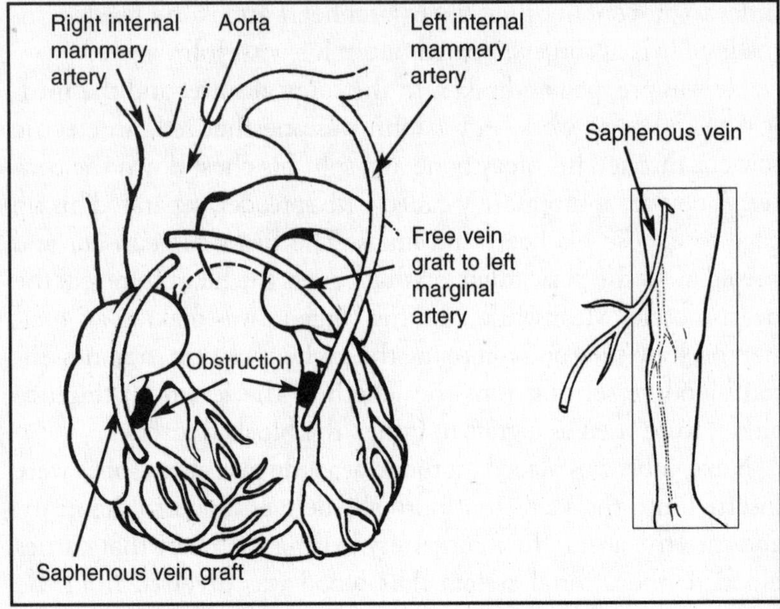

FIGURE 6: Bypass Surgery

It doesn't get much more dramatic than this, does it? But just because coronary artery bypass surgery has all the elements of high drama doesn't mean that it's an effective therapy.

A HISTORICAL PERSPECTIVE

Prior to the 1960s the treatment of survivors of heart attacks consisted of little more than bedrest and large doses of hope and prayer. At the same time, more and more people were dying from heart disease every year, so the race was on to develop new treatments. Dozens of different surgical procedures were performed in an attempt to relieve angina. The vast majority of them underwent no controlled studies to see whether they really helped patients, and the few that were scientifically scrutinized failed miserably.[2]

In 1967 coronary artery bypass graft surgery came onto the scene. The original intent of this operation was to relieve angina, and it did indeed alleviate chest pain. With this first blush of success, many physicians arbitrarily assumed that the operation would also prevent heart attacks and prolong life. They also presumed that since the rate of death from heart disease began falling in the 1970s, the same time bypass surgery was gaining a foothold, the surgery was saving lives. Despite the lack of any evidence to support these assumptions, bypass surgery rapidly grew in popularity.

Bypass surgery was universally accepted before it was subjected to any clinical trials at all to determine its safety and to see if it really helped patients. And when these well-controlled studies demonstrated that for the vast majority of patients the surgery did not save lives or prevent future heart attacks, it didn't make any difference at all! The heart surgery industry, as I will show you later in this chapter, had become so entwined in the economics and culture of medicine that the results of these studies were ignored altogether.

THE VETERANS ADMINISTRATION COOPERATIVE STUDY

It wasn't until the early seventies that the scientific community decided it was time to evaluate bypass surgery, since by then it was being performed on tens of thousands of patients every year. In order to assess the efficacy of bypass, it would have to be compared with another therapy, and both would have to be administered to patients with similar severity of disease, age, and other factors that might influence the study's outcome. The treatment group would have bypass, while the other, the control group, would be treated with appropriate drugs and medical follow-up.

The first of these studies was the Veterans Administration Cooperative Study, which involved physicians and researchers at thirteen VA hospitals across the country. Five hundred and ninety-six patients with heart disease characterized by stable angina (chest pain that came on predictably with exercise) that had not changed significantly over six months, were randomly placed in one of two groups. The 286 patients in one group received bypass surgery, while the 310 patients in the other group were treated simply with standard heart drugs.

The results of this study were completely unexpected. When the VA study was published in 1977, coronary artery bypass graft was well on its way to becoming the most popular surgical procedure in medical history. It had already developed a following among both cardiologists and surgeons, and everyone figured that this study would demonstrate its benefits and justify the near-billion-dollar industry that had emerged. What they found instead was that with the exception of a small subset of patients, surgery conferred no significant advantages. After three years, the death and heart attack rates in the patients treated with surgery and those treated more conservatively were about the same.[3] In other words, for the majority of patients, coronary artery bypass graft did not save lives or provide any long-term benefits.

Yet many cardiologists were so committed to heart surgery that they paid little heed to the results of this well-controlled study. One who did was Eugene Braunwald, M.D., of Harvard Medical School, who warned:

> An even more insidious problem is that what might be considered an industry is being built around this operation: the creation of facilities for open heart operations in community hospitals in which no other cardiac procedures are performed, and the enlargement of surgical facilities in teaching hospitals, the proliferation of catheterization and angiographic suites as well as facilities for performing screening exercise electrocardiograms, and expansion and development of training op-

> portunities, clinical cardiology, cardiovascular surgery, and cardiovascular radiology. This rapidly growing enterprise is developing a momentum and constituency of its own, and as time passes it will be progressively more difficult and costly to curtail it materially if the results of carefully designed studies of its efficacy prove this step to be necessary.[4]

In spite of this study and Dr. Braunwald's warning, rapid growth of bypass continued unchecked. Two subsequent studies involving VA participants provided even more damning evidence that the surgery was largely ineffective. In a 1988 follow-up study, researchers evaluated the coronary arteries of 119 of the nonsurgically treated patients and 109 of the patients who had had bypass years earlier. The results strengthened the original findings. Although the overall rate of progression of atherosclerosis was comparable between the two groups, atherosclerosis was actually accelerated in the arteries that had been grafted![5] And an eight-year follow-up of VA study subjects made an even worse case for bypass surgery. Except for very high-risk patients (with three-vessel disease or a low ejection fraction indicative of poor heart function), mortality rates were twice as high for patients who had had bypass (32.2 percent), compared to those treated conservatively (16.8 percent).[6]

THE CORONARY ARTERY SURGERY STUDY

Following on the heels of the initial Veterans Administration Study was the Coronary Artery Surgery Study (CASS), surely the most important study of the benefits of bypass surgery ever undertaken. Funded by the National Heart, Lung and Blood Institute at a cost of more than $24 million and involving eleven different surgical centers, it included 780 patients carefully selected from a registry of 16,626 patients. The inclusion criteria were the presence of stable angina, good heart function, and a significant blockage in one, two, or three of the major arteries supplying blood to the heart. The patients were further divided into subgroups based on the number of arteries involved (single-, double-, and triple-vessel disease). Then half of the patients underwent surgery, while the other half was treated with medications and other conservative measures.

The first of the CASS papers was published in 1983, after five years of follow-up. Like the VA study, the results ran counter to expectations. Bypass surgery did virtually nothing to improve longevity or reduce heart attacks, compared to treatment with medication, even in patients with three-vessel disease. In fact, the death rate of patients treated conservatively was so low that bypass surgery could do little to improve on it. The annual mortality rate of patients treated simply with medications was only 1.6 percent, compared to 1.1 percent for those who had bypass surgery—a difference so small as to be statistically insignificant. Even in what was considered to be a particularly high-risk group of patients, those with triple-vessel disease, medical therapy had a mortality rate of only 2.1 percent.[7]

Let's look at what these numbers really mean in terms of lives saved. To simplify things, let's assume that bypass surgery reduced the death rate by 50 percent—cut it in half—from 2 percent to 1 percent. While this may sound like a lot, when we're talking about the difference between 1 and 2 percent, it isn't much. In order for bypass surgery to save just one life per year, 100 patients would have to undergo surgery, with all its potential risks and complications. In reality, in the CASS study this difference was not 50 percent but only 0.5 percent—a statistical toss-up. Patients who did not have bypass surgery had a 98.4 percent chance of surviving five years, odds that are hard to beat.

CASS also compared the frequency of nonfatal heart attacks between the two groups and found it to be virtually identical: 11 percent in the medical group and 14 percent in the surgery group.

The conclusion of the CASS researchers was, "As compared with medical therapy, coronary artery bypass surgery appears to neither prolong life nor to prevent myocardial infarction."[8]

The CASS team followed up their study participants again after ten years, and about 80 percent of them in each group were still alive. (Mortality rates were 21.8 percent in the medical group and 19.2 percent in the surgical group.) Among survivors there was little difference in quality-of-life markers, such as presence of angina, use of medications, frequency of heart failure and hospitalization, and employment and activity limitations. Based on these findings, the researchers concluded that there was little long-term advantage to the surgical approach and recommended that medical therapy be initially used in the majority of patients.[9] These same findings were seen again in CASS's fifteen-year follow-up study. With the exception of a subgroup of very high-risk patients (those with left main coronary artery disease) survival rates were similar in the medical and surgical groups.[10]

I cannot overemphasize the importance of CASS. It remains the most expensive, comprehensive and carefully designed study of its kind. You would think that such a study would have had a huge impact on the practice of cardiology. Yet coronary artery bypass surgery remains the treatment of choice for hundreds of thousands of patients with heart disease.

OTHER STUDIES ON CORONARY ARTERY BYPASS

Although these were the best and most enduring studies comparing coronary artery bypass surgery to conservative treatment, there have been other randomized trials, including the large European Coronary Artery Surgery Study (EuroCASS). In a review study that analyzed data from all the patients enrolled in EuroCASS plus four smaller trials, the consensus was the same as the VA study and CASS: Bypass did not save lives or prevent heart attacks. In fact, according to this study, although patients in very high-risk groups had some benefit from bypass, those with one- or two-vessel disease and a well-functioning heart (which encompasses most patients undergoing bypass) had a *greater* risk of heart attack and death when treated with surgery, compared to a conservative strategy.[11]

There is one more study I want to tell you about. VANQWISH (Veterans Affairs Non-Q-Wave Infarction Strategies in Hospital) was begun in 1993 to determine the best treatment for patients who have had non-Q-wave myocardial infarctions. More than half of all heart attacks in this country are of this type, and they are considered to be pretty serious, as they are often followed by angina and repeat heart attacks. Consequently, treatment has become increasingly aggressive, with a greater push toward bypass and angioplasty. The purpose of this study was to see if such aggressive treatment is warranted. William E. Boden, M.D., and colleagues enrolled 920 patients in medical centers across the country who had experienced an acute non-Q-wave myocardial infarction. Half of these patients were randomly assigned to an invasive strategy of angiography followed by bypass surgery or angioplasty. The other half were assigned to a conservative management program with noninvasive testing and medication. The patients were then followed for an average of twenty-three months.

The results came as no surprise to me. Patients who underwent surgery did worse. During the first nine days, twenty-one patients in the invasive strategy group died, compared to only six in the medical group. The in-hospital death or heart attack rates were more than twice as high—214 percent—in the surgical group compared to the conservative treatment group. And this trend held during the first twelve months of the study. At the end of the first month it remained 165 percent higher, and after the first year, 116 percent higher. Dr. Boden's team concluded that there was no evidence that aggressive treatment helped patients who

Who Benefits from Bypass Surgery?

There is no question that patients with clearly defined and significant blockages in the left main coronary artery benefit from coronary artery bypass surgery. The left main coronary artery, which is sometimes called the "widow maker," is only an inch or so long, but it is the trunk artery that branches into the two arteries that supply blood to the left side of the heart muscle. Because this artery is the source of blood for such a significant portion of the heart, blockages here are indeed very dangerous and a clear indication for bypass surgery.

Patients with severe, incapacitating chest pain that limits activity and is unresponsive to medications may also be appropriate candidates for surgery. Stable angina, the common, predictable chest pain that comes on with exercise or stress and is relieved with medication, is not an indication for invasive therapy.

If a patient has significant blockages in three coronary arteries *plus* a low ejection fraction indicative of poor left ventricular function, invasive interventions may be necessary. (A normal ejection fraction is greater than or equal to 50 percent.) Severe blockages—even in three vessels—are no reason to rush into surgery, provided that left ventricular function is not compromised. There may be other combinations of risk factors that would suggest the need for an invasive course. However, a second opinion from an independent physician is always recommended prior to consenting to any invasive procedure.

had had non-Q-wave myocardial infarctions. On the contrary, it actually harmed them.[12]

Three years later, in 2001, this research group examined 115 patients who were considered to be at very high risk because they had had a non-Q-wave myocardial infarction after receiving thrombolytic, or clot-busting, therapy. Again, this is a group that is often rushed into angiography, frequently followed by surgery. As in the previous study, they were randomly assigned to a conservative or an aggressive treatment group and followed for an average of twenty-three months. During that time, 33 percent of the patients in the invasive management group (who had bypass surgery and angioplasty in equal numbers) died or had a nonfatal heart attack, compared with 19 percent of those in the conservative strategy group, and there were more deaths in the invasive group (11 versus 2). The researchers concluded: "Routine invasive management may be associated with an increased risk of death."[13]

All these studies clearly demonstrate that the aggressive approach often does more harm than good. Why, then, do so many physicians continue to shuttle millions of trusting and frightened patients into these unnecessary procedures?

BYPASS SURGERY AND PAIN RELIEF

One thing you do have to hand to bypass is that it does relieve angina. Exactly how it does this is not clearly understood. The explanation most doctors give is that it increases circulation. Blood now courses through the graft around the blockage, nourishing the heart that had been crying out for lack of oxygen-rich blood. A second, though rarely mentioned reason for pain relief is damage to the heart during surgery. Heart attacks during bypass, known as perioperative infarctions, occur more frequently than you would imagine. Like any heart attack, they result in the death of heart tissue. If the section of the heart muscle that dies is the area responsible for angina, no more pain! Pain relief or not, this is not a good thing. According to Dr. E. D. Mundth: "Although some patients may be benefited in terms of relief of angina by perioperative infarction, the occurrence of an infarction has a definite adverse effect in the long-term. . . ."[14]

A third way in which bypass might relieve chest pain is by disrupting the nerves of the heart. The heart is covered with a thin membranous sac called the pericardium, and in this sac are nerves that transmit pain signals from the heart. The pericardium and its nerves are cut during surgery to expose the heart. Therefore, substantial pain relief likely results from this nerve resection. Relieving the pain this way is like relieving pain in your foot by cutting nerves in your leg. The injury to the foot is still there, but you don't feel it.

The fourth and perhaps the most significant explanation for the pain relief associated with bypass surgery has to do with the placebo effect. A placebo is an intervention that has no real effect—but because the individual receiving it strongly believes that it is helping, benefits do occur. We often think of a placebo as a sugar pill, but surgical procedures are the most powerful placebos ever, because of the patients' emotional involvement. Dr. Thomas Preston, professor of medicine at the University of Washington and director of cardiology at the U.S. Public Health Service Hospital, Seattle, Washington, describes how surgery achieves this seemingly magical effect:

> Patients today undergo the same sort of ceremony [as in ancient faith-healing rituals] when they have coronary bypass surgery. They spend several days at the temple (hospital) prior to the ultimate healing act. During this time they are given much encouragement; they are told of how they will be cured; they are prepared with special diets and purging; they read pamphlets . . . describing the cure; and they receive news of the cure from patients who have preceded them. On the night before the cure they are taken to the scene of the ceremony, the method of the cure is described to them, and they are shown where they will awaken afterwards. There are very few patients who are not convinced that they will be cured by the

eve of their bypass operation. When it is time for the operation they are taken to the inner chamber of the temple and put to sleep. They awaken healed.[15]

Regardless of how bypass surgery relieves pain, patients typically respond with overwhelming gratitude, convinced that they have been resurrected by their surgeon. Unfortunately, this one genuine effect of bypass surgery, pain relief, is fleeting. Since the surgery doesn't slow the process of atherosclerosis (in fact, it actually accelerates it), the disease progresses and the chest pain returns at a predictable rate. The CASS researchers confirmed this. When they surveyed patients five years after their initial therapy, they found that although the group of patients who had had surgery required less medication after surgery, there were no significant differences in their recreational or occupational activities in comparison to the group treated without surgery.[16] In other words, they had no greater tolerance for exercise. And as I mentioned above, in the ten-year follow-up CASS study, there was virtually no difference in angina or medication requirements.[17]

These results have been replicated in other studies. Dr. Stuart F. Seides, associate professor of medicine and cardiology at George Washington University and consultant to the National Institutes of Health, studied records of patients for a period averaging five years after bypass. Three to nine months after surgery, 73 percent of the patients were pain free and 27 percent had only mild symptoms. After five years, however, only 23 percent were pain free, 45 percent had mild symptoms, and 32 percent had severe symptoms that had not been present at all a few months after surgery.[18] The overall trend noted in studies on long-term follow-up of bypass patients is significant deterioration with time and a return of pain at rates between 5 and 15 percent per year. It is a disappointed patient who finds himself back in the cardiologist's office with the same pain in his chest only two or three years after the great drama of bypass surgery.

BYPASS SURGERY ACCELERATES ATHEROSCLEROSIS

The fact that coronary artery bypass graft surgery does not ameliorate angina over the long run is bad news, but there's worse. Arteries that have received grafts undergo an accelerated degree of atherosclerosis, caused at least in part by the changes and disruptions in blood flow brought on by the graft itself. Dr. B. J. Maurer, of the University of Alabama Medical Center in Birmingham, found that total occlusion, or blockage, was sixteen times more frequent in arteries that had received bypass grafts than in arteries that had been left alone.[19] Dr. L.S.C. Griffith, of Johns Hopkins Medical Center, reported that arteries with grafts developed complete blockages in 40 percent of cases studied, while those without grafts went on to total blockage in only 6 percent.[20]

When heart surgeons don't let well enough alone and operate on patients with only minimal disease, they are setting their patients up for future problems. Drs. Linda W. Cashin and David Blankenhorn from the University of Southern California School of Medicine studied 85 men who had undergone coronary artery bypass surgery. Thirty-seven of the bypassed arteries had minimal atherosclerosis, defined as being less than 50 percent blocked. After an average of thirty-seven months, they reexamined the arteries and found that those that had been bypassed had significant progression of atherosclerosis ten times more frequently than arteries with similar blockages that had not been bypassed. In other words, had these minimally atherosclerotic arteries been left alone, they would have been in much better shape.[21]

What is the fate of the bypass grafts themselves? Grafts are usually segments of saphenous vein that are sewn onto sick arteries. Veins lack the flexible muscular walls that arteries have and are therefore more rigid. They also have valves to prevent backflow, so in order to stay open they need a brisk flow of blood. Therefore, if the artery receiving blood from the graft is diseased and impedes blood flow through the graft, the graft may close within the first few months after surgery. Even when put into place by top surgeons, many grafts close within the first year. Because of this perennial problem, more and more surgeons are using internal mammary artery grafts, which are more resistant to obstruction.

Grafts are also subject to the same process of atherosclerosis that takes place in the arteries. Unless steps are taken to radically reduce the patient's risk factors for atherosclerosis, the graft will close at the same rate as, if not faster than, the coronary arteries.

WHAT ARE THE RISKS OF THE SURGERY?

As with any surgery, there is always the possibility of wound infection, and blood transfusions and hospitalization carry risks of their own. Abnormalities in heart rhythm following bypass are not uncommon, nor are strokes or heart attacks during or after surgery.

Another potential complication of bypass surgery is what is known as the "post-pump syndrome": damage to the lungs, liver, kidney, and brain as a consequence of being hooked up to a heart-lung machine. Your blood carries antibodies called immunoglobulins that rally against viruses, bacteria, and other foreign substances. When blood is circulated through the heart-lung machine, these immunoglobulins may become activated and, like mutinous soldiers, damage normal cells. Dennis E. Chenoweth, Ph.D., measured the level of activated immunoglobulins in patients after bypass surgery and found them to be dramatically increased.[22] Immunoglobulins aren't the only immune cells that are activated. There are huge increases in other markers of inflammation as well that may be the underlying cause of post-pump syndrome.

Obviously there is a risk of death with any surgical procedure. The risk of death from coronary artery bypass graft surgery in the best medical centers that do a tremendous number of these surgeries every year ranges from as low as 1 percent to as much as 5 percent. However, most bypass surgeries are done in community hospitals across the country. Although these hospitals will never have the volume of surgery that the large university centers have, their patients are generally told that their risk is the same as that reported in the medical literature for the busiest surgical centers.

This is highly unlikely. It is very well documented that the medical centers that perform the most of any given surgery are the safest, most proficient, and have the lowest rates of death and complications. With surgery as with most things in life, practice makes perfect, and this is particularly true of such a complicated procedure as bypass surgery, which involves a closely knit team of surgical personnel. Unfortunately, we do not know the surgical death rates in community hospitals, for unlike the large university centers, their statistics are rarely published. At least one study, published in 2000, reported that the top cardiovascular programs beat out others by 4.7 to 31 percent in eight measures of clinical quality and efficiency.[23] The moral? If you must undergo coronary artery bypass graft surgery, select a high-volume hospital and a high-volume surgeon.

BRAIN DAMAGE—WIDELY SUFFERED, OFTEN OVERLOOKED

Patients who survive bypass surgery and leave the hospital aren't necessarily in the clear—neurological complications are extremely common. A patient of mine whom I'll call Joe came to me after having coronary artery bypass surgery. He was the police chief in a small southern California town and had received several commendations for his job performance. Since his surgery, however, things weren't going so well. He was forgetful. He would give conflicting orders, asking one person to do something, then telling another to do something entirely different. He had trouble doing mental math and focusing his attention. Before the surgery he had been a much-sought-after public speaker. Now he had to search for words and no longer felt confident in front of a group. Furthermore, there were marked changes in his temperament. Before he had been even-tempered, but now he was prone to such outbursts that he had to warn people around him not to take it personally. In short, his professional and social life had been abruptly and dramatically altered.

Patients who have undergone bypass surgery and their families frequently report similar problems: difficulty following directions and doing mental tasks, subtle personality changes, mood swings, and increased irritability. Yet until recently these complaints were swept under the rug. Cardiologists are highly skilled specialists who focus on the heart. They are rarely tuned into the mental changes experienced by patients after bypass surgery.

According to a 2001 editorial in the *New England Journal of Medicine*, 1.5 to 5.2 percent of patients have a stroke while on the operating table, resulting in damage to the brain, sometimes fatal and often permanent. Another 10 to 30 percent of bypass patients have a period of disorientation immediately following surgery that may include hallucinations, seizures, or other evidence of central nervous system dysfunction. Known as postoperative delirium, it is believed to be related at least in part to anesthesia.

Less severe changes in cognitive function occur to some degree in an astounding 50 to 80 percent of patients after bypass. For most patients, this appears to be temporary. Within six weeks, fewer than half remain obviously mentally impaired, and by six months this figure hovers between 10 and 30 percent.[24] Long-term problems have always been thought to be blessedly rare.

Yet a 2001 study by researchers at Duke University Medical School confirms what millions of patients and their families already knew. Lasting cognitive impairment after bypass surgery is quite common. Mark F. Newman, M.D., and colleagues followed 261 patients who had undergone bypass surgery and administered tests of cognitive function before bypass, after discharge, and then six weeks, six months, and five years after surgery. There was a high incidence of cognitive decline at discharge. More than half of the patients scored significantly worse on cognitive tests a few days after surgery than they did before surgery. Overall, mental function appeared to improve at six weeks (only one-third of the patients still exhibited deficits) and at six months (one-quarter remained affected). The finding that has taken everyone by storm, however, is that when these patients were retested five years after their coronary artery bypass surgery, 42 percent showed signs of mental impairment![25]

There may be several explanations for this. Ill effects of anesthesia, as I mentioned earlier, may be a factor. Inflammatory chemicals released during surgery in massive quantities throughout the body, including the brain, likely have adverse effects as well. However, the primary culprit appears to be the heart-lung machine. Blood is routed out of the body to the machine, oxygen is bubbled into it, and it is returned back into the body via the aorta. This may introduce air bubbles into the bloodstream that can interfere with blood flow in the brain. Even worse, messing with the aorta frees embolic matter (bits of plaque and blood clots), which can travel up the carotid arteries in the neck, lodge in the blood vessels of the brain, and disrupt oxygen delivery.

Indeed, there is ultrasonic evidence to suggest that this is a common occurrence. Dr. Leif Henriksen of the Department of Neurology and Thoracic Surgery, State University Hospital in

Copenhagen, Denmark, measured blood flow in the brains in 37 patients before and after bypass surgery. He found in every case a reduction in blood flow following surgery. He made identical measurements in patients who underwent chest surgery but were not put on the heart-lung machine and found no reduction in brain blood flow.[26] In one very dramatic case history, D. L. Price, M.D., of the Department of Neurology at Harvard Medical School, reported on the autopsy findings of a bypass patient who never regained consciousness after surgery and died shortly thereafter. Thirty-five percent of his brain had been destroyed by a shower of embolic material.[27]

WHY IS CORONARY ARTERY BYPASS SURGERY SO POPULAR?

Given its lack of proven benefits and its potential for harm, you might wonder why bypass surgery has remained so popular. One obvious answer is that it appeals to both patients and physicians who want to do something immediate and dramatic about heart disease. Coronary artery bypass surgery looks great on paper. When a patient reviews his or her own angiogram and sees the location of the blockages, it is hard not to believe that well-placed grafts would solve the problem. As Robert A. Buccino, M.D., of the Watson Clinic in Lakeland, Florida, points out:

> Most cardiologists favor an activist course of treatment. Consultants are brought in at an early stage often before simple measures are applied. Cardiologists have a tendency to encourage excessive performance of special tests and procedures thus justifying their involvement in the case and satisfying expectations of the patient, family, and referring physician. There is a bias to interpret borderline data at each point of evaluation by erring on the side of safety—by doing more

rather than less. The path of least resistance leads ultimately to the operation suite.[28]

A second reason for its popularity is that yesterday's assumptions have become today's beliefs. The claims of early proponents, even though now discredited for the most part, are nevertheless believed by the majority of physicians trained in the use of bypass surgery, and today this includes physicians in almost every community in this country. Once a therapy is commonplace, the burden of proof of efficacy is lifted—and for the large number of physicians who have spent several years and thousands of hours learning and perfecting this therapy, curtailing its use would seem inconceivable.

Third, bypass surgery generates billions of dollars a year. The profit motive is at work in every industry, and the heart surgery industry is no exception. Every step along the way, from screening to hospitalization to the actual operation, is a moneymaker for someone in the system. Given the data indicating that as many as 90 percent of all patients who have bypass surgery are not medically appropriate candidates for the procedure, do you think that the frequency of this procedure would be the same if it were not profitable?

Finally, I believe that fear is a major factor in the popularity of this procedure. To put it bluntly, physicians frighten patients into having unnecessary surgery. Sure, a minority of patients may insist on aggressive management, believing bypass surgery to be "state of the art." But where do they get this idea? From their doctors and surgeons, most likely. The demand for invasive procedures is created by physicians who terrorize their patients with frightening phrases like "You're a walking time bomb" or "Without surgery you'll be dead in six months."[29]

M. S. Bates summed up all these explanations for the popularity of bypass surgery in a compelling and thoughtful 1990 article. He wrote:

> How can we understand the behavior of physicians and surgeons who ignore the readily available evidence of CABG surgery . . . ? The development and continued use of CABG demonstrates how medical and surgical practice in the U.S. is shaped more by socio-cultural, political, and economic forces than by unbiased, value-free, 'scientific' facts or by an overriding concern for the health and welfare of the American public.[30]

IS THERE A BETTER WAY?

The heart surgery industry has seen some significant changes since the first bypass surgery was performed in 1967. More sophisticated diagnostic tools are available, as well as improved surgical techniques, instruments, and drugs. Surgeons and supporting staff are better trained today, and many hospitals have much better track records, compared to the early days of surgery. Yet as I hope I have made clear in this chapter, people still die on the table and in the hospital after surgery. They still have strokes and repeat heart attacks and brain damage, and their bypassed arteries still close up. And patients—now they number in the hundreds of thousands every year—are still being inappropriately recommended for bypass surgery.

Today's potential bypass recipients should realize that they do have options. Of course, the one you will hear about most is angioplasty, which we will cover in the next chapter. You may not get as much information from your doctor on the treatment of heart disease with lifestyle changes and medical management, but this approach is extremely successful for most patients.

A research team from Harvard Medical School reported their experience with 212 patients whose exercise stress tests indicated they had severe heart disease. The overwhelming majority of cardiologists in the country would have referred almost all of these patients for an angiogram, which would have led many of them into the operating room. The Harvard group, however, treated these patients with exercise and a dietary program (similar to the diet I will describe in Part III), as well as appropriate medications, and they did well. The yearly death rate among these patients was only 1.4 percent—lower than the death rate from surgery! These researchers concluded: "There is rarely a need to resort to cardiac surgery; medical management is highly successful and associated with a low mortality."[31]

GET A SECOND OPINION

If you ever find yourself or a loved one in the position of deciding whether or not to have coronary artery bypass surgery, review the information in this chapter with your cardiologist. Every study is referenced, and each of them can be obtained at any medical library. (The CASS studies are particularly important.) It may take several hours for you to read them in their entirety, but certainly less time to read only their summaries and conclusions. Ask your physician how your particular condition compares to that of the patients described in the studies, and politely request reprints of scientific studies that form the basis of his or her decision.

Also, get a second opinion, and get it from someone outside your doctor's medical practice. The most important study ever published on second opinions for bypass surgery was spearheaded by Harvard Medical School cardiologist Thomas B. Graboys, M.D. (who also conducted the second-opinion study on angiography I told you about in the previous chapter). In this study Dr. Graboys and his colleagues demonstrated how a patient's risk of heart attack could be predicted accurately, and how that risk could then be compared to the risks of surgery.

They outlined a protocol for the noninvasive evaluation of coronary risk that is as reliable today as it was when this study was published. Included in the criteria that defined a low-risk patient, who would do well on a conservative course of treatment, were the following: 1) absence of impaired ventricular function (i.e., a normal ejection fraction); 2) angina brought on by exercise or stress that could be relieved with medications (as opposed to unpredictable, uncontrollable angina); 3) reasonable performance on exercise stress testing; 4) ease of instituting a medical program that the patient would adhere to; and 5) absence of critical blockage of the left main coronary artery.

Using this protocol, the Graboys team rendered a second opinion for 88 patients who had been recommended by a cardiologist to have bypass surgery. In their determination, 74 of the 88 patients did not need surgery, even though their angiograms had shown significant blockages. Sixty of these patients went with the second opinion and elected not to have surgery, and after two years they were all alive—living evidence of the accuracy of this protocol and the inappropriateness of most recommendations for bypass.[32]

I have been giving second opinions to patients referred for invasive heart procedures for more than twenty years, utilizing the Graboys protocol. Like the Harvard physicians, in most cases I recommend the nonsurgical approach. I then encourage my patients to take their time, review my findings with their cardiologist, and carefully evaluate their options. After all, the decision is theirs, not mine or any other doctor's. Such an important decision should be made by a well-informed patient with a clear understanding of all the risks and benefits.

Regardless of whether or not a patient decides to undergo bypass or angioplasty, I also stress the importance of an "aggressive conservative approach," consisting of a low-fat diet, an exercise program, large doses of vitamins and minerals, and other noninvasive therapies, as indicated. This is the crux of my program for reversing heart disease, which we will cover in Part III.

CHAPTER 8

Angioplasty and Coronary Artery Stenting: Overrated and Overused

IN 1978 SWISS PHYSICIAN ANDREAS R. GREUNTZIG, M.D., DEscribed a new procedure for the treatment of coronary artery disease: percutaneous transluminal coronary angioplasty (PTCA). Dr. Greuntzig had been experimenting with this for several years, applying a procedure used since the 1960s to open up femoral arteries in the legs. He perfected his technique first on animals and then on cadavers, and he was now reporting the results of his first patients.[1] Although Dr. Greuntzig's results were less than spectacular (4 percent died in the first year, 14 percent had to undergo emergency bypass surgery, and 6 percent had to have a repeat angioplasty), a star was born.[2]

The popularity of angioplasty, which is also called balloon angioplasty, took off like a helium-filled balloon. Here was a therapy for heart disease that was less invasive than bypass surgery and apparently safer. Within five years 32,000 angioplasties were performed in the United States every year. By 1985 this number had exploded to 118,000 a year (a 372 percent increase in just two years). Yet it would be seven more years before this blockbuster procedure was scientifically evaluated.

In a chain of events uncomfortably similar to those surrounding coronary artery bypass graft surgery, angioplasty has failed to live up to its promise. Three randomized controlled trials comparing angioplasty with conservative medical therapy have found that the procedure does not reduce rates of death or incidence of heart attacks. As with any invasive procedure, there is a risk of complications. And treated patients have a high likelihood of needing repeat procedures in the future. Most disturbing, it is evident that the majority of the 600,000[3] patients who undergo angioplasty every year are at very low risk of death or heart attack and should not be subjected to an invasive procedure of any kind.

WHAT IS ANGIOPLASTY?

In order for you to understand exactly what angioplasty entails, let me tell you about the experience of my patient Benjamin. This healthy sixty-five-year-old had a true passion for exercise. For thirty years he had exercised almost every day during his lunch hour, jogging, swimming, or working out in the gym, and he played golf every chance he got. After he retired, he concentrated on swimming, tennis, and golf—and he often walked the course and carried his own clubs. With the exception of some pain in his knees, which he attributed to all those years of jogging, he felt great. Over the course of four or five months, however, he noticed increasing fatigue during his workouts. When Ben mentioned this to his physician during a routine checkup, he was immediately referred to a cardiologist, who gave him an exercise stress test, then recommended an angiogram. When the angiogram revealed a blockage in one of his coronary arteries, he was told that he needed to have an angioplasty right away. The doctor made it sound urgent, so Ben consented. His father had died of a heart attack, and he wanted to do everything he could to avoid the same fate.

He was admitted to the hospital and taken to the angioplasty lab, where, after receiving local anesthesia and IV drugs to discourage excessive clotting of the blood, a sheath was placed in his femoral artery, a large artery in the groin. A catheter with a small inflatable balloon on its tip was inserted into the sheath and threaded up through the artery and into the blocked coronary artery. Assisted by images projected on a screen made visible by dye injected through the catheter, the cardiologist guided the catheter to the area of blockage. Once it was in the proper position, the balloon was inflated for two or three minutes, pressing the plaque against the walls of the artery and opening it up. The catheter was removed and another angiogram was obtained to confirm that the blockage had been adequately opened. Ben was observed for several hours, the femoral artery sheath was removed, and the bleeding stopped by pressing on the puncture site. He was required to rest in bed overnight and was discharged the next day.

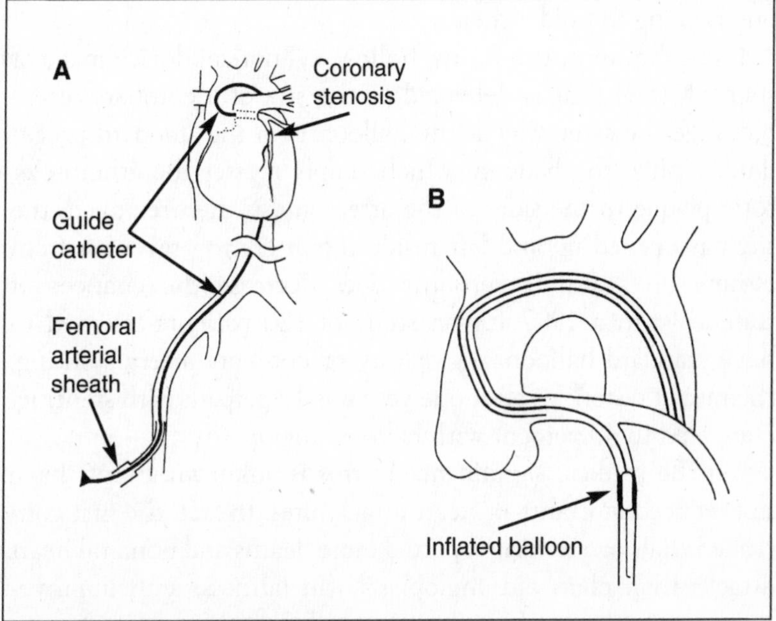

FIGURE 7: Coronary Angioplasty

CORONARY ARTERY STENTING

Ben's angioplasty was done in the late 1980s. Had it been done today, he would likely have had a coronary artery stent inserted. Since the coronary stent was introduced in the early 1990s and approved for elective implantation in 1994, its surge in popularity has been meteoric, going from essentially zero in 1994 to almost half a million in 1998.[4] Stents are now used in almost 70 percent of all angioplasties. The idea behind the stent is to strengthen the newly opened artery wall since, as we will discuss later, arteries that have been treated with balloon angioplasty are extremely prone to closing back up. This is called restenosis, and it is the Achilles' heel of angioplasty. Within six months, restenosis occurs in 30 to 40 percent of all arteries, and when this happens, you're back where you started.[5] This is why so many patients require repeat procedures—with no guarantee that this one is going to hold either.

Enter the stent. It is a tiny, hollow, cylindrical device made of stainless steel that is delivered to the site of a coronary artery blockage the same way as the balloon is in the standard procedure. Unlike the balloon, which simply presses the atherosclerotic plaque to the sides of the artery and is then removed, the stent is opened up and left inside the artery to prevent it from closing up again. It certainly does decrease the chances of restenosis. In a 1997 Italian study of 120 patients assigned to have standard balloon angioplasty or coronary artery stenting, the rate of restenosis after one year was 19 percent with stenting, compared to 40 percent with balloon angioplasty.[6]

Yet the medical significance of this is unknown. Stents have not reduced mortality or heart attack rates. In fact, the first controlled trials on stenting reported more deaths and nonfatal heart attacks than plain old angioplasty. (In fairness, with improvements in implantation techniques and the stents themselves in recent years, this is no longer the case.) Eric J. Topol, M.D., editor of the *New England Journal of Medicine*, lambastes the medical community for embracing coronary artery stenting prematurely, stating that "interventional cardiologists have been appropriately characterized as 'medical-technology junkies who thrive on the latest and best products.' Ideally, the use of these devices will be driven by the latest and best data."[7] Despite the popularity of this technique data justifying extensive use of stenting is yet to come.

ANGIOPLASTY DOES NOT SAVE LIVES OR PREVENT HEART ATTACKS

Let's take a look at the three randomized controlled studies that have compared angioplasty to conservative medical therapy. These studies did report more significant decreases in angina in the angioplasty-treated patients, compared to those taking medications, but this was most pronounced in patients with moderate to severe pain. And in one of these studies, a large European trial, the differences in levels of angina between the two groups diminished in three years.[8] Furthermore, there were more serious cardiac events and deaths in the interventional group: Thirty-two patients who underwent angioplasty suffered a heart attack or died, compared to only seventeen who received drugs.[9]

One of the most recent clinical trials on angioplasty, a multicenter study published in 1999, enrolled 341 patients with stable angina, normal left ventricular function, and high LDL cholesterol. These patients were randomly assigned to angioplasty (with or without stenting) plus standard medications or to an aggressive regimen of cholesterol-lowering drugs. They were followed for eighteen months. At the study's conclusion there was no significant difference between the two groups in numbers of deaths or nonfatal heart attacks, although there was a trend toward fewer heart-related events in the patients treated solely with medication.[10]

COMPLICATIONS OF ANGIOPLASTY AND CORONARY ARTERY STENTING

For patients with a 1 to 2 percent chance of having a heart attack or dying from heart disease in a given year—the vast majority of patients who submit to these procedures—having an angioplasty or coronary artery stenting, is like playing Russian roulette. The research clearly demonstrates that neither of these procedures will improve your already-excellent odds of making it through the next year without major heart problems, so why take a chance?

I know exactly why. All too often, you have not been informed about the true benefits and real risks of these invasive procedures. According to a recent survey, three-quarters of patients about to undergo angioplasty erroneously believed it would prevent heart attacks and likely save their lives, while fewer than half of them could name even one possible complication of the procedure, and 25 percent had heard nothing about potential problems.[11]

Although angioplasty is safer than bypass surgery, patients do die during the procedure. Kailash Meta was recommended to undergo angioplasty after an angiogram revealed a blockage in one of her coronary arteries. She had no symptoms of heart disease, but her doctors assured her that this would help her avoid future problems. During the procedure her cardiologist made three attempts to clear the blockage. On the third try, the artery burst. She was rushed into emergency bypass, but it was too late. She had already suffered heart failure and severe brain damage, and she lapsed into a coma from which she never awoke. She died nine weeks later.

Artery rupture, dissection, and perforation are blessedly rare. Bleeding of the plaque, injury to the endothelium, and clot formation are not. Although drugs are now routinely administered during angioplasty to reduce the incidence of these complications, they still occur. So do heart attacks, in 3 to 5 percent of patients during angioplasty. In another 2 to 8 percent, the vessel abruptly closes, generally within minutes. This is frequently associated with heart attack, and it calls for repeat angioplasty or emergency bypass surgery to open the occluded artery. An estimated 3 to 7 percent of patients require emergency bypass for this and other complications.

As with bypass surgery, there is a very strong inverse relationship between in-hospital death and complication rates and volume of procedures performed. A survey of thirty-one hospitals in New York State found that mortality rates were greatest when angioplasty was done in hospitals where fewer than six hundred of these procedures were performed each year, and by cardiologists who did fewer than seventy-five angioplasties annually.[12] If you elect to have an angioplasty, do your homework and select a hospital in which the procedure is done routinely by a physician with a lot of experience under his or her belt.

The most common adverse consequence of balloon angioplasty is restenosis. The purpose of this procedure is to compress atherosclerotic plaque against the walls of the artery, widening its lumen, or interior. During angioplasty, arterial plaque is split, stretched, and compacted against the sides of the artery. But it doesn't always stay put. Flaps of the plaque return to the lumen, and blockage recurs. The artery that was opened closes back up in 30 to 40 percent of all cases—and in 60 percent of chronically occluded arteries—within the first six months. Coronary artery stenting has lowered the incidence of restenosis but has not eliminated it—20 to 30 percent of stents are also affected, and more than half of those that close up once do so a second time. Restenosis is such a common problem that the FDA has recently approved the use of radiation to the area in an effort to inhibit the proliferation of cells that cause restenosis.[13, 14]

Another thing that worries me about angioplasty isn't talked about very much. What do you suppose happens to the artery itself during the procedure? It is being poked and prodded, stretched, and, in a not insignificant number of patients, actually damaged.[15]

Not only does injury to the artery accelerate restenosis, but, as we discussed in Chapter 2, anytime you harm the endothelial cells lining the arteries, you turn on the response-to-injury cascade that results in atherosclerosis. There is no way you can poke around the insides of an artery without doing physical damage to the delicate endothelium and furthering the process of atherosclerosis. You're just asking for trouble, if not now, then down the road.

Although coronary artery stenting reduces the incidence of restenosis, it surely disrupts the endothelium as well—perhaps even more significantly over the long haul, since a foreign body remains in the artery. A compelling 2000 report suggests that stainless steel stents may trigger allergic reactions in some patients. It has been documented that patients who test positive for sensitivity to nickel or molybdenum, metals in stainless steel, are highly prone to stent restenosis.[16] These substances may also leach out of the stent into the body, and what implications this might have for systemic health are unknown.

Finally, I want to address vulnerable plaques, the small, inflamed lesions that are the culprit in the majority of heart attacks. Although these small plaques are not picked up on angiography, they are far more likely to rupture and set into motion the chain of events that results in a heart attack. Isn't it possible that catheters and balloons and metal stents might disrupt the thin caps covering these plaques? Isn't it likely that since angioplasty and bypass attack large, stable plaques, we're fighting the wrong battle? Think about it. This area of reseach is still in its infancy, but I suspect its significance will be more widely recognized in the future.

COMPARISON WITH CORONARY ARTERY BYPASS GRAFT SURGERY

Some patients are forced to make the decision between angioplasty and coronary artery bypass graft surgery. Which is better?

Angioplasty has been pitted against coronary artery bypass graft surgery in at least nine controlled trials. The consensus of the studies is that in patients with low to moderate risk (one- or two-vessel disease, good heart function, and no left main coronary artery involvement), the odds are pretty even in terms of mortality and nonfatal heart attacks. (Keep in mind, however, that these odds are greater than the 1 to 2 percent with conservative therapy.)

Bypass surgery, of course, brings with it all manner of initial complications—prolonged hospitalization, risk of death, neurological damage, and the other problems we talked about in the previous chapter. Yet given the high incidence of restenosis, angioplasty is for all intents and purposes a temporary fix. It is unlikely that future clinical trials—unless they are on an extremely large scale—will shed much more light on this.[17] So perhaps the more important question patients should be asking is: Do I need any invasive treatment at all?

DOES ANYONE NEED ANGIOPLASTY?

The average patient who is considered to be a good candidate for angioplasty has one or two blocked arteries, is in generally good health, and has a well-functioning heart. As you saw in the previous chapter on bypass surgery, this is precisely the type of patient who does very well on a conservative course of treatment—without bypass surgery *or* angioplasty. According to CASS, which compared medical therapy to bypass, such patients treated with medication and perhaps some lifestyle changes had an annual death rate of less than 2 percent. This means that with good medical care, 98 out of 100 patients with one, two, or even three blocked vessels and good left ventricular function would survive each year.[18] Why subject such patients, who already have an excellent prognosis, to the potential complications of angioplasty, where there is little chance that it will prolong their life or reduce their risk of heart attack?

In summary, I believe that angioplasty, like bypass surgery, should be used only in rare cases. The overwhelming majority of patients can be safely treated with a vigorous trial of diet, exercise, and appropriate medications. If and only if this conservative regimen fails to reduce symptoms should angioplasty or another invasive technique be considered.

CHAPTER 9

A Smorgasbord of Drugs

THE PREVAILING BELIEF IN CARDIOLOGY THAT HEART ATTACKS ARE caused by large blockages in the coronary arteries has fueled unbridled growth of the heart surgery industry, as we have seen in previous chapters. Yet recent discoveries about the nature of atherosclerotic plaque and the myriad factors contributing to heart disease have challenged this paradigm. Although these new findings have yet to make much of a dent in interventional cardiology—heart surgeons needn't worry about being out of a job—they have spawned another multibillion-dollar industry: pharmaceutical drugs to treat heart disease.

Drugs that address the underlying biochemical processes involved in atherosclerosis are far superior to the jackhammer approach of bypass and angioplasty. However, because they are unnatural agents that force the system into directions it has never gone before, all drugs have a dark side. While they may engender benefits, they inevitably have a host of adverse side effects as well.[1]

Don't get me wrong. I am not opposed to the use of drugs in the treatment of heart disease. What I am opposed to is conventional medicine's blind acceptance and overuse of drugs. If drugs are so wonderful, why are heart attacks still our principal cause of death? Why do 50 million of us have high blood pressure and 4 million suffer strokes each year? And why do drugs themselves cause so much suffering and so many deaths? The

106,000 Americans who die from adverse effects of prescription drugs every year were not overdosing.[2] They were not taking their spouse's or their friend's medication. They were using prescription drugs exactly as instructed by their physician.

It isn't as if there are no alternatives to drugs other than surgery. As I made clear in Part I and will return to in detail in Part III, adopting a healthy diet, exercising regularly, keeping a lid on stress, and taking targeted nutritional supplements dramatically reduce your risk of heart disease. Public health officials declare that you can slash your risk by an astounding 80 percent by taking these simple steps, and clinical studies have demonstrated that similar measures can reverse existing heart disease as well. If we could put the benefits of lifestyle changes in a bottle, even if we slapped on a $1,000-a-year price tag—comparable to the cost of many heart medications—we would decimate our number one killer.

Let's look at the major classes of drugs that are currently available for the treatment of heart disease. I suggest you read this chapter carefully, for it is unlikely that you will get all of this information from your physician. Just as most people think their bypass or angioplasty saved them from death and heart attack, many believe that their heart drugs are keeping them alive.

DRUGS LOWER CHOLESTEROL, BUT . . .

Drugs to lower cholesterol are enormously popular. We have known for decades that a high cholesterol level is predictive of heart attack—people with a high cholesterol level are far more likely to have a heart attack than those whose level is 200 or lower, and the risk increases as the cholesterol level rises. Nonetheless, it wasn't until the mid-1970s that the National Institutes of Health undertook the first study to determine if lowering cholesterol levels decreased this risk. NIH researchers recruited 3,800 volunteers who had no history of heart disease but a cholesterol level of 265 or higher. They contemplated utilizing dietary changes in this study but ruled against it because the study was designed to last seven years. They felt that even though a low-fat diet would lower cholesterol, it would be difficult for study subjects to stick to it for that length of time. They also wanted this to be a double-blind study—neither the volunteers nor the researchers themselves would know who was receiving the active therapy and who was getting a placebo. Obviously it would be easy for volunteers and researchers to figure who was on the low-fat diet.

They decided instead to use a cholesterol-lowering drug, Questran. The volunteers were randomly divided into two groups, half receiving Questran, the other half receiving a placebo. Both groups were put on a moderate cholesterol-lowering diet. The results of this seven-year study were truly astounding. The group taking Questran had a definite reduction in cholesterol levels in comparison to the control group—8.5 percent lower, translating into a 24 percent reduction in death rate and a 19 percent reduction in risk of heart attack. Those taking the cholesterol-lowering drug also had 20 percent less angina, 25 percent fewer positive exercise stress tests, and 21 percent fewer bypass surgeries, compared to the control group.[3]

The researchers involved in the study were quick to point out that even though a cholesterol-lowering drug had been used, these same results could be expected if cholesterol were reduced by diet rather than drugs, but nobody listened. Instead, this study inspired the race to come up with newer and better drugs to attack cholesterol—a race that continues to this day. There are now three major classes of lipid-lowering drugs, two aimed at cholesterol and one at triglycerides. (Niacin is also listed with prescription drugs for lowering cholesterol, but since it is a natural agent, we will discuss it in Chapter 14.) While all of these drugs do indeed cause a drop in blood lipids, they do so at a cost.

Bile Acid Sequestrants

Cholestyramine (Questran), the drug used in the study cited previously, and colestipol (Colestid) belong to the oldest class of cholesterol-lowering drugs, bile acid sequestrants. They are powders that bind to bile acids in the intestinal tract and block their reabsorption. The reason these drugs affect cholesterol levels is because bile acids, which facilitate the digestion and absorption of fat, are produced in the liver from cholesterol. If they are prevented from being reabsorbed from the intestines and are instead excreted, then cholesterol is excreted at the same time.

One problem with bile acid sequestrants is that they bind to and thus reduce the absorption of fat-soluble nutrients, such as vitamins A, D, E, and K. Long-term use can create problems, most notably bleeding disorders from a deficiency of vitamin K (which is necessary for normal blood clotting) and visual disturbances from vitamin A deficiency. The drugs also inhibit the absorption of thyroid drugs, antibiotics, and several heart drugs. Furthermore, as you might expect, they can cause substantial constipation and other gastrointestinal problems, such as abdominal discomfort, flatulence, nausea, and vomiting.

This is a class of drugs I would never prescribe because there is a very effective, safe, natural alternative that also binds to and removes cholesterol: dietary fiber. (More on this in Chapter 12.)

Fibric Acid Derivatives

The fibric acid derivatives gemfibrozil (Lopid) and clofibrate (Atromid-S) are primarily prescribed for patients with very high triglycerides. Although they may reduce LDL or raise HDL cholesterol to some degree, they are generally aimed at lowering VLDL cholesterol and thus triglyceride levels. Some studies also suggest that fibric acid derivatives may also slightly reduce the blood's tendency to clot and lower some markers of inflammation. Nobody knows exactly how these drugs work, but they appear to inhibit the liver's release of VLDL. They have a number of side effects, such as nausea, loose stools, flatulence, and other gastrointestinal effects. Headache, dizziness, fatigue, muscle cramps, rashes, and other problems with the skin and hair have also been reported.

These drugs have an even darker side. The World Health Organization conducted a six-year placebo-controlled study involving 10,000 patients which found that Atromid-S actually increased the overall death rate by 44 percent, compared to the placebo.[4] It did lower triglycerides enough to effect a reduction in heart attacks, but the increased mortality from other causes more than canceled this benefit. These excessive deaths were associated with gallbladder disease (the drug substantially increases the risk of gallstones), cancer, and pancreatitis. Lopid has actions similar to Atromid-S, and, according to the *Physicians' Desk Reference*, similar side effects.[5] These drugs interact adversely with blood thinners and with statin drugs (described below), and they should not be taken by anyone with gallbladder, liver, or kidney problems. They are so hard on the liver that liver function must be monitored while taking them.

I could never recommend any medication with such a high potential for adverse effects. Anyway, elevated triglycerides—even when levels are in the thousands—are relatively easy to treat with dietary changes. As we will discuss in Chapters 12 and 14, they respond to elimination of sugar and other refined carbohydrates and to high-dose fish oil.

Statins

The statin drugs, more formally known as HMG-CoA reductase inhibitors, are by far the most popular class of cholesterol-lowering drugs. They include some of America's best-selling drugs: atorvastatin (Lipitor), simvastatin (Zocor), lovastatin (Mevacor), pravastatin (Pravachol), and fluvastatin (Lescol). (See why they're commonly called statins?) They inhibit the action of an enzyme called 3-hydroxy-3-methylglutaryl coenzyme A (HMG-CoA), which is required for the synthesis of cholesterol in the liver. It was recently discovered that in addition to lowering cholesterol, statins lower levels of C-reactive protein, an inflammatory marker for heart disease.[6] They also appear to improve endothelial function, likely by increasing production of nitric oxide.[7]

Scores of studies have demonstrated that statin drugs reduce cholesterol and decrease the risk of heart disease and death from heart attack. There have been at least five major randomized controlled trials on statins, averaging 5.4 years in length and involving a total of 30,817 participants, all with elevated cholesterol levels and two-thirds with a history of heart disease. A 1999 analysis of these studies showed that statin drugs raised HDL cholesterol by 5 percent, while lowering total cholesterol by 20 percent, LDL cholesterol by 28 percent, and triglycerides by 13 percent. The risk reduction for major coronary events such as heart attacks was 31 percent, and for deaths from all causes, 21 percent. The findings were similar for men and women, and for both elderly and middle-aged people.[8] Pretty impressive, isn't it?

So impressive that the medical community has gone overboard recommending these drugs. In 1999 the FDA actually approved one statin, Mevacor, for people with normal cholesterol levels and no symptoms of heart disease! Simply having below-average HDL cholesterol is enough to get you a prescription for this drug. Of course, the drug's manufacturer, Merck & Co., notes that it should be used in addition to diet and lifestyle changes, but the "big gun" here is obviously Mevacor.[9] There are doctors out there who feel that statins will benefit most everybody and that these drugs can reduce the risk of everything from osteoporosis to dementia. (One expert jokingly suggested that we should put them in our drinking water.) Some predict that half the population will be taking them in the future, and there has even been a push to reclassify some of them from prescription to over-the-counter status.[10] The latest guidelines of the National Cholesterol Education Program include recommendations for aggressive drug therapy. If they were fully implemented, 36 million Americans—one in every five adults—would be taking cholesterol-lowering drugs.

Statin drugs are useful for patients with highly elevated cholesterol levels when, and only when, lifestyle changes and natural therapies fail to normalize blood lipids. Despite conventional medicine's current infatuation with these drugs, they are not without risks. Side effects include liver toxicity (like the fibric acid derivatives, they require frequent monitoring of liver function), gastrointestinal symptoms, rashes, blurred vision, muscle inflammation and weakness, and rhabdomyolysis, a condition involving muscle breakdown.

These side effects can be fatal. One statin drug, cerivastatin (Baycol), was voluntarily recalled in August 2001 after being linked to 31 deaths from rhabdomyolysis.[11] For the other statin drugs, it is business as usual—and big business at that, since 11 million Americans are currently taking these drugs. In my opinion, all the statin drugs require closer scrutiny. While Baycol may have been the most dangerous of the bunch, every one of the drugs in this class works in a similar manner and has similar side effects. According to Public Citizen, a Washington, D.C., consumer group, other statin drugs have killed an additional eighty-one Americans.[12]

There is another adverse effect of the statin drugs that hardly anybody talks about—and which I believe contributed to the deaths from rhabdomyolysis. It is not listed in the *Physicians' Desk Reference* and it is not printed in the drug inserts, but it is the most chilling of all of the statin side effects. Because the enzyme these drugs inhibit in order to lower cholesterol is also involved in the manufacture of coenzyme Q10 (CoQ10), these drugs also reduce levels of this vital compound. CoQ10 is essential for energy production in the mitochondria of our cells—it is to cellular function what spark plugs are to an engine. Statins deplete the body of CoQ10 by as much as 40 percent according to one double-blind placebo-controlled trial, slowly but surely draining the batteries that fuel the heart muscle and other cells.[13]

The heart, the busiest of all muscles, has extreme energy requirements and thus is hardest hit by shortages of coenzyme Q10.

Several studies have shown that patients with heart failure have measurable deficiencies in CoQ10, and the degree of disease progression correlates directly with the degree of deficiency—the lower the CoQ10 level, the greater the heart dysfunction. I cannot fathom using a drug that reduces production of this essential coenzyme. It is like using a gas additive that burns holes in your gas tank. In fact, I consider the CoQ10 deficiencies caused by the growing use of statin drugs to be in large part responsible for our current epidemic of heart failure. The pharmaceutical giant Merck & Co., which first brought statin drugs to market in 1987, appears to know this as well.

In 1990 Merck & Co. sought and received two patents for Mevacor and other statin drugs formulated with up to 1,000 mg of coenzyme Q10. This is, according to the patent, "for the avoidance of myopathy as well as the amelioration of myopathy." (Myopathy, specifically cardiomyopathy, is a common cause of congestive heart failure.) The company holds a second patent for the same formulation "for the avoidance of liver damage . . . as well as the amelioration of said damage." Merck has not brought these combination products to market despite their potential benefit. Nor has the company educated physicians on the importance of supplementing CoQ10 to offset the dangers of statins to the liver and heart. And patients who take these drugs are paying with their health.

Let me tell you about Sam. In 1987, forty-year-old Sam was a busy dentist who was in great health except for a slight elevation in cholesterol. His doctor prescribed Mevacor, which Sam took for ten years. In 1997, at age fifty, he wound up in a cardiologist's office with life-threatening congestive heart failure. His coenzyme Q10 level was found to be exceptionally low. Since Sam had no other risk factors, it is obvious to me that this statin drug played a role in this once-vigorous individual's developing near-fatal congestive heart failure. Sam was treated successfully with coenzyme Q10, and his Mevacor was immediately discontinued.

Noted cardiologist Peter H. Langsjoen, M.D., warns that this problem is only going to get worse: "The concern over the long-term consequences of statin-induced CoQ10 deficiency is heightened by the rapidly increasing number of patients treated and the increasing dosages and potencies of the statin drugs."[14]

I urge you not to fall prey to all the hype surrounding the statins. Simple dietary changes, including lowering intake of fat, were demonstrated in the very well-controlled Finnish Mental Hospital study to dramatically lower cholesterol levels and reduce risk of death from heart disease by 53 percent in men,[15] and these same dietary changes, as well as fiber, fish oil, red yeast rice, and other supplements can lower cholesterol as effectively as drugs in most people. If you have no option but to take a statin drug, it is imperative that you take at least 200 milligrams of coenzyme Q10 every day to protect yourself from inevitable deficiencies.

NITROGLYCERIN EASES ANGINA

Nitroglycerin is the oldest and one of the most effective of the heart drugs, and surely there is no other drug with a more bizarre history. An Italian chemist first used it in 1836 to create a highly explosive and very unstable liquid. The formula was refined over the years and in 1863 Alfred Nobel brought it out in a paste he called dynamite. At the same time, a German homeopath named Constantine Hering, who was testing all kinds of substances, noticed that nitroglycerin caused headaches, and homeopaths soon began using it as a treatment for that malady. (The "like-cures-like" homeopathic philosophy is to treat symptoms with minute quantities of substances that cause those symptoms.) Observations of the unexpected effects of nitroglycerin on the heart led to further research, and it was first used to treat angina in 1879.[16]

Nitroglycerin comes in more forms than any other drug—oral, sublingual, buccal (dissolving in the cheek), patches, transdermal ointments, oral sprays, and IV. It is delivered to the smooth muscle cells of the blood vessels, where it is converted to nitric oxide. As you may recall from Chapter 2, nitric oxide is a potent vasodilator. It relaxes and dilates the blood vessels, thereby increasing blood flow and reducing the amount of work the heart has to do. In this way it lessens the oxygen requirements of the heart muscle and relieves angina. Some speculate that nitroglycerin might also improve blood flow through collateral channels, the vessels that grow around and naturally bypass coronary blockages. In addition, it may discourage the aggregation of platelets.[17]

This drug gets to work fast and in most cases relieves chest pain rapidly, but repeat doses are sometimes required. It is generally administered when symptoms arise, although some forms are taken to prevent symptoms—prior to exercise, for example. Patients must be careful not to overdose on nitroglycerin, lest they become tolerant of the drug and it loses its effectiveness. The best way to avoid this is by taking a ten- to twelve-hour break from nitroglycerin every day.

Headache is a very common side effect of nitroglycerin, as is low blood pressure. Patients taking the drug also report flushing, restlessness, insomnia, and nightmares. One drug that does not mix well with nitroglycerin and all nitrate-containing drugs is Viagra, the popular pill for erectile dysfunction. Both work on a similar principle, the release of nitric oxide. Using these drugs in tandem can result in dangerously low blood pressure and has been associated with several deaths.

BETA BLOCKERS: NOT FOR LONG-TERM USE

Another very popular class of drugs for patients with heart disease is beta blockers. There are so many of them that I'll list only a few of the most popular: atenolol (Tenormin), metoprolol (Lopressor and Toprol XL), nadolol (Corgard), and propranolol (Inderal and Inderal LA). They are prescribed for chest pain (chronic stable angina), high blood pressure, congestive heart failure, and to patients who have had a heart attack. Beta blockers are so named because they bind to beta adrenergic receptors in the heart and blood vessels, blocking their response to norepinephrine (also called noradrenaline), a hormone that signals the arteries to constrict and the heart to beat faster. By reducing the heart rate and relaxing the blood vessels, blood pressure falls and more blood and oxygen are delivered to the heart. These drugs also inhibit the kidneys' release of renin, an enzyme that sets into motion a cascade of chemical reactions that results in sodium retention and increases in blood pressure.

Beta blockers are beneficial for temporary relief from chest pain and for short-term control of blood pressure, but that is not how they are used in conventional medicine. Virtually every doctor prescribes these drugs with instructions to take them indefinitely, despite the fact that these drugs have more side effects than any other heart medication. They impair circulation and cause cold extremities, fatigue, dizziness, insomnia, and nausea. They are notorious for lowering libido and contributing to sexual dysfunction and depression. They constrict the bronchi in the lungs and precipitate asthma attacks in some patients. More worrisome for patients with heart disease, beta blockers often raise triglyceride levels, lower HDL cholesterol, and cause palpitations. Furthermore, these drugs limit the ability to exercise, which is one of the best therapies for patients with heart disease.

But the most serious charge that can be made about these drugs is that they may contribute to heart failure. Here's what the *Physicians' Desk Reference* says about one beta blocker, Lopressor:

WARNINGS

Cardiac Failure: Sympathetic stimulation is a vital component supporting circulatory function in congestive heart failure, and a beta blockade carries the potential hazard of further depressing myocardial contractility and of precipitating more severe failure. . . .

In Patients Without a History of Cardiac Failure: Continued depression of the myocardium with beta-blocking agents over a period of time can, in some cases, lead to cardiac failure. . . .

ADVERSE REACTIONS

Cardiovascular: Shortness of breath and bradycardia [heart rate below 60] have occurred in approximately 3 of 100 patients. Cold extremities; arterial insufficiency, usually of the Raynaud type; palpitations; congestive heart failure; peripheral edema; and hypotension have been reported in about 1 of 100 patients.[18]

Beta blockers should never be abruptly discontinued, as this may result in severe angina and even heart attack. Withdrawal should be done gradually, while implementing the program described in Part III, and only under the supervision of a physician.

CALCIUM CHANNEL BLOCKERS ARE LOSING THEIR LUSTER

Calcium channels are tiny conduits in the smooth muscle cells of the arteries. When calcium flows into these channels, the muscles contract and the arteries constrict, impeding circulation and raising blood pressure. Drugs known as calcium channel blockers, or calcium antagonists, enter these channels and prevent excess calcium from flowing in. The arteries thus relax and dilate, resulting in lower blood pressure, improvements in circulation, and decreased demands on the heart. Some of the calcium channel blockers also slow the heart rate.

This class of drugs is prescribed mainly for patients with hypertension, angina, and arrhythmias. There are actually two types of calcium channel blockers. The short-acting drugs work quickly, usually within thirty minutes, but their effects are transient, so they must be taken several times a day. They are less popular than the longer-acting calcium channel blockers, which have more sustained actions. These include nifedipine (Adalat CC, Procardia XL), verapamil (Calan SR, Covera HS, Isoptin SR, and Verelan), and diltiazem (Cardizem CD, Cardizem SR, Dilacor XR, and Tiazac), to mention a few.

Side effects of calcium channel blockers include headache, flushing, constipation, nausea, potassium loss, elevated serum cholesterol, swelling in the lower extremities, and low blood pressure. These drugs also stress the liver and interfere with normal carbohydrate metabolism, which is why I strongly discourage diabetics from using them. But these side effects are minor compared to those found in a 1995 study sponsored by the National Institutes of Medicine. In this study, Bruce M. Psaty, M.D., and colleagues compared 623 hypertensive patients who had had a heart attack to a control group of 2,032 patients with hypertension but no history of heart attack. They found that those taking calcium channel blockers experienced a 60 percent increase in heart attack, compared to patients who had been treated with other blood pressure medications.[19]

Not surprisingly, the pharmaceutical companies that manufactured these drugs cried foul and immediately got to work to discredit the study. Their tactics were so aggressive that they prompted the publication of an article in the *New England Journal of Medicine* chastising authors regarding their "published positions on the safety of calcium-channel antagonists and their financial relationships with pharmaceutical manufacturers. The medical profession needs to develop a more complete disclosure of relationships."[20]

Perhaps the most damning study of all was a 2000 review of randomized controlled trials on calcium channel blockers. Nine trials involving 27,743 participants pitting calcium channel blockers against other antihypertensive drugs were analyzed. The researchers found that patients taking calcium channel blockers had a significantly higher risk of heart attack, congestive heart failure, and other cardiovascular events. They concluded: "Calcium antagonists are inferior to other types of antihypertensive drugs as first-line agents in reducing the risks of several major complications of hypertension."[21]

A number of studies have also linked these drugs with an increased risk of cancer. Researchers at the Catholic University in Rome evaluated 5,052 hypertensive patients aged seventy-one and older, and found that individuals taking calcium channel blockers developed cancer at about twice the rate of those using other blood-pressure-lowering drugs. Most prevalent were cancers of the lung, urinary tract, colon, prostate, and breast.[22] Following on the heels of this damaging study was another involving 1,198 women who were at least sixty-five years old and were taking drugs for high blood pressure. The women in this study group who were taking calcium channel blockers were more than twice as likely to have breast cancer, and if they were taking estrogen plus an immediate-release calcium channel blocker, the risk was 8.38 times greater than for women taking other blood-pressure-lowering drugs.[23]

If you are using a calcium channel blocker, make sure you avoid grapefruit juice for at least two hours before and after taking your medication. Naringenin, a natural flavonoid in grapefruit juice, interferes with the liver's ability to detoxify and eliminate these drugs. This intensifies the drugs' effects and they stay in your system longer. No other citrus juices have this effect.

Also discuss alternatives with your doctor. Magnesium acts remarkably similar to calcium channel blockers, as I will explain in Chapter 14, and the only side effect of this nontoxic mineral is loose stools when taken in very large amounts.

ACE INHIBITORS: THE BEST OF THE BUNCH?

Angiotensin-converting enzyme (ACE) inhibitors have been used for years to treat hypertension and congestive heart failure. Recent research suggests that they also decrease the risk of heart attack, stroke, and even diabetes. Drugs in this class include ramipril (Altace), quinapril (Accupril), captopril (Capoten), lisinopril (Prinivil and Zestril), enalapril (Vasotec), and benazepril (Lotensin). They work by inhibiting the action of ACE, the enzyme that converts angiotensin I into angiotensin II. While angiotensin I has no ill effects, when blood levels of the powerful vasoconstrictor angiotensin II rise, the blood vessels become chronically tense, causing blood pressure to climb and the heart to work harder. By blocking the action of ACE, less angiotensin II is produced. The arteries relax and dilate slightly, blood pressure falls, oxygen demands of the heart decrease, and cardiac output (the amount of blood pumped by the heart) increases.

Among the most recent research on ACE inhibitors is a 2000 Canadian study of more than 1,400 patients fifty-five years of age and older, with heart disease. These patients were considered to be at high risk for heart attack because they had at least one additional risk factor, such as hypertension, elevated total or LDL cholesterol, or cigarette smoking. They were randomly assigned to take either an ACE inhibitor (in this study it was ramipril) or a placebo every day. After five years, patients taking the ACE inhibitor had fewer heart attacks, strokes, problems with heart failure, angioplasties, and deaths from cardiovascular disease. There was also a reduced incidence of new-onset diabetes and diabetic complications in the group taking the ACE inhibitor, suggesting that the drug may have an effect on insulin sensitivity.[24]

ACE inhibitors appear to be less dangerous than other heart medications. Their most common side effect is an annoying, persistent dry cough. This is caused by elevations in blood levels of bradykinin, a naturally occurring protein that can trigger contractions of the smooth muscles of the bronchioles. This same mechanism can also, though infrequently, cause dangerous constriction of the bronchioles and asthmatic symptoms. (Angiotensin II inhibitors are a related class of drugs that do not raise levels of bradykinin and therefore do not cause cough or breathing difficulties. They are sometimes given to patients who cannot tolerate ACE inhibitors.)

Other common side effects of these drugs are altered sense of taste and reduced appetite. A rare side effect is acute swelling of the face, tongue, lips, vocal cords, and extremities. Alterations in levels of important trace minerals such as selenium, zinc, and copper; kidney damage; and reduced white blood cell count have also been reported. Patients with lung or kidney disease should avoid ACE inhibitors.

ANTITHROMBOTIC DRUGS THIN THE BLOOD

Patients with heart disease are also treated with antithrombotic agents. These drugs are aimed at preventing the formation of blood clots by inhibiting different aspects of the natural coagulation cascade we talked about in Chapter 3. Such agents are almost always used in patients with unstable angina (the type that comes on unpredictably or persists, rather than being triggered by exertion or stress), atrial fibrillation (a chaotic rhythm of the heart), or artificial heart valves. But they are also used by some patients with less severe coronary artery disease, and milder antithrombotic drugs, such as aspirin, are even used for preventive purposes.

There are two types of antithrombotic agents. The first are antiplatelet drugs. These drugs discourage the aggregation or clumping together of platelets, which are involved in clotting. Aspirin is the best-known antiplatelet drug, although ticlopidine (Ticlid), clopidogrel (Plavix), and other prescription antiplatelet drugs are also effective in reducing platelet aggregation.

The other class of antithrombotic drugs are anticoagulants such as warfarin (Coumadin) and heparin. They inhibit the production of fibrin, the "net" that holds platelets together to form a blood clot. Heparin is administered intravenously or by injection, so its use is usually limited to a medical setting. Warfarin is taken orally, and although it is certainly a lifesaver for some patients, it is, in my opinion, overprescribed. It has numerous side effects and potential complications, the most serious of which is a high risk of bleeding. For this reason, blood clotting time must be monitored frequently to make sure the dose is in the safe but therapeutic range. This drug also interacts with a very long list of medications, herbs, and even foods. If you are taking warfarin, it is worth asking your physician if you have other options.

ASPIRIN: A 100-YEAR-OLD WONDER DRUG

Aspirin, or acetylsalicylic acid, is an inexpensive over-the-counter drug that has been used for more than a century to treat pain and inflammation. It is also a powerful agent for preventing heart attacks and improving odds of survival after a heart attack. Aspirin suppresses the production of a very powerful platelet aggregator and vasoconstrictor called thromboxane A2. It relaxes and widens the arteries, discourages clot formation, and improves blood flow. In addition, it hampers the activity of prostaglandins involved in inflammation. As we discussed in Chapter 3, inflammation as evidenced by elevated levels of C-reactive protein is a significant risk factor for heart disease. A 1997 study suggests that this may be aspirin's most most significant mode of action.[25]

Charles Hennekens, M.D., professor at Harvard Medical School and chief of the Division of Preventive Medicine at Brigham and Women's Hospital in Boston, has been the principal investigator in three long-term studies of the effects of aspirin in preventing heart attacks. In one of these studies, 22,071 male physicians aged forty to eighty-four were assigned to one of two protocols: 325 mg of aspirin every other day or a placebo. Aspirin's clear and obvious benefits were recognized early on. In fact, the study was stopped almost six years sooner than scheduled because the men taking aspirin had a 44 percent reduction in heart attacks![26] Similar results have been obtained in other large long-term studies, both in the United States and Europe. All have shown that small, regular doses of aspirin reduce heart attack rates by 20 to 44 percent.

Aspirin also improves survival when taken at the first sign of a heart attack. In the Second International Study of Infarct Survival, which followed 17,187 patients seen in a hospital within twenty-four hours of the onset of a heart attack, those given aspirin at that time and for thirty days thereafter had a 23 percent lower death rate than those receiving no aspirin.[27] Aspirin's effectiveness is comparable to that of conventional clot-busting therapies used in hospitals, and the cost savings of using aspirin at the time of a heart attack instead of these newer drugs are astronomical. Yet physicians routinely select the more high-tech treatments. According to Dr. Hennekens, "If aspirin was only half as effective, but ten times more expensive and available only by prescription, people would take it more seriously."[28]

The American Heart Association recommends aspirin for patients who have unstable angina or have already had a heart attack, stroke, or transient ischemic attack (TIA or "mini-stroke"). Unfortunately, only one in four who would benefit from aspirin actually takes it.[29] Aspirin has some very serious side effects, including the potential to cause ulcers and gastrointestinal bleeding. It puts tens of thousands of people in the hospital every year and kills thousands.[30] These problems generally occur with higher doses than those recommended for cardiovascular disease and can be largely avoided by taking aspirin with a meal and sticking with a low dose—one-half of a regular 325 mg aspirin (162.5 mg) every other day, or one baby aspirin (81 mg) every day.

If you suspect that you or anyone you know is having a heart attack, a regular-strength aspirin (325 mg) should be taken at once, and a doctor's help sought immediately.

THE DOWNSIDE OF DIURETICS

I want to touch briefly on diuretics, for they are a very popular treatment for high blood pressure, which afflicts many patients with heart disease. Diuretics reduce blood pressure by decreasing blood volume and thus pressure against the arteries. They stimulate the kidneys to absorb less sodium, so sodium and water are excreted through the urine. Unfortunately, other essential nutrients are excreted at the same time.

One of the minerals lost is potassium, and the repercussions can be severe. The Multiple Risk Factor Intervention Trial (MRFIT), a double-blind, placebo-controlled study involving more than 12,800 men with high blood pressure, compared the effects of aggressive drug treatment (primarily a class of diuretics called thiazides) with minimal drug treatment. MRFIT found that although stepped-up drug treatment did lower blood pressure, it did not decrease deaths from heart disease. Even worse, aggressive drug therapy for men with borderline hypertension caused potassium deficiencies that prompted wildly irregular heartbeat, actually increasing the risk of sudden cardiac death.[31] These drugs also raise blood sugar, cholesterol, and triglycerides—not a good thing for patients whose elevated blood pressure already puts them at risk of heart attack.

Pharmaceutical companies have come out with "potassium-sparing" diuretics, which stem potassium losses. However, no diuretic addresses the losses of other water-soluble nutrients that are critically important in heart disease, such as magnesium. Volumes of research prove that lifestyle changes could eliminate high blood pressure in a majority of patients. Nevertheless, the treatment approach of many physicians is to immediately start patients with hypertension on a lifelong regimen of diuretics and other drugs.

DRUGS AREN'T ALWAYS THE ANSWER

People come to the Whitaker Wellness Institute for many different medical conditions, but one common goal shared by our patients is the desire to get off some of their prescription drugs. We have patients walk into the clinic on ten, twelve, fifteen different drugs. One of my patients, Louise, is a case in point. Louise's initial complaint twelve years earlier was heart disease, and she was started on a drug. Over the years, more and more drugs were added as her health deteriorated. When I first saw Louise, she was so sick and on so many drugs—twenty different medications, sixteen of them prescription drugs—that it was obvious to me that a lot of her problems were caused by the cocktail of drugs she was taking. Just reducing her medication load dramatically improved Louise's health.

If you are taking any drugs for heart disease, I suggest that you discuss potential problems and possible alternatives with your physician. There are safer, equally, if not more, effective natural options to every drug we have covered in this chapter. We are quite successful at the Whitaker Wellness Institute in helping our patients eliminate their dependency on drugs, including medications they were told would be required for a lifetime. We don't do anything extraordinary—we simply stress the importance of lifestyle changes in alleviating the underlying causes of disease. It is the patients themselves who do the real healing when they embrace the recommended program of diet, exercise, and nutritional supplementation you will learn about in the next section.

Part III

The Whitaker Wellness Institute Program for Reversing Heart Disease

CHAPTER 10

Heart Disease Is Reversible

GENE, A SUCCESSFUL CONTRACTOR, WAS DIAGNOSED WITH HYPERtension when he was in his late fifties. His doctor immediately put him on a blood-pressure-lowering medication. He was not told that hypertension was a significant risk factor for heart disease, nor was he given any advice about diet, exercise, or any other measures he might take to protect himself.

Over the next few years Gene began to have occasional chest pain. Because he was so heavily involved in his work, he dismissed it as a minor annoyance—until it became so severe that merely walking across the living room brought it on. He was given heavy doses of a beta-blocker drug, nitroglycerin tablets, and a nitroglycerin patch to wear on his chest.

He was also referred for an angiogram, which showed that one of his coronary arteries was completely blocked and two others had severe blockages. His doctor recommended immediate coronary artery bypass surgery.

Had he not had a cold, Gene probably would have had surgery; however, because of it his surgery was postponed a few days. While he was getting over the cold, a friend who had heard me lecture on alternatives to bypass surgery encouraged him to check out the Whitaker Wellness Institute. Gene called, and he expressed his doubts and fears. "Doctors in the hospital scheduled me for a major operation on my heart like they were making an appointment for a haircut. I just felt something was wrong in the way I was being rushed." He was told about the program we offer patients at the institute, which is designed not only to slow the progression of heart disease but to actually reverse it, and about our considerable success in relieving angina and other symptoms of heart disease.

Gene came to the institute to undergo our treatment program. He had a complete physical examination, blood tests, and an exercise stress test. We went over his test results and discussed the research on bypass, which shows that except for small, select subgroups of patients, surgery does not prevent heart attacks, stop the progression of heart disease, or prolong life. I told him that because his angina was so severe, he might be one of those rare patients who truly does need surgery. However, I suggested that he try our program before resorting to heart surgery.

Since this approach requires active participation of patients—it is you, not your doctor, who has to eat right and exercise—we spend a lot of time on patient education. Gene joined a group of patients with heart disease and other health problems, attended lectures, and received personalized instruction in the particulars of a heart-healthy diet, a moderate exercise program, and appropriate nutritional supplementation. The patients ate together, exercised together, and received specialized therapies together. They shared their health challenges and triumphs and served as keen motivators for one another.

Within days Gene began to notice changes. When he arrived, his chest pain was so severe that he couldn't walk two hundred yards, and he was taking more than a dozen nitroglycerin tablets a day. After a week at the institute he was walking two miles and taking only three to five nitroglycerin tablets. Dosages of his other medications were also cut back, and he felt more energetic than he had in years. Gene returned home with a program he thought he could live with and more hope than he ever imagined.

He continued to improve. Within eighteen months Gene had

lost 25 pounds, his cholesterol level dropped to 155, his blood pressure stabilized, he was off all medications, and he had not had angina in over a year. An exercise stress test and thallium scan done at that time showed that his heart function was completely normal. Four years later, at age sixty-nine, Gene built a home gym so he could intensify his exercise program. He continued to be off all drugs, his blood pressure and weight were stable, and he hadn't had chest pain in more than three years. He had returned to his former vigorous and productive life and had just completed building a sixty-unit condominium complex while working out daily and sticking to his diet.

Gene got a lot out of our program, and let me say that the credit is largely his. This is not one of those situations where the doctor "fixes" a passive patient, like a plumber fixing a stopped sink. In our program for reversing heart disease the doctor guides and teaches while the patient learns the hows and whys of the program. We provide a network of support during the early stages as patients step into their new lifestyle. Then they continue to live wisely, effecting their own cures. The doctor is almost entirely a teacher: It is the patient who carries out the course of treatment.

In this section I will outline for you the Whitaker Wellness Institute treatment program that Gene so successfully used to reverse his heart disease. While Gene spent some time at the institute—and that is certainly an option for interested patients—the purpose of this book is to provide you with all the information you will need to implement a safe, effective program for reversing heart disease on your own.

WHERE'S THE PROOF?

The idea of reversing a condition as serious as heart disease with natural therapies such as diet, exercise, and nutritional supplements generates heated controversy. Cardiologists who are enthralled with high-tech interventions like bypass, angioplasty, and the latest medications quite naturally discount the value of this more conservative approach. Yet the scientific data supporting the effectiveness of lifestyle measures in reversing atherosclerosis is there, and ironically, some of it is more valid than the data used to support bypass and other conventional therapies. Here is a brief overview of the research.

Early Animal Experiments

Scientists have been trying to figure out the mechanisms underlying atherosclerosis for centuries. Something was damaging the arteries, but what? In the early twentieth century, European scientists attempted to find out by injecting irritating substances into the arteries of rabbits. In time the rabbits were sacrificed and their arteries sliced open. Clean. No trace of atherosclerosis in these vegetarian creatures. No matter what irritants their arteries were exposed to, atherosclerosis did not occur.

The culprit was discovered by accident. In 1909 a Russian scientist was studying the effects of a high-protein diet on rabbit kidneys by feeding the animals meat, milk, and eggs. In due time the rabbits were dissected and, while kidney damage was nil, severe atherosclerosis was found in their arteries.[1] The study was repeated with the same results, and a debate ensued. Was it the protein in these foods that was damaging the animals' arteries or was it the fat? Another Russian researcher settled the dispute in 1913 by producing severe atherosclerosis in rabbits with a high–saturated-fat, protein-free diet.[2]

Since that time the routine way to produce atherosclerosis in lab animals for study purposes has been to feed them saturated fat—it never fails to damage and clog up the arteries. No other method consistently produces coronary artery disease in animals. According to Dr. William E. Connor of the University of Oregon, "If ever a human disease can be produced in animals, it is atherosclerosis, and if ever the requirements of that disease have been isolated it is fat and cholesterol in the diet."

But what about reversing heart disease? The excitement really begins when these animals with diet-induced blockages in their arteries are put back on their natural low-fat diets. Atherosclerosis begins to reverse![3] This has been demonstrated not only in rabbits but in monkeys and other primates as well. Dr. Draga Vesselinovitch of the University of Chicago reported a 50 percent reduction of artery damage in monkeys after eighteen months on a low-fat diet. Not only did blockages regress, but the linings of arteries showed signs of regeneration.[4]

The medical literature on atherosclerosis in animals would fill a library, and it clearly points to a high-fat diet as a major culprit in heart disease. You may have heard that experiments on animals are not conclusive for humans, and that is true. Human beings are very different from rabbits and we can't always apply to our own systems what we learn from rabbit experiments. Even though monkeys are close to us in organ structure and function, and experimental results with them must be taken seriously, they cannot be definitively applied to humans. However, these animal studies did point the way for research that is consequential for humans.

Epidemiological Observations

Epidemiology is the study of the "interrelationships of the host, agent, and environment in causing disease."[5] Researchers compare disease rates among groups of people with different diets and other lifestyle factors and try to sort out which factors contribute to disease. It was epidemiological research that first linked a fatty diet to heart disease in humans, and some of the earliest studies came out of war-ravaged Europe.

During World War I and World War II, Europeans endured drastic food shortages, the most noticeable being meat, eggs, milk, butter, cheese, and lard. The complex industry of raising and slaughtering livestock and processing, storing, transporting, and distributing these foods was disrupted by war. People fell back on potatoes, vegetables, fruits, and grains, which are easier to grow and can be stored for prolonged periods.

A few astute scientists observed that the effects of privation might have been a blessing in disguise. Dr. T. Ashoff reported that during and just after World War I, there was a significant reduction of plaque in the arteries of the civilian population, which he attributed to the reduced consumption of high-fat foods.[6] More conclusive evidence was gathered during World War II. In Finland, Drs. Ilmari Vartiainen and Karl Kanerva documented a 67 percent drop in deaths from heart disease in the civilian population compared with prewar days.[7] The Norwegian government reported similar findings during the war and the austere period following it, and routine autopsies on civilians showed marked reduction of atherosclerosis.[8, 9] All of these researchers concluded that the decline in the heart disease death rate was associated with reduced consumption of meat, butter, and other foods rich in fat and cholesterol.

William Castelli, M.D., initial director of the Framingham Study, which, as we discussed earlier in this book, was the first study to conclusively show an elevated blood cholesterol level to be a major risk factor for heart disease, received his medical training in Belgium in the early 1950s. He had a crusty pathology professor, Dr. Eugene Picard, who amused students by walking around mumbling, "They're coming back." Someone asked him who "they" were, and Dr. Picard replied, "Cholesterol deposits in the arteries." Sure enough, atherosclerosis was again showing up in cadavers as Belgians returned to their rich peacetime eating habits.[10]

All this splendid wartime documentation is ignored today by those who say that we have had no definitive, controlled, large-scale studies proving that a shift to a low-fat diet dramatically reduces atherosclerosis in humans. These wartime observations may be the best data we'll ever have. Think about it. When and how could scientists ever persuade 50 million people to shift to a low-fat diet for four years? What kind of test would rival the wartime experience of Europe for conclusive results?

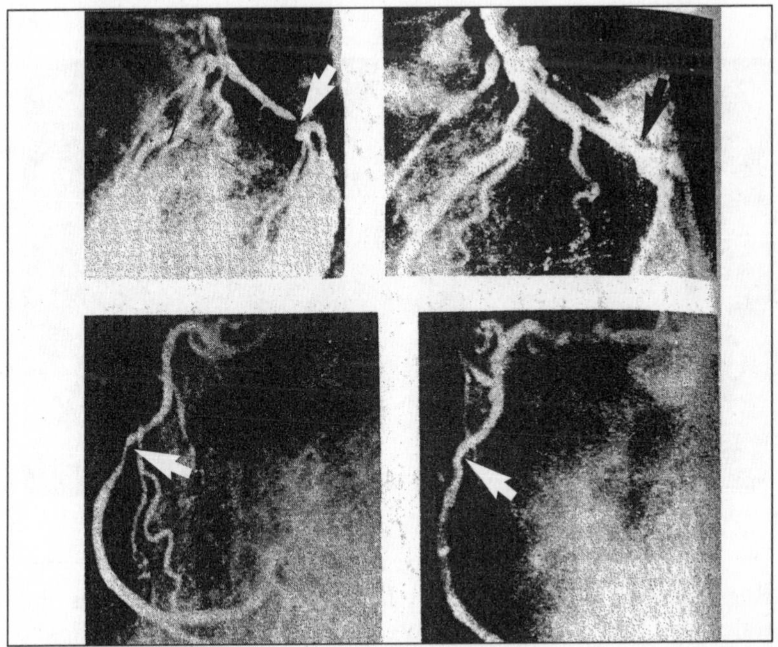

Regression of Atherosclerosis: These before-and-after pictures, obtained by angiography, show distinct changes in degree of atherosclerosis of two coronary arteries. The arrows in the pictures on the left point to visible arterial blockages with restriction of blood flow. In the pictures on the right, taken after the patient began an intensive exercise program, you can see marked widening of arterial diameter and restoration of blood flow.[11]

Case Studies

Case studies have also shed light on the reversal of atherosclerosis through lifestyle changes. Well-documented histories of patients using one or more clearly identified therapies are an excellent way of determining therapeutic efficacy. There are volumes of case histories of proven, documented reversal of atherosclerosis attributed to diet, exercise, and other lifestyle factors, and I want to share a few of them with you.

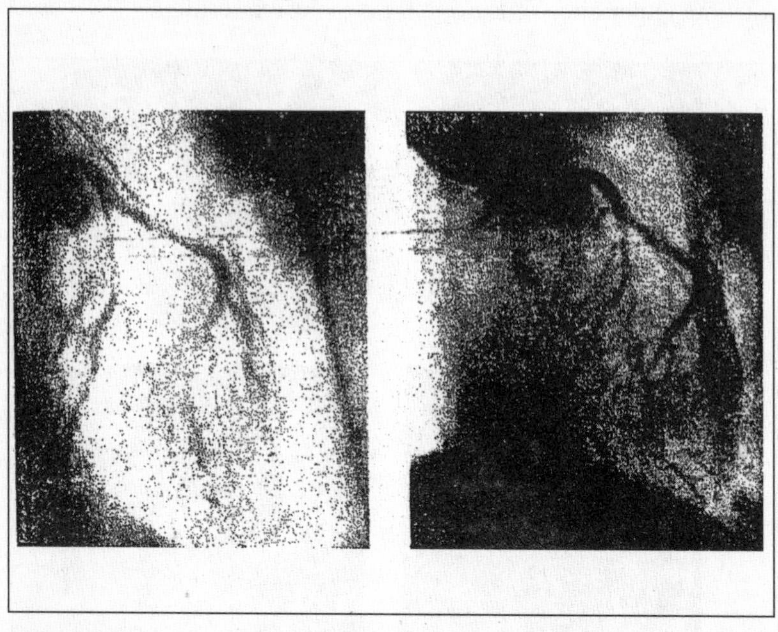

Regression of Coronary Artery Disease. These two pictures illustrate the differences in blood flow through the coronary arteries before the patient went on a diet and exercise program. Note the darker color, indicating greater circulation, plus the greater number of vessels receiving blood flow in the "after" picture on the right.[12]

Dr. Thomas Bassler reported the case of a sixty-one-year-old man who had endured angina for thirteen years. Angiography revealed that one of his coronary arteries was blocked 95 percent and another had a 75 percent blockage. Although he was considered to be an ideal bypass candidate, the man decided to take matters into his own hands by increasing his daily walking from two miles to six, and he started to do some slow jogging. His angina went away in about two months. He kept up his program and at the age of sixty-eight repeat angiography showed that the larger blockage had shrunk from 95 to 50 percent and the smaller one from 75 to 30 percent.[13]

Dr. D. Roth of the University Hospital of London, Ontario, followed a forty-six-year-old attorney who was admitted to the hospital with severe chest pain and an eight-month history of angina brought on by exertion. An exercise stress test and thallium scan showed inadequate blood flow to certain areas of the heart, and an angiogram revealed a large blockage in a major artery. Told he would benefit from surgery, the patient instead went home, cut down his meat and dairy intake, and increased his exercise. Six months later his chest pain was completely gone, his cholesterol level had dropped from 269 to 209, and his triglycerides went from 205 to 93. A year later his heart was functioning normally and a repeat angiogram showed that the blockage had unquestionably been reversed.[14]

These and hundreds of other very compelling case studies are often overlooked by physicians. Several years ago I was scheduled for an interview on a Los Angeles TV station to talk about reversing heart disease. The day before, a prominent cardiovascular surgeon was on the same show, discussing bypass surgery and how reversibility of atherosclerotic blockages in the coronary arteries using conservative therapies had never been demonstrated by angiography. Well, I appeared the next day on the same program with several angiograms showing blockages in the coronary arteries that had been reversed. These examples had been published in the medical literature and were easily available.

Dr. Castelli commented in a lecture at Loma Linda University that he ran into this bias all the time. He has presented at numerous medical centers before-and-after angiograms of coronary arteries showing that arterial blockages evident at one point in time had disappeared with conservative treatment. He was always amused that after his talks, many cardiologists and heart surgeons would form a line at the microphone to state that the blockages on the original angiograms were not plaque, but an involuntary spasm of the artery that only looked like a blockage. Dr. Castelli quipped that if this were the case, a lot of patients were having bypass surgery for spasms of the arteries, not actual blockages!

Controlled Clinical Trials

As I mentioned earlier, the problem with animal research is that we can't be entirely sure that study findings will apply to humans. Case studies are interesting and instructional, particularly when many of them point to the same cause and effect, but again, extrapolating from individual cases to larger populations is difficult. Epidemiological studies have the advantage of large numbers of people, but it is impossible to control all the variables. Therefore, controlled clinical trials that pit one therapy against another in similar groups of patients are considered the gold standard—the most reliable way of determining the efficacy of any therapy.

One of the pioneers in this type of research regarding the effects of lifestyle changes on atherosclerosis is Dean Ornish, M.D. He was the first physician to prove in a controlled clinical trial that heart disease can be reversed with lifestyle measures. In his first study of this nature, Dr. Ornish enrolled 23 patients with heart disease in a twenty-four-day in-hospital lifestyle program. These were sick patients. Roughly a third of them had already had a heart attack, all of them were taking heart medications, and they were having an average of ten attacks of angina per week. Each had been identified by angiography as having blockages of greater than 50 percent in one or more major coronary arteries.

These patients were placed on an extremely low-fat vegetarian diet and stress-reduction techniques as their major therapy. Their results were compared to another group of similarly ill patients who received standard medical treatment. After twenty-four days on the lifestyle regimen, patients experienced an average drop in cholesterol of 20.5 percent. They were able to exercise longer on follow-up stress tests, and their hearts functioned better as well. Furthermore, there was a 91 percent reduction in frequency of angina. Attacks were reduced from an average of almost two per day to less than one a week.[15]

When these results were published in 1983 I was excited. I had long followed the work of Nathan Pritikin, who was having success reversing heart disease with a program of low-fat diet and exercise. Now with Dr. Ornish's research, we had clinical proof that it was effective. Skeptics were quick to criticize. They pointed out that this might work in a clinical setting for a short period such as twenty-four days, but they were certain that patients would not make appropriate changes in their diet on their own over the long haul. Dean Ornish decided to prove them wrong.

He mounted a one-year study of patients with heart disease called the Lifestyle Heart Trial. Twenty-eight of these patients were instructed in a low-fat vegetarian diet, smoking cessation, stress management training, and moderate exercise, while 20 served as a control group receiving standard medical care. All patients underwent angiography to determine the degree of blockages in their coronary arteries before the study and again at the study's conclusion. The lifestyle group then spent a week in a residence program to learn the basics of the program, and throughout the remainder of the study, they met regularly in support groups to help them stay on track.

After one year, cholesterol levels in the lifestyle group fell by 24.3 percent and LDL cholesterol by 37.4 percent—without the use of cholesterol-lowering drugs. Angina symptoms also improved dramatically. There was a 28 percent reduction in severity, a 42 percent reduction in duration, and an astounding 91 percent reduction in frequency of angina. The most important finding, however, was that the lifestyle regimen actually reversed blockages in the arteries. The average blockage decreased from 40 percent at the study's onset to 37.8 percent, and improvements were even greater in the more severely blocked arteries. In comparison, the control group of heart patients on a standard fare of medications got worse, with measurable progression of arterial blockages.[16]

Dr. Ornish has since published several other studies along this same line. In one of them, he followed patients on a lifestyle regimen for five years and, as expected, noted even more regression of coronary atherosclerosis. During those five years, more than twice as many cardiac events (heart attack, angioplasty, bypass, etc.) occurred in patients in the control group receiving standard medical care than in those who were eating a low-fat diet, exercising regularly, and managing their stress.[17]

PROGRAM OVERVIEW

As you can see, the use of nutrition, exercise, and stress management to reverse atherosclerosis is not a fanciful theory but a solid, proven alternative to invasive procedures and heavy drug regimens. Hundreds of other studies have evaluated the individual components of such a treatment program, and we will cover some of them as we work our way through the next few chapters. For now I want to give you a preview of the Whitaker Wellness Institute program for reversing heart disease.

1. Eat a Heart-Healthy Diet

Americans have made substantial modifications in their diets since the mid-sixties, when heart disease rates were at their peak. We eat less red meat, and our consumption of whole milk, cream, and butter is considerably lower. This is a step in the right direction, but we still have a long way to go. We eat more sugar than ever and indulge in foods laden with unhealthy oils and white flour. Quick convenience foods and take-out fare have become more common than meals made with whole foods. Food preferences are a societal phenomenon, and the cultural influences that have addicted us to our current diet are a formidable obstacle to change.

However, a good diet is without a doubt the foundation of health, and the diet I describe in Chapters 11 and 12 will have a positive impact on virtually all the risk factors for heart disease. While implementing dietary changes requires some effort and discipline on your part, rest assured that our diet for reversing heart disease is not one of deprivation or unappealing "health foods." You will be pleasantly surprised at the variety, tastiness, and ease of preparation of the meal plans and recipes in Part IV. Furthermore, this diet will be a boon not only to your heart but to all aspects of your health.

2. Take Targeted Nutritional Supplements

A 2001 British study found that people with the highest blood levels of vitamin C had half the risk of dying from heart disease as those with the lowest levels of this vitamin.[18] Harvard researchers demonstrated that women who took supplemental vitamin E had a 46 percent lower risk of heart disease, compared to women who took no vitamin E.[19] Low blood levels of B-complex vitamins are associated with increased risk of heart disease. Magnesium, selenium, and other nutrients we will discuss in detail are also directly linked to the health of the heart and blood vessels.

Yes, you can theoretically get the requisite vitamins, minerals, and other nutrients from the food you eat. However, as you will see in Chapter 13, it is a hit-or-miss proposition. The only way to ensure that you are getting adequate levels of these therapeutic nutrients is to take them in supplement form on a daily basis. Nutritional supplementation is a cornerstone of my program for reversing heart disease. Although many physicians ignore the contribution of nutritional supplementation, I will show you in Chapter 14 how this simple step can provide tremendous protection against the multiple processes that ravage the cardiovascular system.

3. Exercise Regularly

People are much more conscious of the benefits of physical activity than they were twenty years ago. Health clubs have proliferated and professional athletes are among the most admired men and women in America. Unfortunately, we talk the talk, but we don't walk the walk. Fewer than two out of ten adults in this country exercise on a regular basis. It's easy to understand why—exercise is hard work. But that's the whole point.

Only by working out hard enough to get your heart beating faster, your lungs taking in more oxygen, and your muscles moving vigorously will you improve the health of your cardiovascular system and indeed of your entire body. Exercise is highly protective against heart disease. And if you've already had a heart attack, beginning an exercise program will increase your odds of avoiding a repeat heart attack or surviving if you do suffer a second heart attack.[20] In Chapter 15 we will talk about the benefits of exercise, and I will provide you with a safe and detailed exercise program to optimize heart health.

4. Get a Handle on Negative Emotions

Our hearts pound with anxiety and jump out of our chests with fear. Grief and depression leave us sick at heart. A strong emotional response is heart-wrenching, and anger makes our blood boil. Have you ever noticed how so many references to the heart crop up in our descriptions of intense emotion? This is no accident. Strong emotional responses have immediate, powerful, and long-lasting effects on the cardiovascular system.

Everyone experiences intense emotions every now and then—it's part of being human. However, reacting with anger, anxiety, or depression to all of life's hills and valleys takes it toll on your heart and arteries. As I will explain in Chapter 16, the root of this damage is the biochemical changes that are part and parcel of the stress response. We will discuss exactly how negative emotions affect your cardiovascular system, and I will give you ten easy-to-implement antidotes for chronic stress.

5. Consider Hormone Replacement Therapy

You know that estrogen and progesterone relieve menopausal symptoms, and testosterone builds muscle mass and improves libido in men. But hormones and the heart? Decades-old research proves that supplementing with certain hormones can lower cholesterol, improve blood flow, strengthen the heart muscle, lower body fat, and help regulate heart rhythm. Not that you will ever hear about this from your physician. For some reason, with the exception of estrogen and progesterone for postmenopausal women and thyroid for people with low thyroid function, hormone therapy is generally ignored by conventional physicians. And when you do hear about hormone replacement therapy, it is often with a warning of its potential dangers.

This is unfortunate, because patients are missing out on an entire category of therapeutic agents that when used appropriately can make a real difference in their health. At the Whitaker Wellness Institute we use a wide variety of natural hormones to treat specific medical conditions, and cardiovascular disease is one of them. In Chapter 17, we will go over the most effective hormones for the treatment of heart disease.

6. Intensive Therapies for Advanced Disease

In addition to the lifestyle elements that are the basis of my treatment program for reversing heart disease, we have three "big guns" at the Whitaker Wellness Institute that we pull out for patients with serious heart disease. One of them, enhanced external counterpulsation (EECP), is the closest thing going to bypass surgery—without the surgery. It is such an effective treatment for chest pain associated with heart disease that Medicare now reimburses for it. Another is EDTA chelation therapy, an intravenous treatment that removes toxic metals from the bloodstream and arterial walls, thus protecting the arteries by reducing their free-radical load. Finally, there is hyperbaric oxygen therapy, which forces healing oxygen into the tissues, even those deprived of adequate circulation by atherosclerosis. I will explain the benefits of these unique therapies in Chapter 18.

7. If You Smoke, Stop

In the past thirty-five years there has been a greater than 30 percent reduction in use of tobacco, most of it among men over the age of thirty, who are especially vulnerable to heart disease. This has played a huge role in the declining rate of death from heart disease and other tobacco-related illnesses. However, we're not nearly out of the woods yet. Forty-seven million adults in this country continue to smoke, and the numbers of teenage, particularly female, smokers are actually increasing.[21] Smoking is unequivocally associated with heart disease. Of the 400,000 Americans who die every year as a direct result of tobacco use, a majority of them die not from lung cancer but from heart disease. Perhaps even more tragic are the 40,000 deaths from cardiovascular disease of nonsmokers attributed to secondhand smoke.

Tobacco smoke contains hundreds of chemicals that damage the arteries, hamper blood flow, and dramatically raise the risk of heart attack. Smokers have more than twice the risk of heart attack as nonsmokers and two to four times the risk of sudden cardiac arrest.[22] Don't think you're off the hook if you smoke cigars or use smokeless tobacco. You are still at increased risk. I recognize how hard it is to stop smoking. However, this is one lifestyle change that is just not negotiable.

YOU CAN DO IT

We have spent the bulk of this book thus far laying the groundwork for my program for reversing heart disease. Now let's get down to the business of actually implementing the program. If prevention is your primary concern because of a family history of the disease or other risk factors, you are doing yourself and your loved ones a huge service by protecting your health. I have great admiration for anyone who takes the bull by the horns—prevention is much easier than reversal, and your chances of success are close to 100 percent!

If you are already struggling with heart disease, kudos to you as well. It is the intelligent, proactive patient who looks for solutions outside the box, who does his or her own research and makes truly informed decisions. This program for overcoming heart disease can be added to your current treatment. It is not a quick fix—there is no such thing. But it does offer hope to people who know the pain and anxiety of heart disease and want to avoid the surgery route. Of course, you should work closely with your doctor, particularly if you are taking medications for your heart. (The majority of patients who give this program a serious go are able to discontinue or dramatically reduce their prescription drugs. However, this should be done only under a doctor's supervision.)

Whatever your motive, this program will help you increase your chances of survival to a ripe old age, improve the quality of the rest of your life, and even reverse the deterioration of your arteries. All this without surgery, and likely without heavy medication. What I propose for you is entirely doable—and enjoyable. Once you get started on this program, you'll know that you have never lived better. You *can* do it, but it's up to you to take that first step on the road to optimal health.

CHAPTER 11

Diet and Health

"YOU ARE WHAT YOU EAT." YOU'VE PROBABLY HEARD THIS TRITE phrase dozens of times, but have you ever really considered its wisdom? When it comes to heart disease, it's right on the money. Atherosclerosis is a multifaceted disease, and multiple factors contribute to its initiation and progression. Chief among them are the things you put in your mouth every day.

Although most healthcare professionals would agree that a healthy diet is important for people with heart disease, there is a lack of consensus as to what a healthy diet is. At one end of the spectrum are the advocates of a high-fat, high-protein diet. These folks claim that eating lots of meat, eggs, cheese, and other fatty foods will control weight and all the diseases associated with excess weight. At the other end are the proponents of an extremely low-fat, primarily vegetarian diet who forbid even fish and lean poultry. Then there are the niche diets that are all over the map. Juicing, raw foods, eating for your blood type, getting into the zone, shunning carbohydrates—you name it and there's a book out there extolling its merits.

If you're like the patients who come to the Whitaker Wellness Institute seeking help in getting well and reversing or preventing disease, you're not looking for the next fad diet but a program you can live with for the rest of your life. You want something that is healthful yet doesn't require keeping copious records, making complex mathematical calculations, or measuring out portions before eating. In these next two chapters I am going to lay the groundwork for the Whitaker Wellness Institute diet for reversing heart disease. (I have devoted a special section of this book, Part IV, to the more practical aspects of the diet: tips for shopping and cooking, meal plans, and recipes.) I will explain the underlying rationale for the diet and show you solid research published in the most prestigious medical journals that supports its benefits. This will take some time and space, but it has been my experience that if you truly understand the particulars of every aspect of this treatment program for heart disease, you will be much more likely to stick with it, and the improvements in your health will be all the more striking.

WHAT ARE HUMANS DESIGNED TO EAT?

Let's start by comparing the human digestive system to that of other animals. Mammals can be separated into three different classes based upon their natural diets: meat eaters (carnivores such as lions, tigers, dogs, and cats), leaf and grass eaters (herbivores such as horses, cows, antelopes, and other large herding mammals), and fruit and vegetable eaters (monkeys, apes, and chimpanzees).

The digestive tract of each of these groups is uniquely suited to its diet. For example, the mouth of a carnivore is a keen tool for hunting and defense. It has sharp, pointed canine fangs ideal for piercing hide and tearing chunks of flesh from a carcass. The meat eater has no molars or grinding teeth to chew food, for it swallows chunks of meat whole. It produces only insignificant amounts of digestive enzymes in the saliva, as these enzymes are involved in the breakdown of carbohydrates, which carnivores just don't eat.

In contrast, fruit and vegetable eaters have no sharp fangs, as they do not use their mouths for hunting. This is true of humans as well—our first recourse in defense or aggression is to use our hands, not our mouths. Again, like the fruit-and-vegetable-eating animals, human have well-developed molars in the back of the mouth, which are needed to grind vegetables and fruits and mix them with the enzymes present in saliva that begin the digestion of carbohydrates.

Strong acid is necessary for the rapid digestion of animal flesh, and the stomach of meat eaters complies, producing twenty times the hydrochloric acid of the human stomach, for fruit and vegetable digestion requires much less hydrochloric acid. Furthermore, because meat spoils rapidly, producing toxic substances in the gut, meat eaters' intestinal tracts are very short, only three times the length of the body. This short gut is designed to rapidly digest meat and quickly eliminate the decaying toxic waste products. Plant foods, on the other hand, do not putrefy quickly. Consider how nicely fruits and vegetables keep for days without refrigeration, then imagine eating ground beef that has been sitting on your windowsill for four or five days. The intestinal tract of the fruit and vegetable eater is twelve times the length of the body to allow for the slow trip necessary for complete digestion of high-fiber plant foods.

When man's physical characteristics are compared to those of other animals, it is obvious that the human body is designed to eat plant foods.

MAN, THE MIGHTY HUNTER?

Contrary to popular belief, early man was not a mighty hunter. He could be described as an "opportunistic omnivore," eating primarily wild fruits, vegetables, roots, nuts, and seeds, and whatever small or easily hunted animals he encountered while foraging for food. Weapons needed for killing prey evolved late in human history, and without them man was in no position to play a predatory role. Humans are among the slowest mammals on earth, outrun by almost every other species except the three-toed sloth of South America. Indeed, even if man did catch and kill something, he would be quickly run off by stronger, more aggressive carnivores. A human without a weapon is no match for a 25-pound dog, much less a hungry leopard, cheetah, or wolf.

What's more, humans lack the instinctual drive to acquire large amounts of meat. If meat were natural to the human diet, we would stalk animals in the field, catch them with our hands, bite them to death, and feast on their warm, bleeding carcasses. Instead, we have someone else do the killing, and we boil, bake, or fry the meat and disguise it with all kinds of sauces and spices so that it bears little resemblance to the flesh of an animal. Most people would be sickened if they had to stalk and kill their meat themselves. If you don't believe me, visit a slaughterhouse or meat-processing plant. If everyone did this a couple of times a year, I believe that meat consumption would be sharply curtailed. For many, one visit would be enough to swear off meat altogether.

If we would resist our cultural conditioning and eat the foods that our bodies are designed to eat, we would be so much the better for it. Vaughn Bryant, associate professor of anthropology at Texas A & M University, researched the diet of Paleolithic man and determined that it was likely primarily vegetarian (with an occasional grasshopper), very low in fat, and high in carbohydrates and fiber. At the age of thirty—and 30 pounds overweight—Professor Bryant went on a modified caveman diet by eliminating meat, eggs, butter, oil, and simple sugars. Instead, he ate whole-grain bread, fruit, vegetables, rice, and a little fish. Within months he lost the 30 extra pounds and noted a marked increase in his energy and well-being.

Rarely does a civilized person voluntarily return to the primitive state, but it occasionally happens by accident. You may remember the story of the lone Japanese soldier who was marooned on an out-of-the-way island in the South Pacific and maintained a vigilant state of preparedness for thirty years after the end of World War II. He was forced to forage for his food, living on whatever edible leaves, roots, fruits, and vegetables he could gather. When he was found and returned to civilization, doctors were amazed at his robust health. Although he was close to sixty, he looked and tested out on all manner of medical examinations at not a day over forty.

CULTURAL FOOD PREFERENCES

If our bodies are meant to be fueled with fruits and vegetables, why are we drawn to ice cream and hamburgers? Food preferences are an interesting phenomenon. Animal behavior, unless it has been modified by man, is largely instinctive and universal. Most species of animals in the wild eat the same kinds of food regardless of where they live. Human beings, on the other hand, have developed myriad cultures with customs and food preferences that differ markedly from one place to another. Though they may seem natural, these preferences are the result of cultural conditioning.

Like other cultural characteristics, dietary preferences follow distinctive patterns from country to country. Tastes are acquired in childhood and reinforced by habit. While Americans are revolted at the thought of fried insects, they are a delicacy in some cultures. Such ingrained food preferences do not arise because they are natural or healthful. They are simply habits that are later rationalized with scientific-sounding explanations.

Take for example the four basic food groups of the American diet: milk, meat, fruits and vegetables, breads and cereals. Most of us learned about this concept of nutrition as children. We grew up feeling that this "balanced diet," in which milk and meat were the undisputed stars, was passed down with the Ten Commandments, etched in stone. Yet the four food groups came into being only in 1956. The milk and meat industries volunteered to educate the public through the school system, and their biased brainwashing has been so effective that millions of Americans remain convinced to this day that milk is nature's perfect food. The four food groups have been replaced with the newer food pyramid, and our children and grandchildren are growing up with a similarly erroneous belief that the starchy foods such as breads and refined grains that form the base of the pyramid are the epitome of health.

DIETARY VARIATIONS AFFECT HEALTH

If you had to select one quintessential American food, it would likely be the hamburger. For Italians, you'd probably choose pasta. Chinese and rice, French and wine, Japanese and fish: Distinct food preferences are associated with various cultures. And these dietary differences are accompanied by marked variations in rates of heart disease and other diseases. The nations in North America and Europe that eat the typical Western diet, with lots of meat, dairy, eggs, white flour, and sugar, have the highest rates of heart disease in the world (for reasons we will discuss in the next chapter). The traditional cuisine of Japan, China, and other Asian countries includes lots of rice, vegetables, and fish, and among these people heart disease is rare. Disease rates among the Mediterranean populations, whose diet is comprised of some meat but lots of vegetables, fruits, grains, and olive oil, are almost as low as Asians'.

The best example of how these cultural food preferences affect health is the experience of Japanese immigrants. Native Japanese have one of the longest life expectancies and lowest rate of cardiovascular disease, cancer, and other maladies on earth. When they move to the United States and switch from their low-fat, high-fiber, largely vegetarian diet and begin eating more meat, processed foods, and other fare typical of the Western diet, their cholesterol levels and other markers of heart disease begin to rise. They are more likely to suffer with cardiovascular disease and similar Western ills than their relatives in Japan, and their children and grandchildren, who grow up eating the diet of their adopted country, have exactly the same risk of disease as any other American.

EVOLUTION OF THE DIET FOR REVERSING HEART DISEASE

The dietary recommendations that I give to my patients with heart disease—indeed, to all my patients—are not based on principles I learned as a medical student. Medical school included very little instruction in nutrition. Only a few hours during our entire four years were devoted to diet, and all we got was a superficial description of the general properties of fat, protein, and carbohydrates. The health implications of diet were never discussed. I came out of medical school in the 1970s knowing little more about nutrition than what I had learned in grade school about the four food groups.

After graduation, as I started exploring new avenues of medicine, I was amazed at the amount of nutritional research that had been done. Hundreds of studies, some of it decades old, revealed the therapeutic effects of various dietary components. Why had we medical students never been told about this research? I spent most of my free time over the next few years in the medical library, rediscovering forgotten studies that in my opinion should have been part of the medical school curriculum. As I explained in the introduction to this book, it was during this period that I decided to take the road less traveled in medicine and help patients overcome serious diseases with diet and other powerful, natural therapeutic tools.

When I opened the Whitaker Wellness Institute in 1979, the diet we offered was what was known at the time as the Pritikin diet. Before opening the institute I had worked for a time with the developer of this diet, Nathan Pritikin, and saw firsthand how it relieved angina, lowered blood pressure, improved cholesterol and blood sugar levels, and promoted weight loss. The Pritikin diet was very low in fat, no more than 10 percent of total calories, and with the exception of egg whites and a little fat-free milk and yogurt, no animal products were allowed. It was based on whole, natural foods with avoidance of the fried, processed, salty, sugary things that make up such a large part of the American diet.

My patients did well on this diet. However, as the years went by and new research came out, I began to realize that the Pritikin diet needed some adjustments. The importance of the essential fatty acids, which we will discuss in the next chapter, was demonstrated, and I realized that I needed to put some of these important fats back in the diet. Important new findings on carbohydrates were also emerging. It became evident to me that all carbohydrates are not created equal, and I began restricting intake of starchy carbohydrates such as bread and potatoes.

I am very happy with the Whitaker Wellness Institute diet in its present incarnation. I have retained the best of the original diet—it still emphasizes vegetables, fruits, legumes, and whole grains—but made it more healthful, palatable, and easier to follow by adding moderate amounts of fish, lean poultry, eggs, and olive oil and flaxseed oil. There is a lot of variety, enough to satisfy all but the most die-hard meat-and-potatoes eaters. And recognizing the power of the sweet tooth, it even includes healthy desserts.

Of course, there is no one diet that is perfect in every way for everyone. You may have a food allergy, for example, that prohibits you from eating some of the recommended foods. You may dislike eggplant with a passion, or you may live in a small town where fresh asparagus is hard to come by. It's okay. I encourage you to make modifications to suit your lifestyle and personal preferences. But I promise you that if you follow the general guidelines of this diet, you will feel better for it.

FOOD IS POWERFUL MEDICINE

Unlike drugs that squelch one symptom or another, the right kinds of food provide your body with the nutrients it needs to heal itself. By eating the life-sustaining foods that comprise my diet for reversing heart disease, you will see improvements in all of the risk factors for heart disease we discussed in Part I.

- Blood pressure normalizes when you eat more potassium-rich fruits and vegetables and less sodium.
- Extra pounds are shed as you cut out high-caloric junk food, saturated fat, and excess sugar.
- Insulin resistance and diabetes recede as you concentrate on the proper types of carbohydrates and avoid foods that drive up blood sugar.
- Free radical damage to the arteries and LDL cholesterol is inhibited by antioxidants in fruits and vegetables.
- Homocysteine levels are kept in check by the B-complex vitamins in grains and lean animal protein.
- Inflammatory compounds decrease and blood flow is enhanced when you eat the healthful fats in fish and flaxseed.
- Cholesterol and triglyceride levels are lowered by eating adequate fiber and cutting back on saturated fat and very starchy carbohydrates.

The beauty of this diet is that because it supports the body's innate ability to heal itself, you will see improvements in other aspects of your health as well. While some physicians support the

American Heart Association diet for patients with heart disease, the American Diabetes Association diet for diabetics, and other targeted diets, we at the Whitaker Wellness Institute believe that there are underlying factors common to all diseases. Free-radical damage isn't involved only in atherosclerosis; it is implicated in cancer, arthritis, diabetes, and even aging. Elevated homocysteine, in addition to damaging your arteries, also harms your brain and weakens your bones. High blood pressure doesn't present a risk only for heart disease but also for stroke and memory loss. A diet that addresses the basic mechanisms of disease doesn't just work on one problem—it engenders total health.

I'd like to close this chapter with a letter I recently received from Franceen. It is a powerful testimony to the multiple benefits of this program for reversing heart disease.

> *When I first came to the Whitaker Wellness Institute I was not well. I had high blood pressure, triglycerides, cholesterol, and blood sugar, not to mention I was overweight. My emotional health was very poor as well. My hormones were off balance and I was feeling very discouraged.*
>
> *My doctor set me up on a wonderful life-changing program of herbs and vitamins as well as a diet to help me control my medical problems, change my eating habits, and lose weight. Everyone at the institute—from the doctors to the nurses to the nutritionist—gave me instructions, assistance, and encouragement throughout, and I left with a clear plan for regaining my health.*
>
> *Now, six months later, I have the physical and emotional control I was searching for. My blood pressure, triglycerides, cholesterol, and blood sugar levels are all normal. My hormones are balanced, and my eating habits are finally under control. I have a new lifestyle! I have lost 18 pounds and I am still losing. I went from a dress size 16 to a size 10. I exercise daily and have never felt better. Thanks to all!*

CHAPTER 12

The Diet for Reversing Heart Disease

WE HAVE A LOT TO COVER IN THIS CHAPTER. WE WILL EXPLORE in detail the three primary dietary components—fat, protein, and carbohydrate—and how they affect the health of the heart and arteries. We will also touch on other items in the diet such as coffee and alcohol, and I'll provide you with a list of the "all-star" foods for patients with heart disease. Let's begin with fat.

A HIGH-FAT DIET PROMOTES HEART DISEASE

A diet high in certain types of fats is detrimental to the cardiovascular system for several reasons. First and foremost, it deprives the cells of oxygen. Oxygen is transported through the bloodstream on a special protein called hemoglobin that makes up the bulk of our red blood cells (erythrocytes). Once it reaches the smallest blood vessels in the body, the capillaries and capillary beds, it diffuses through these tiny, thin-walled vessels and is transferred to the adjacent cells. The oxygen-depleted blood then picks up a load of carbon dioxide and begins its journey back to the heart and lungs, where it gets rid of the carbon dioxide and picks up more oxygen.

Capillaries are minuscule, some of them a mere five microns in diameter (a micron is one ten-thousandth of a centimeter).

Red blood cells are about seven microns across. Therefore, in order to pass through the smaller capillaries, they must line up single file—and scrunch up a bit at that. This might seem like poor planning, but as with most things in our magnificently engineered bodies, it serves a purpose. Red blood cells are shaped like shallow soup bowls, a configuration that gives them a third more surface area than a spherical cell of similar size so they can carry more oxygen. Their flexibility allows them to bend and contort to pass through small capillaries, and the weak electromagnetic charge they carry slightly repels each cell from its neighbors so they don't clump together but flow smoothly, one after the other. The large surface area of the red blood cells coupled with the snug fit allows them to cozy right up to the cells on the other side of the capillaries to facilitate oxygen exchange.

Unfortunately, a fatty meal throws a wrench into the works.

Excess Fat Deprives the Heart and Arteries of Oxygen

You know how fat feels to the touch—greasy and sticky. This is essentially the state fat is in when it enters the bloodstream after a meal. It is emulsified by bile acids and broken down by enzymes in the intestine into tiny units of fat called triglycerides. Triglycerides, as you may recall from Chapter 3, are carried by chylomicrons, a type of lipoprotein formed in the intestines, after you eat. They are first absorbed by the lymphatic system, which dumps the fatty triglycerides into the bloodstream. Following a high-fat meal, you will have an excessive amount of triglycerides in your blood. Triglyceride levels may also remain elevated, even when you are fasting. This occurs when the liver produces excesses of triglyceride-carrying VLDL, prompted by insulin resistance or other factors common in people with heart disease.

However it gets there, too much fat in the bloodstream gums up circulation. It coats the red blood cells and causes them to stick together like a roll of gummy poker chips. (This is called rouleaux formation, after the French word for roll. It is also referred to as red

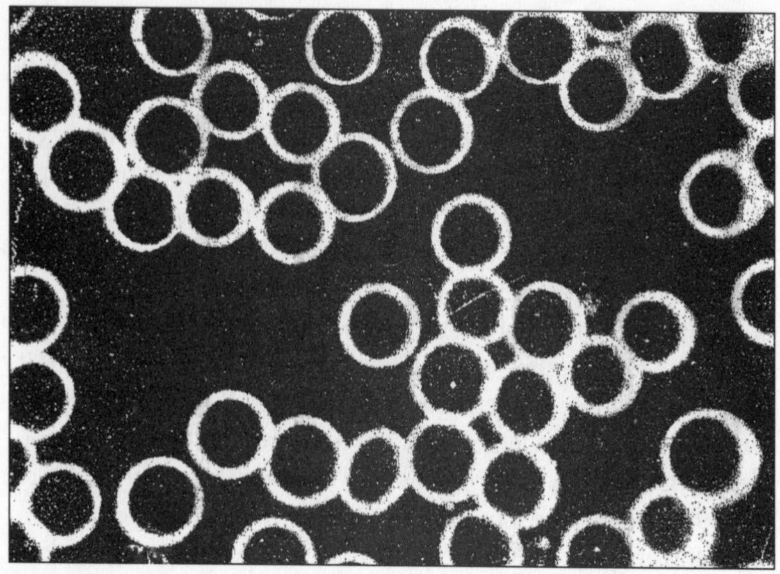

Blood cells normally space themselves and flow in single file.

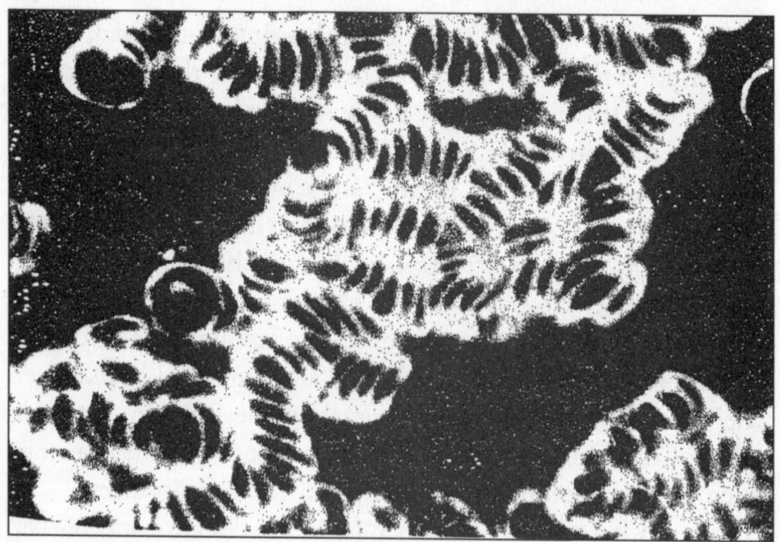

After a high-fat meal, blood cells clump together. This impedes blood flow and oxygen delivery.

blood cell aggregation.) When triglyceride levels are high, you end up with masses of sticky red blood cells that simply can't get through the capillaries. This causes a serious reduction in the oxygen supply to the tissues—including the heart.

In the cardiovascular research laboratories at Wayne State University College of Medicine, Timothy Regan, M.D., studied the way a single high-fat meal impeded the supply of oxygen to the heart tissue. He fed healthy volunteers a fat-laden meal and then measured their oxygen uptake. At peak levels of fat in the blood, the oxygen uptake by the heart was reduced by one-fifth. Once the blood was cleared of excess fat, oxygen uptake by the heart tissues returned to normal.[1]

For patients with heart disease, a high-fat meal can bring on angina, suffocating pain that occurs when the heart isn't getting enough oxygen. Several years ago, Peter T. Kuo, M.D., from the University of Pennsylvania published a study showing that commonly eaten high-fat foods could, by themselves, bring on angina. He gathered 14 patients who suffered from angina attacks during exercise for a simple but very illuminating experiment. Dr. Kuo measured the triglyceride levels in their blood, gave each of them a glass of cream to drink, then measured their triglycerides again. Of course, they rose dramatically. Not only that, six of the 14 patients had chest pains identical to those they experienced while climbing stairs or with other kinds of exercise. Of these six patients, four had changes on EKG indicating that their hearts weren't getting enough oxygen.[2]

In addition to restricting blood flow, excess fat in the blood also harms the arteries. It unleashes free radical damage on the endothelial cells that line the blood vessel walls and decreases the availability of nitric oxide, which relaxes and protects the arteries.[3] In addition, it deprives the endothelium of oxygen. Because the endothelium has no blood supply of its own, it is dependent upon diffusion of oxygen from red blood cells traveling through the arteries. When excessive fat in the blood causes

Coffee, Tea, and Heart Disease

Americans drink more than 100 billion cups of coffee every year, yet many drink it with some trepidation. There have been so many conflicting reports about the pros and cons of this popular beverage that you may not be sure if you should feel good or guilty about your caffeine habit. Coffee does have proven benefits. It gives you a boost of energy, improves exercise endurance, quickens reaction time, and promotes alertness. A cup of strong coffee can stop a migraine headache and relieve symptoms of asthma. Coffee consumption decreases the risk of gallstones, Parkinson's disease, and colon cancer. Too much coffee, on the other hand, can cause headaches, tremors, and indigestion. Excessive intake is linked with osteoporosis, rheumatoid arthritis, urinary incontinence, and infertility.

Scores of studies have looked at coffee's effects on the cardiovascular system. Excessive intake of caffeine from any source stimulates the central nervous system and can speed up the heartbeat and cause heart palpitations. According to a 1999 review of eleven controlled clinical trials, coffee can also elevate blood pressure—five cups a day was associated with an average 2.4/1.2 mm Hg increase.[4] However, more pronounced elevations in blood pressure tend to occur only in people who are not habitual coffee drinkers.[5] Although coffee has been linked to elevated cholesterol in a number of studies, it turns out that only coffee that has been prepared by boiling or steaming has this effect. The cholesterol-raising oils are removed if you brew coffee through a paper filter, which is the way most Americans prepare their coffee.

One definite downside of coffee is that it can raise homocysteine levels. As I explained in Chapter 3, this toxic by-product of protein metabolism damages the lining of the arteries, encourages the formation of blood clots, and sets the stage for atherosclerosis. If you have heart disease, this is one very valid reason to go easy on coffee, and if your homocysteine level is high, avoid it altogether.

What about tea? According to Chinese legend, tea is a gift from God, and its health benefits support this belief. Tea contains scores of compounds that help the heart, such as catechins, tannins, and flavonoids. Several studies have shown that people who drink tea regularly have a lower risk of heart attack.[6] Heart specialist Michael Gaziano, M.D., and colleagues tracked the coffee- and tea-drinking habits of 680 men and women in Boston, half of whom had previously suffered a heart attack. After one year, they found that those who drank one or more cups of tea a day slashed their risk of heart attack by 44 percent, compared to those who did not drink tea. Regular and decaffeinated coffee had no effect on heart attack risk.[7]

Green tea and the lesser-known white tea are the Cadillacs of teas because they contains more antioxidants and catechins than the more popular black tea. However, green, white, and black tea all have proven benefits for heart health. My secretary makes a big thermos of green tea sweetened with stevia, a calorie-free herbal sweetener, every morning, and I sip it throughout the day. If you are a big coffee drinker, try substituting this healthier beverage. If you have osteoporosis, hypertension, or an elevated homocysteine level, or if you are prone to anxiety and depression (more on this in Chapter 16), pregnant or breastfeeding, or taking medications such as beta-blockers or theophylline (an asthma drug), you should probably avoid coffee, tea, and other sources of caffeine such as colas and sodas. Regardless of your state of health, limit coffee intake to one or two cups per day.

---

the red blood cells to stick together, oxygen diffusion is inhibited, and the endothelium cannot function normally.

Fat-induced endothelial damage and dysfunction have been demonstrated in a number of studies. In one, researchers from the University of Maryland measured changes in the ability of the endothelium to signal the arteries to dilate or constrict, a key process in maintaining blood pressure. Before study subjects ate a 900-calorie meal containing 50 grams of fat (about the amount found in a Big Mac and an order of fries), their arteries were able to dilate or widen by 21 percent. Afterward, however, as levels of triglycerides rose, their arteries were much less responsive, dilating only 10 to 11 percent.[8] Other studies have demonstrated that a single high-fat meal suppresses endothelial function in the coronary arteries for hours!

It should be obvious to you by now that excessive intake of dietary fat bodes very poorly for your health. It contributes to endothelial damage, and it reduces the oxygen-carrying capacity of the red blood cells, depriving the heart of oxygen and, in some cases, causing angina. Our high-fat diet plays a role in many other serious disorders, including obesity, diabetes, high blood pressure, and some types of cancer. Eating less fat will reduce your risk not only of heart disease but of these other degenerative conditions as well.

FATS IN THE DIET

You obviously need some fat in your diet. Fat cushions your organs and serves as a backup energy source. It is required for the absorption of fat-soluble nutrients, it serves as an essential component of cellular membranes, and it is the precursor of chemical messengers called prostaglandins. (More on this in Chapter 14.)

How much fat should you eat? My dietary guidelines are not as restrictive as you might expect. As I explained in the previous chapter, I used to belong to the extremely low-fat school, recommending that patients eat no more than 10 percent of their total calories as fat. Patients who followed this diet did well in many aspects—cholesterol levels and blood pressure went down, and angina and exercise tolerance improved. Yet few patients were able to adhere to such a strict diet for prolonged periods. The food they were permitted didn't taste as good as the food they were used to—fat is a powerful flavor enhancer and brings out the natural flavors in food. These patients also reported that they found themselves eating more, which isn't surprising, since fat prolongs feelings of fullness. It is well documented that people on an extremely low-fat diet eat more of the foods they perceive to be healthier, such as fat-free, high-carbohydrate snack foods, which are in reality a dietary disaster.

The fat intake I recommend my patients aim for is about 20 percent of total calories. Much more important than the precise percentages however is the quality of the fat you eat. Not all fats are bad—some are absolutely essential for health. Others, however, you should avoid like the plague.

Bad Fats: Saturated Fats

Saturated fats are the dominant fats in meat, eggs, and dairy products, as well as tropical oils such as palm and coconut. These fats are solid at room temperature because, as their name implies, their molecular structure is "saturated," or loaded, with hydrogen. This makes them very stable, so they are not prone to oxidation or rancidity. Unfortunately, that's about the only good thing you can say about saturated fats.

Saturated fat is a primary dietary contributor to heart disease. It causes the red blood cells to stick together, impairing circulation, decreasing oxygen delivery, and increasing your risk of heart attack. These fats may be stored in adipose, or fat, cells and deposited within your organs, contributing to obesity, heart disease, and other degenerative conditions. Saturated fat also raises cholesterol levels. For many years it was assumed that dietary cholesterol was responsible for the high cholesterol levels in the American population, and that cutting back on or eliminating cholesterol-laden foods was an effective therapy for lowering cholesterol. Numerous studies dating as far back as the late 1950s demonstrated that when people ate a lot of high-cholesterol meat, eggs, and dairy foods, their blood cholesterol rose dramatically.

We now know that while a diet loaded with these foods does indeed raise cholesterol levels, it is not the cholesterol per se that causes this elevation. In 1997 researchers from the University of Arizona in Tucson analyzed data from 224 studies involving more than 8,000 people. They found that lowering dietary cholesterol to 100 milligrams a day (the amount found in half an egg) reduced blood cholesterol levels only by 2.2 mg/dl. A far more efficient way of lowering blood cholesterol, researchers found, was to cut back on saturated fat. In fact, they discovered that each 1 percent reduction in saturated fat intake resulted in a 1 percent fall in the blood cholesterol level.[9]

It's not that the earlier researchers were wrong about which foods raised cholesterol—they were just focusing on the wrong component of these foods. When J.M.R. Beveridge, M.D., of Queens University in Kingston, Ontario, fed 93 college students a fat-free, cholesterol-free diet back in 1960 and saw their average blood cholesterol level plummet from 201 to 146 in only eight days, he very logically concluded was that this was caused by the absence of dietary cholesterol.[10] Hundreds of researchers after him came to the same conclusion.

It is small wonder that research all those years took us down the wrong path. After all, most foods that contain saturated fat, such as meat, eggs, and high-fat dairy products, also contain cholesterol. (There is no cholesterol in plants.) Today we know that one of the most important things you can do to keep your cholesterol level in check and reduce your risk of heart disease is to avoid saturated fat. I'm not suggesting that you become vegetarian—fish and skinless poultry are fine, and occasional indulgences are part of life. But I do recommend that you dramatically cut back on red meat. And if you consume dairy products, choose only fat-free varieties.

What about another legendary dietary villain: the egg? According to a 1999 study, eggs are not as bad as they've been cracked up to be. Researchers analyzed data from two long-term and ongoing studies involving 117,933 men and women who were initially free of cardiovascular disease, high cholesterol, diabetes, and cancer. They followed these people for a number of years, tracked the incidence of heart disease and stroke, and correlated it with egg consumption. Much to their surprise, they found no significant association between the two for the majority of people. The one exception was an increased risk of heart disease in diabetics who ate lots of eggs. For everyone else, eating up to seven eggs a week had virtually no impact on their risk of heart attack.[11] Eggs are a good source of protein, brain-nurturing choline, and eye-enriching carotenoids. Unless you are diabetic, feel free to eat up to seven eggs a week. If you want more eggs, stick with egg whites, which are pure protein.

Worse Fats: Hydrogenated Fats and Trans Fatty Acids

If saturated fats are the bad boys of dietary fats, then hydrogenated fats and trans fatty acids are the hardened criminals. Hydrogenated fats have been around since the early 1900s, when Procter & Gamble took liquid cottonseed oil, subjected it to a process called hydrogenation, and came up with Crisco. Hydrogenation, which involves high temperatures and harsh chemicals, alters the chemical structure of polyunsaturated oils like corn, sunflower, or soy oil by forcing hydrogen atoms onto their molecules. This makes them more like saturated fats: stable, unlikely to go rancid, and solid at room temperature. This is great for food manufacturers, but really, really bad for you.

The molecules that are created during hydrogenation, called trans fatty acids, are like nothing Mother Nature has ever seen. These altered fats raise the risk of heart disease even more significantly than saturated fats, for in addition to elevating total cholesterol, they also lower protective HDL cholesterol. Trans fats have been implicated in cancer, diabetes, immune dysfunction, and infertility. Harvard School of Public Health researchers Walter Willett, M.D., and Alberto Ascherio, M.D., estimate that 30,000 premature deaths every year are attributable to our consumption of trans fats.[12]

Whenever you see the words *hydrogenated* or *partially hydrogenated* on a label, steer clear. Trans fatty acids are abundant in solid vegetable shortening and most margarines, and since these are the fats used in most commercially baked goods, you'll find them in pastries, cookies, and cakes as well. The biggest source of trans fatty acids in our diet is fast food. Most fast-food restaurants boast that they use "cholesterol-free" oils. What this really means is partially hydrogenated vegetable oils. Those big vats of hot oil used to fry French fries and chicken contain a witches' brew of trans fatty acids, toxic free radicals, and other harmful compounds. Stay away from them.[13]

Good Fats: Monounsaturated Fats

The chemical structure of monounsaturated fatty acids differs only slightly from that of saturated fatty acids. They contain one "double bond" (*mono* means "one") in place of two hydrogen atoms, which leaves a gap in their structure. This gap is like a joint, enabling the monounsaturated fat to flex a bit more easily, and it increases its chemical reactivity. Because monounsaturated fatty acids have only one double bond, they are still relatively stable and resistant to oxidation and rancidity. This makes them a good choice for cooking and a healthful addition to your diet.

The shining star of the monounsaturated oils is olive oil, which contains 74 percent monounsaturated fatty acids, along with hundreds of other beneficial compounds. It is a rich source of vitamin E as well as other powerful antioxidants such as ferulic acid and caffeic acid that shield LDL cholesterol from oxidation. It also contains polyphenols, which have been demonstrated to enhance production of artery-protective nitric oxide, and squalene, a unique compound with multiple health benefits, including lowering cholesterol.

Unlike saturated fat, olive oil helps keep the blood fluid and prevents platelets from sticking together. It can also lower blood pressure. In a 2000 Italian study, patients treated with medications for moderately high blood pressure were assigned to diets containing either sunflower oil or olive oil. After six months, they were switched over to the other oil for another six months. During the time that each group was eating olive oil, their blood pressure fell so much that they were able to lower their antihypertensive drugs an average of 48 percent.[14] All told, olive oil is very potent protection against heart disease.

Olive oil is a mainstay of the Mediterranean diet, which consists of whole grains, pasta, legumes, vegetables, fruits, fish, and limited amounts of meat and dairy. The Mediterranean populations enjoy one of the lowest rates of heart disease in the world. For people who have already suffered a heart attack, eating a Mediterranean diet with ample amounts of olive oil offers similar protection. The Lyon Diet Heart Study found that individuals who followed such a diet for four years after their initial heart attacks fared better than a similar group of patients who were on a relatively low-fat Western diet. In the Mediterranean diet group there were fewer fatal and nonfatal heart attacks and episodes of angina, and lower levels of cholesterol and triglycerides.[15]

Although canola oil is another primarily monounsaturated oil (it is 59 percent monounsaturated), I cannot recommend it as enthusiastically because of the way it is processed. Olives are soft and their oil is extracted through an organic, cold-pressing process that has been used for thousands of years. Canola, on the other hand, requires extensive processing in order to extract its oil and remove its strong flavor. (The canola plant is a relative of mustard.) Any time you expose oils to high temperatures and chemical solvents and bleaches, you alter their healthful properties and create some pretty scary, unnatural compounds. For this reason, I suggest that olive oil be your cooking oil of choice.

Heard It Through the Grapevine

Another important and healthful component of the Mediterranean diet is wine. That alcohol lowers the risk of heart disease is hardly news. The "French paradox," which postulated that the high alcohol consumption by the French may be responsible for their low risk of heart disease, was first proposed in 1987. Since then, hundreds of studies have confirmed the protective effects of alcohol on the cardiovascular system.

What is new is our understanding of this phenomenon. It is now clear that the protective benefits of alcohol are not derived from the proanthocyanidins in red grapes or the B vitamins in beer, but from ethanol, the "alcohol" in alcohol. In addition to raising protective HDL cholesterol levels, ethanol inhibits the formation of blood clots that may lead to a heart attack. It does this by increasing the breakdown of fibrin, the protein described in Chapter 3 that entangles platelets to make clots, and by lowering levels of plasminogen activator inhibitor-1, which retards the breakup of blood clots.

Ethanol has also recently been discovered to improve insulin sensitivity, which is a concern for the millions of people in this country who suffer with both heart disease and insulin resistance. (For more on this, see Chapter 4.) Furthermore, it slows down the production of advanced glycation end products (AGEs), which are formed when sugars bind to proteins, alter their structure and function, and accelerate atherosclerosis by damaging arterial walls. AGEs are particularly problematic for diabetics and are partially responsible for the atherosclerosis that plagues so many of these patients.

When it comes to alcohol, like most things in life, moderation is key. Approximately 10 percent of the population is afflicted with alcoholism. For them, no amount of alcohol is

healthful. However, if you partake of an occasional alcoholic beverage, enjoy it with the knowledge that it is helping your cardiovascular health. Women should not exceed one or two drinks a day, and men two or three. *À votre santé!*

Best Fats: Essential Fatty Acids

Essential fatty acids (EFAs) are polyunsaturated fats that cannot be produced by the body and must be obtained from the diet or from supplemental sources. As their name suggests (*poly* means "many"), polyunsaturated fats contain multiple double bonds, which makes them the most chemically active of all the fats. This is a mixed blessing. On the one hand, their unique chemical structure enables them to flex and bend and perform functions in the body that no other fats are able to do. On the other hand, their relative instability compared to other fats means that they are the most readily subject to oxidative damage.

There are two types of EFAs: omega-3 and omega-6 (so-named because of the location of their first double bond). While both of these fatty acids are crucial for optimal health, the omega-3s are particularly important for cardiovascular health—so important that I suggest you not only make sure they are part of your diet but also take them in supplement form. Two members of the omega-3 family, eicosapentaenoic acid (EPA) and docosahexaenoic acid (DHA), protect the cardiovascular system in numerous ways. They improve circulation and lower levels of inflammatory compounds and clotting factors in the blood. They enhance endothelial function, relax the arteries, and help prevent dangerous rhythm disturbances. Believe it or not, these fats even lower blood fat levels, particularly triglycerides, and, to a lesser degree, cholesterol. I have had patients with exceptionally high triglycerides—in the 2,000 to 3,000 range (normal is less than 150)—watch their blood fats plummet by hundreds of points while taking high doses of omega-3s.

Most Americans get plenty of omega-6s in their diet, for they are found in grains, vegetables, nuts, seeds, and most of the polyunsaturated oils we consume. However, because the richest sources of the omega-3s are fatty cold-water fish and flaxseed, deficiencies of these fats are very common. In the MRFIT study, a large study that examined risk factors for heart disease, 60 percent of the 6,000 participants had almost *zero* omega-3 intake![16] The best way to remedy this deficiency is to eat salmon, mackerel, sardines, tuna, trout, anchovies, and other fatty fish several times a week. I also suggest that you get acquainted with flaxseed and flaxseed oil. A quarter cup of freshly ground flaxseed or one to two tablespoons of flaxseed oil will provide you with an abundance of omega-3 fatty acids. Supplementing with fish oil capsules is an even simpler option, and we will cover this further in Chapter 14.

I want to conclude this discussion of fats with a few words about the other polyunsaturated oils. It would seem that all vegetable oils would be good choices. While it is true that corn, safflower, peanuts, sunflower seeds, and other nuts, seeds, and grains in their natural state contain wonderful, heart-healthy polyunsaturated fats, these oils are very fragile and easily damaged by heat, air, light, and chemicals. Unfortunately, like canola oil, virtually all of the oils sold in your supermarket have been extracted with harsh chemicals at high temperatures, bleached, and otherwise altered, and they contain the same toxic by-products of processing that canola oil has. Stay away from these processed vegetable oils. Shop instead in your health food store and purchase only cold-pressed, unrefined oils. Store them in your refrigerator and do not expose them to high temperatures during cooking. Baking is acceptable, since temperatures do not get terribly high, but sautéing and frying are not recommended with polyunsaturated oils.

WHERE WILL I GET MY PROTEIN?

Ask the average American where they get their protein and they will tell you from meat. Americans eat an average of 68 pounds of beef and 93 pounds of poultry every year.[17] Patients who are advised to reduce their consumption of meat, dairy, and other high-fat animal foods often ask, "Where will I get my protein?" The idea that we need to eat lots of meat and other animal products to meet protein requirements is firmly ingrained, along with the belief that without these foods we can expect health problems. The mere suggestion of eliminating or cutting back on meat and dairy products is often met with resistance. Ironically, these are the very foods that have put so many in their current state of ill health. Let's look closely at what protein can and cannot do for your health, and then establish what your actual protein requirements are.

If a person were suffering from protein deficiency, what might the symptoms be? Anemia? No, anemia results from blood loss, inadequate iron replacement, or vitamin B12 or folic acid deficiency, not from protein deficiency. Muscle deterioration? Weight-bearing exercise, not excessive protein, builds and maintains bulky muscles. And if you're talking about the systemic deterioration that occurs with starvation, it is caused by overall caloric deprivation, not an isolated protein deficiency. Loss of energy? This myth has led to all manner of high-protein concoctions that are supposed to boost energy, but protein is rarely used for energy. Even in the throes of starvation, when protein is burned for energy, it is first converted into glucose before it is utilized. Protein deficiencies in this country are very rare indeed. The irrational fear of such, however, perpetuates our excessive consumption of high-fat meat and dairy products, the foods that contribute to heart disease, high blood pressure, diabetes, stroke, and a host of other conditions.

You obviously need some protein in your diet. Protein is required for growth and tissue formation and repair. Protein and its component amino acids are the building blocks of enzymes, hormones, neurotransmitters, blood plasma, sperm, and saliva. It is a common misconception, however, that just because the majority of your tissues are made of protein, you need to eat a lot of protein. Your body is very efficient at using and reusing available protein. Even during periods of growth, the amount of protein required is much smaller than generally imagined.

The Food and Drug Administration has set the recommended daily intake of protein (for a 2,000-calorie-a-day diet) at 50 grams. Most Americans get much more than that. The average man eats an additional 52 percent above this level, and the average woman, an additional 27 percent.[18] The World Health Organization has established protein recommendations based on body weight, and they are even lower: approximately one-half gram of protein per kilogram of body weight for adults. Therefore, an adult weighing 150 pounds (70 kilograms) would require about 35 grams of protein per day.[19] As you can see, our problems do not lie with inadequate protein intake.

It is commonly believed that vegetarianism leads to protein deficiencies because many plant foods lack some of the essential amino acids, the building blocks of protein that cannot be synthesized in the body. This myth is so persistent that it frightens many away from the idea of giving up meat and causes vegetarians to take great pains with their diet. The reality is that every plant food contains all of the essential amino acids, although some contain lower concentrations of certain amino acids than others. (Where do you suppose horses, cows, and other grazing animals get their protein since all they eat is grass?) As long as a vegetarian eats a variety of plant foods, protein needs will be met. Grains, cereals, nuts, beans, and legumes are not only carbohydrates, but also excellent sources of protein.

Excess Protein Stresses the Kidneys

The real problem in our diet is not too little protein but too much. To understand the problems with excessive protein, let's review how the body handles fats, carbohydrates, and protein. Fat is used for energy when needed, and excesses are stored in the adipose, or fat, cells of the body. Carbohydrates are broken down into glucose, which is utilized to meet energy needs, or stored in the liver and muscles for later use. (If too much glucose is circulating in the blood, it may be converted to fat and stored in the adipose cells.) Carbohydrates and fats are made up of hydrogen, oxygen, and carbon, and when they are burned for energy, the primary breakdown products are carbon dioxide, which is eliminated through the lungs, and water, which is used by the body or easily excreted through the kidneys.

The body handles protein very differently. Protein contains not only carbon, hydrogen, and oxygen, but also nitrogen, and among the breakdown products of protein metabolism are nitrogen-containing compounds that the body has no means of storing. Therefore, these compounds must be converted into urea and eliminated through the kidneys. When you eat lots of excess protein, your metabolic systems are stressed by the overload, and your kidneys take the worst beating. Thanksgiving may be a holiday for you, but your kidneys work overtime. In fact, the accepted way of assessing how well a patient's kidneys are functioning is to measure the amount of protein breakdown products circulating in the blood. Levels of blood urea nitrogen (BUN) and creatinine are low when the kidneys are healthy. When the kidneys begin to fail, levels of these markers of kidney function rise.

The kidneys are remarkable organs with a lot of reserve capacity and they are generally able to handle the excesses. However, when these crucial organs are already functioning at subnormal levels, damaged by diabetes, hypertension, or other diseases, excess protein speeds up kidney failure. Patients with these disorders may suffer complete kidney failure and require chronic dialysis or kidney transplant. This disaster could be delayed or perhaps prevented altogether if such patients were started early on low-protein diets.

Protein and Calcium Loss

Excessive protein intake also creates an acidic condition in the blood. In order to neutralize this acid, bicarbonate is mobilized from the bones and, along with it, calcium. Once the pH of the blood is returned to normal, the calcium is not returned to the bone but eliminated in the urine. Over a lifetime, a high-protein diet robs the bones of this essential mineral, seriously weakening them. Excessive protein intake is one of the reasons for our country's current epidemic of osteoporosis.

Some of the early work in this area was done by Richard B. Mazess, M.D., of the University of Wisconsin. He studied a group of 217 Alaskan Eskimos living on their traditional high-protein diet of fish, marine mammals, and caribou. These people consumed up to three times the amount of protein that the average American consumes. By the age of forty, this high protein intake had caused enough calcium loss to reduce their bone density by 10 to 15 percent.[20]

More recently University of California at San Francisco researchers observed the diets of more than 1,000 women. They discovered that compared to women who ate low-acid diets, those whose diets contained lots of high-acid (i.e., protein) foods had three times more bone loss and 3.7 times more hip fractures. Other studies have demonstrated that women who eat more than 95 grams of protein per day are at increased risk of fracture, compared to women who eat less than 68 grams.[21]

Ruth M. Walker, M.D., of the Department of Nutritional Sciences, University of Wisconsin, showed how excessive protein consumption causes calcium loss even in healthy young men. She assigned volunteers to diets containing adequate calcium (800 milligrams) and one of three levels of protein: 47 grams, 95 grams, or 145 grams. Dr. Walker then measured their calcium balance, comparing the amount of calcium ingested with the amount excreted. Men on the low-protein diet were in positive calcium balance, retaining 12 milligrams of calcium per day from their 800 milligram intake. Those on a moderate-protein diet retained much less calcium—an average of 1 milligram daily.

But men on the high-protein diet (145 grams) had a serious calcium imbalance. These healthy young men were losing 85 milligrams more calcium than they were taking in. The excessive protein they ate was leeching calcium from their bones at such a rate that in forty years they would have lost 75 percent of the calcium in their skeletons![22] It is clear from all these studies that the body's calcium stores are as much, if not more, a function of protein intake as of calcium intake. This means that if you are on a high-protein diet you could be losing calcium from your bones regardless of how much calcium you ingest.

Your next question may reasonably be "Where will I get my calcium if I cut back on dairy products?" We have been brainwashed by the dairy industry into believing that milk is the only source of calcium in our diet. Leafy green vegetables such as parsley, watercress, and kale are excellent sources of calcium. In fact, the rate of calcium absorption from kale is superior to that of milk. Furthermore, calcium derived from vegetable sources is not accompanied by the massive amounts of protein that cause calcium loss, so even if you're taking in less calcium, your bones are likely retaining more of it. Rather than encouraging people to consume dairy products, we should educate them about the importance of reducing their protein intake and increasing their intake of calcium-rich plant foods.

Milk, Nature's Imperfect Food

Of all the nutritional myths, the belief that milk is the perfect food is one of the most absurd. American parents unwittingly pass this myth on to their children, and celebrities reinforce it in a multimillion-dollar advertising campaign sponsored by the dairy industry. In reality, milk and other high-protein dairy products weaken the bones and accelerate osteoporosis by promoting calcium loss, as described above. But that's not the only downside of milk.

While eating fruits, vegetables, and whole grains has been documented to lower the risk of heart attack and high blood pressure, the consumption of dairy products has been linked to increased risk of heart disease. Most of you know that whole milk, butter, and cheese are significant sources of saturated fat, which raises cholesterol levels and the risk of heart disease. However, William B. Grant, Ph.D., has amassed evidence that nonfat milk is also a major player in bringing on heart disease. He points out that nonfat milk, which contains substantial amounts of protein, is very low in B-complex vitamins. The metabolism of all this protein in the absence of B vitamins contributes to the buildup of homocysteine, a marker for heart disease I told you about in Chapter 3.[23]

Now that the FDA allows dairy farmers to treat cows with recombinant bovine somatotropin (rBST), a genetically engineered hormone that increases milk production, milk is less wholesome than ever. Milk from treated cows contains elevated levels of insulin-like growth factor-1 (IGF-1), a powerful growth factor. Recent studies have found a sevenfold increase in the risk of breast cancer in women with the highest IGF-1 levels, and a fourfold increase in prostate cancer in men with the highest levels. Furthermore, cows treated with rBST require more antibiotics to stave off udder infections, so higher traces of these drugs, as well as pus and bacteria from infected udders, are found in their milk.[24] A little bit of organic rBST-free milk in your coffee or on your cereal is acceptable, but discard the idea that drinking a glass of milk with every meal is healthy.

PLANT FOODS: CORNUCOPIA OF HEART-HEALTHY NUTRIENTS

Although Americans are eating more plant foods than they did ten years ago, even today fewer than half of us meet the recommended daily minimum of five servings of fruits and vegetables.

Furthermore, our choices are less than spectacular. The most popular vegetable in this country is iceberg lettuce, which is little more than a pale bundle of water and fiber. The second most popular is the tomato, a healthy choice except when consumed as sugar-laden ketchup, and the third—get ready for this—is French-fried potatoes![25] We fare no better when it comes to grains. Rather than eating whole grains, we indulge in donuts for breakfast, sandwiches on white bread for lunch, and snack on pretzels and buttered popcorn.

The reason plant foods are so important in the human diet is that they contain things vital for health that are simply not found in any other foods. Vegetables, fruits, grains, beans, and other plants contain thousands of vitamins, minerals, amino acids, and phytonutrients that protect us against heart disease. Brightly colored fruits and vegetables are the most concentrated sources of beta-carotene and other carotenoids. Vitamin E is found in nuts, seeds, whole grains, and vegetable oils. Citrus fruits, peppers, guavas, and greens supply us with vitamin C, while nuts, seeds, and grains give us homocysteine-lowering B-complex vitamins. Calcium and magnesium are abundant in leafy greens. Chromium, which helps improves insulin sensitivity, is found in whole grains.

Then there are the phytonutrients unique to specific plants. The quercetin in onions has been shown to protect LDL cholesterol from oxidation, inhibit blood clotting, and preserve nitric oxide. The catechins in tea protect the blood vessels, reduce cholesterol, and prevent atherosclerosis. The proanthocyanidins in berries strengthen the arteries and protect them from free radical damage. The liminoids in citrus fruits raise HDL cholesterol, and the polyphenols in grapes improve blood flow and discourage blood clotting. The terpenoids, kaemperol, and flavonoids in broccoli and other cruciferous vegetables have potent antioxidant effects and other cardioprotective actions. And these are just a few of the thousands of protective phytonutrients.

In addition to the vitamins, minerals, and phytonutrients in plants, there are other components in these foods that are essential for heart health.

Fantastic Fiber

Another important nutrient found only in plant foods is fiber, the indigestible portion of plant cell walls. Fiber is the insoluble "roughage" in vegetables and the skins of grains, fruits, and legumes. It is also the soluble gel-like substance abundant in beans, oats, and fruits. Fiber moves food along our long intestinal tract and prevents constipation and diarrhea as well as other diseases of the colon. It is also protective against several types of cancer, diabetes, obesity, and, as you might expect, heart disease.

One of the best-documented benefits of fiber is its ability to lower cholesterol. Soluble fiber reduces cholesterol by binding to bile acids and causing them to be excreted. With fewer bile acids available in the intestine, less cholesterol is absorbed into the bloodstream. Fiber also slows the manufacture of cholesterol in the liver. If this sounds familiar, it's because soluble fiber works much like the cholesterol-lowering drugs called bile-sequestering agents discussed in Part II—but with none of their side effects and scores of other benefits. Adding just 5 to 10 grams of fiber per day can reduce cholesterol by about 5 points, resulting in a 10 percent drop in risk of heart disease.

Fiber-rich foods will also help you achieve and maintain your ideal weight, a very important goal for anyone with heart disease. Such foods take longer to eat than fiber-free foods—you cannot chow down on apples and broccoli the way you can on chocolate and ice cream. This allows time for the signal of fullness to reach your brain, enabling you to stop eating before you've stuffed yourself. That feeling of satiety stays with you longer too, because fiber slows the rate at which food leaves your stomach. Studies have shown that volunteers fed a high-fiber breakfast eat less at lunch than those who eat a breakfast containing the same number of calories with no fiber. (In fact, in one recent study, people fed a fiber-free breakfast ate as much at lunch as those who had only water for breakfast!)[26] It also prevents the roller-coaster ride of dramatic elevations and just as sudden drops in blood sugar levels that leave you feeling tired and hungry. A fiber-rich lunch can help you resist that midafternoon candy bar. And if you grab an apple instead, chances are you'll eat less at dinner too.

A fiber-rich diet is also one of our most powerful tools for the control of insulin resistance, a significant risk factor for both heart disease and type 2 diabetes. As you will recall from Chapter 4, in patients with insulin resistance, blood sugar remains abnormally elevated, especially after eating. This prompts the release of increasing amounts of insulin from the pancreas, resulting in high levels of insulin in the bloodstream as well. Fiber slows the absorption of sugars in the gastrointestinal tract, promoting a more gradual rise in blood sugar levels, followed by a gradual release in insulin. It also improves the body's sensitivity to insulin, combating insulin resistance and helping this hormone do its job of ushering glucose into the cells. In two large studies involving nearly 100,000 women, a high intake of whole grains and cereal fiber had a dramatic effect on the risk of developing insulin-resistant (type 2) diabetes. Women consuming the most of these fiber-rich foods experienced a 21 to 28 percent decrease in risk compared to women with the lowest intake.[27]

This combination of benefits—lowering cholesterol, maintaining normal weight, and improving insulin sensitivity—adds up to powerful protection against heart disease. Harvard researchers followed the dietary habits of men, ages forty to seventy-five, for six years and found a strong inverse relationship between fiber intake and risk of heart attack. They concluded: "Fiber, independent of fat intake, is an important dietary component for the prevention of coronary disease."[28] A 1999 study found similar protection in women. Among the 68,000 women involved in this study, those who consumed the most dietary fiber, particularly from cereal and grain sources, were significantly less likely to develop heart disease than women who ate the least fiber.[29]

Optimal health requires at least 30 grams of fiber daily. Americans average one-third to one-half this amount. Adding fiber to your diet is easier than you think. The simplest way to ensure you are getting the recommended 30-plus daily grams of fiber is to make plant foods the mainstay of your diet. Start your day with a bowl of bran cereal (8 grams). Snack on an apple (3.5 grams). Have a spinach salad (4 grams) and whole-wheat bread (2 grams) for lunch. Eat half a cup of beans (6 to 8 grams) at dinner. If you need to add a fiber supplement to get enough, good choices include psyllium, citrus pectin, and flaxseed. Be sure to increase your intake of water as you increase your consumption of fiber.

Naturally Low in Sodium, High in Potassium

Everybody "knows" that salt drives up blood pressure, which is one of the most significant risk factors for heart attack. While some sodium is essential for life—it controls fluid volume, aids in nerve impulse transmission, and is involved in cellular energy production—excess sodium attracts and holds water in the bloodstream, and thereby raises blood pressure. It is also an independent risk factor for heart disease and death from all causes, especially in people who are overweight.[30]

Unfortunately, excessive dietary sodium is the norm in this country. Salt is a powerful flavoring agent, and it is added to countless processed and prepared foods—even cereals and ice cream may contain lots of sodium. Couple the sodium in packaged foods and restaurant fare with liberal use of the salt shaker and many Americans consume ten to 15 grams a day—twenty to thirty times the body's need!

Several studies have shown that cutting down on salt intake normalizes blood pressure in many hypertensive patients. Yet for others, restricting sodium is just not enough. Norman Kaplan, M.D., professor of medicine at the University of Texas Southwest

Medical School, points out that for many patients, the degree of salt restriction necessary to significantly reduce blood pressure is so severe as to be impracticable. It leaves patients frustrated and doctors quick to prescribe blood-pressure-lowering drugs.[31]

There is an easier way to naturally regulate blood pressure: Increase your intake of potassium. Dr. Graham A. MacGregor and colleagues at the Department of Medicine, Charing Cross Hospital Medical School in London, demonstrated that giving supplemental potassium to hypertensive patients reduced their average blood pressure by 8 points.[32] While you could increase your potassium intake by taking a potassium supplement or flavoring your food with potassium chloride (No-Salt or Nu-Salt), the best way, in my opinion, is simply to eat more plant foods.

That's exactly what one of my patients, Frank M., did. This fifty-four-year-old airline pilot came to me in desperation. He was three weeks away from a mandatory Federal Aeronautics Administration (FAA) physical exam, and with a blood pressure of 225/115, he was sure to lose his license. Commercial pilots are grounded if they have high blood pressure or are taking medication for it. Frank needed to bring his blood pressure down fast, and we couldn't do it with medications. So we radically altered his diet. He was allowed to eat nothing but fresh fruits, vegetables, and brown rice—but he could eat these foods to his heart's content. This meant he was getting little fat in his diet, minimal sodium, and lots and lots of potassium. After twelve days his blood pressure was 130/84, and a week later he passed his FAA physical with flying colors. When I last spoke to Frank, almost three years after his initial visit, he was still flying. Following the less stringent but still very healthy diet described in this book, his blood pressure had remained at the 120/75 level.

According to government estimates, more than 80 percent of Americans fail to get the recommended 3,500 milligrams of potassium in their daily diet (an amount present in six or seven servings of plant foods).[33] If you suspect that you are one of them, an easy way to get additional potassium is to drink 12 ounces of low-sodium V-8 or tomato juice every day. (See p. 196.)

Good Carbs, Bad Carbs

Carbohydrates are various configurations of sugar molecules, from one-molecule simple sugars to extremely long and complex chains of sugars. They are broken down during the digestive process into glucose, the sugar that is burned in your cells to create the energy that keeps you alive. Although almost all carbohydrates end up as glucose, they are not all metabolized in the same way, and they have differing effects in the body. There are good carbs and there are bad carbs, and it is important that you understand the difference.

The easiest way to avoid the undesirable ones is to eat plant foods in as close to their natural state as possible. This simple rule of thumb will keep you on the straight and narrow 95 percent of the time. Whole wheat, fresh corn, and apples are great. These foods are slowly digested, and their sugars are gradually released into the bloodstream. They fill you up and tide you over, helping you control your caloric intake and maintain optimal weight. And because they are not processed, these whole foods retain the nutrients that protect you from disease.

Wheat that has been finely ground, bleached, and refined into white flour, corn that has been transformed into high-fructose corn syrup and added to a Coke, and apples that have been mixed with sugar and baked into a fatty piecrust are not so good. Not only have they been stripped of nutrients during processing, they are also much more rapidly broken down into their component sugar molecules and absorbed into the bloodstream. They cause the blood sugar to rise quickly, which prompts a large influx of insulin to usher sugar into the cells. This is followed by a similarly rapid fall in blood sugar, which may leave you hungry and, if levels fall too low, cranky and spacey.

Make it a point to eliminate "white foods" from your diet—

anything made with white flour or sugar. The average American eats more than 150 pounds of sugar every year and gorges on white bread. In addition to the excessive calories these white foods pack in (which are a likely reason for the surge in obesity in the past fifteen years), refined, nutrient-deprived carbohydrates raise triglyceride levels, stress your body's blood sugar control mechanisms, and promote insulin resistance. A high sugar intake has been identified as the single most important dietary risk factor for heart disease in women. (Animal fat consumption remains the number one problem for men.) It has been estimated that our out-of-control sugar consumption may be responsible for more than 150,000 premature deaths from heart disease in the United States each year.[34]

Like salt, sugar is hidden in prepared and processed foods. It is added in so many different forms that you need to learn to decipher food labels. Sucrose, dextrose, fructose, lactose, high-fructose corn syrup, and corn, rice, and barley malt syrups, as well as maple syrup and fruit juice concentrates are all names for simple sugars. Unfortunately, honey, molasses, and other "healthy" sweeteners aren't much better—they all rapidly drive up blood sugar levels.

In an effort to cut back on sugar, many people turn to calorie-free artificial sweeteners, the most popular of which is aspartame (NutraSweet and Equal). I recommend you steer clear of aspartame, which is broken down in the body into toxic formaldehyde, formic acid, and methanol. Its component amino acids phenylalanine and aspartic acid can also upset the balance of neurotransmitters in the brain, and not surprisingly, this sweetener has been linked with seizures, mood disorders, and other nervous system problems. I don't recommend other artificial sweeteners such as Sucralose and Acesulfame-K either. There just hasn't been enough research to definitively demonstrate their safety.

What we recommend for our patients at the Whitaker Wellness Institute are the natural sweeteners stevia, xylitol, and brown rice syrup. Stevia is an intensely sweet herbal extract from South America. Available in liquid or powder form, a few drops or sprinkles perk up beverages and cereals. Xylitol, derived from birch trees, looks and tastes like white sugar. Although it is not calorie-free, xylitol is very slowly metabolized, so it does not cause sharp rises and falls in blood sugar. Brown rice syrup, which as its name suggests is derived from brown rice, is likewise not calorie-free, but it is also easier on the system. (More on these sweeteners in Part IV.)

Occasional sweets or breads made with refined carbohydrates are okay, but a steady diet of them contributes to weight gain, insulin resistance, elevated triglyceride levels, and increased risk of heart disease. Most whole, unprocessed carbohydrate-containing foods, on the other hand, are an excellent part of a diet for reversing heart disease. However, there are a few exceptions.

The Glycemic Index

David Jenkins, M.D., and colleagues at the University of Toronto have spent the past twenty-five years analyzing scores of different foods to determine how quickly they are metabolized into glucose, the basic sugar molecule utilized by the cells. Using the blood sugar elevation caused by eating a specific amount of either glucose or white bread as the standard, they and other researchers have assigned various foods a "glycemic index" rating. Items with a high-glycemic rating enter the bloodstream quickly and cause a rapid spike in blood sugar, while those with a low-glycemic rating cause a slower, more sustained rise.

What does this have to do with heart disease? As you recall from Chapter 4, insulin resistance and the complex of conditions called syndrome X (hypertension, low HDL cholesterol, elevated triglycerides, and abdominal obesity) dramatically increase the risk of heart disease. In people with this condition, whenever there is an abrupt rise in glucose, as there is with foods with a high-glycemic rating, the corresponding release of insulin is exceptionally high. This combination of elevated insulin and blood sugar damages the arteries and interferes with fat metabolism. Therefore, avoiding high-glycemic carbohydrates is important for anyone concerned about heart disease.

Swedish researchers compared the effects of these differing types of carbohydrates in patients with type 2 diabetes, a population with extreme insulin resistance and a very high risk of heart disease. These patients were divided into two groups and fed diets that had identical proportions of carbohydrate, protein, fat, and fiber. However, one diet was centered around low-glycemic foods, while the other was based on high-glycemic foods. After twenty-four days, the diets were switched, so the groups spent twenty-four consecutive days on each of the two diets. Throughout the study, blood samples were taken and various markers of heart disease were measured. The researchers determined that while on the low-glycemic diet, study participants had lower LDL cholesterol levels and decreases in PAI-1 (a clotting factor that inhibits the breakup of blood clots, discussed in Chapter 3), suggesting that such a diet confers protection against heart disease.[35]

As you might expect, most fruits, vegetables, beans, and whole grains have a low-glycemic rating and are therefore excellent choices in a diet for reversing heart disease. As you would also likely predict, processed foods made with sugar and white flour are high-glycemic—another reason why these high-calorie foods, which have been stripped of fiber and valuable nutrients, have no place in your diet.

There are, however, a few foods that are exceptions to the "whole foods versus refined foods" general rule. Starchy foods such as white potatoes and most breads, even those made with whole wheat, have a high glycemic index so should be eaten sparingly. Pasta, on the other hand, is considered low glycemic, and can be eaten more frequently. While whole grains such as oatmeal and brown rice are fine, most cold cereals have a very high glycemic rating and should be eaten only in moderation. Most fruits are low on the index and should be a regular part of your diet. Tropical fruits like pineapple and ripe bananas, and most dried fruits however, have a high glycemic rating and are best eaten infrequently.

When patients with heart disease adhere to this particular aspect of the diet for reversing heart disease, they often see dramatic improvements in their blood sugar, cholesterol, and triglyceride levels. One of my patients, Kerry, came to clinic with all the markers of heart disease: a triglyceride level of 5,300 mg/dl (less than 135 is desirable), cholesterol 490 (normal is below 200), and blood sugar 590 (ideal is around 100). I told him to cut out bread, potatoes, and sugary and starchy snack foods that were the bulk of his diet, exercise regularly, and follow a nutritional supplement regimen that included high doses of fish oil. After just one month on this program his triglycerides dropped to 764, his cholesterol to 260, and his blood sugar to 189.

ALL-STAR FOODS FOR HEART DISEASE

The particulars of the Whitaker Wellness diet for reversing heart disease are pretty simple: Cut back on saturated animal fats and trans fatty acids, and dramatically increase your intake of unprocessed plant foods. Now I want to tell you about a few foods that stand out for their protective and therapeutic effects in heart disease.

1. Flaxseed

Flaxseed protects the heart on several fronts. It is the richest plant source of heart-healthy omega-3 essential fatty acids. It also contains soluble fiber, which is particularly effective in lowering cholesterol.[36] James, a sixty-two-year-old from Tennessee, got a wake-up call when his cholesterol measured a scary 288 mg/dl. He had read about the benefits of flaxseed for lowering cholesterol in my monthly newsletter and decided to give it a try. He mixed a quarter cup of ground flaxseed in juice and drank it once a day, an hour before his main meal. After only fifteen days his cholesterol fell to 232, and six months later it plummeted to 188. He also lost 33 pounds and reported improvements in his skin, hair, and energy level.

General improvements such as those James experienced are to be expected, for the omega-3s and soluble fiber contained in flax enhance many aspects of health. Flax also contains an abundance of lignans, plant compounds with potent anticancer activity. Incorporate into your daily diet one-fourth cup of ground flaxseed (grind whole seed in a coffee grinder), mixed in water or sprinkled on cereal or salads. Flaxseed is sold in health food stores or from the mail-order sources listed in the resource section. Although flaxseed oil (1 to 2 tablespoons per day) is an excellent source of omega-3 EFAs, it has no fiber, and so has a much less dramatic effect on cholesterol.

2. Soybeans

Any heart-healthy diet should include soybeans. Soy contains numerous compounds that benefit the cardiovascular system. These include sterols, lecithin, and fiber, which bind to and remove cholesterol, as well as isoflavones, powerful antioxidants that protect the arteries and inhibit LDL oxidation. One particularly potent isoflavone is genistein, which discourages the formation of potentially dangerous blood clots.

Scores of studies have demonstrated that soy protein consumption reduces cholesterol. James W. Anderson, M.D., from the University of Kentucky, reviewed thirty-eight of these studies and found that study subjects who consumed an average of 47 grams (only 3 tablespoons) of soy protein daily had reductions in total cholesterol of 9.3 percent, LDL cholesterol of 12.9 percent, and triglycerides of 0.5 percent. Soy also improved the important total cholesterol to HDL ratio.[37]

Try to eat a little soy—the equivalent of about 50 milligrams of isoflavones—several times a week. Experiment with cooked dried soybeans (½ cup), tofu and tempeh (¾ cup), textured soy protein (¼ cup), soy protein powder (3 to 4 tablespoons), or soy-based meat substitutes. All of these are sold in your health food store.

3. Low-Sodium Tomato Juice

Tomatoes are an abundant source of potassium. As I explained earlier, adequate potassium intake—and in proper balance with sodium—is crucial for the regulation of blood pressure. Unfortunately, most Americans consume too much sodium and not enough potassium. Unless you severely restrict your salt intake or eat copious amounts of fruits, vegetables, and grains, sodium may gain the upper hand. A very easy way to ensure that you get enough potassium is to drink a glass or two of low-sodium tomato juice every day. I know from clinical experience that increasing potassium intake in this way lowers blood pressure. Ted, a longtime patient of mine, reported that after years of moderately high blood pressure readings, his blood pressure has been in the low-normal range since he began drinking low-sodium V-8 juice every day.

Potassium isn't the only good thing about low-sodium tomato juice. Unlike most juices, it is very low in sugar. It also contains antioxidants such as vitamin C, vitamin A, and lycopene. Lycopene has long been known to protect against cancer of the prostate, lung, colon, stomach, and pancreas but was only recently discovered to benefit the heart. A 2000 New Zealand study of men with diabetes found that tomato juice protected LDL cholesterol from free radical damage and lowered levels of C-reactive protein, an inflammatory marker of heart disease.[38] In another 2000 study, men with the highest tissue levels of lycopene had half the risk of heart attack of men with the lowest levels.[39]

I suggest drinking 12 ounces of tomato or V-8 juice every day. It is important that you get the low-sodium variety—look for it in your health food store if you can't find it in the grocery store, or ask your grocer to stock it for you. Regular tomato juice has so much added sodium that it may elevate blood pressure in susceptible individuals.

4. Fatty Fish

Salmon, mackerel, tuna, herring, sardines, anchovies, and trout contain considerably more fat than most species of fish, but it's the best fat around: omega-3 fatty acids. These important fats have myriad benefits for the cardiovascular system. They increase circulation, inhibit the formation of blood clots, protect the arteries, help normalize blood pressure and heart rhythm, and lower cholesterol and triglycerides. Drs. Scott H. Goodnight and W. E. Connor from the University of Oregon fed volunteers a diet that included salmon fillets every day for four weeks and recorded remarkable drops in their blood fats: an average 17 percent drop in cholesterol and a 40 percent drop in triglycerides.[40]

More recent studies have shown that people who eat at least one serving of fatty fish per week have a 60 percent reduction in the risk of developing coronary artery disease compared to those who eat less.[41] Eat a serving of these fatty fish two or three times a week. Your cardiovascular system will certainly benefit—and it just might sharpen your memory, improve your insulin sensitivity, protect against cancer, help you lose weight, and relieve arthritis pain at the same time.

5. Nuts

Nuts are a great source of healthy monounsaturated and polyunsaturated fats that help reduce cholesterol levels. They are also loaded with vitamin E, which prevents LDL cholesterol from being converted to its oxidized, artery-damaging form. Furthermore, nuts contain arginine, an amino acid that the body converts into nitric oxide. As you may recall from Chapter 3, nitric oxide protects against the adherence of plaque, prevents platelets from sticking together, and relaxes the arteries, helping to control blood pressure.

A number of studies have documented the protective effects of nuts on cardiovascular health. The Nurses' Health Study, a fourteen-year study of more than 84,000 female United States nurses, found that eating nuts five times a week reduced heart disease risk by 35 percent—a risk reduction similar to the effects of cholesterol-lowering statin drugs.[42] Most nuts are great, although the best studied for heart health are walnuts. Eat your nuts raw whenever possible, for roasting damages their fragile polyunsaturated fats. And don't go overboard on nuts—they are very calorie-dense.

6. Garlic

Another great food for the heart is garlic (*Allium sativum*). Although most people think of garlic as a cooking herb, its medicinal properties have been recognized for centuries. The active constituents in garlic (allicin and other sulfur compounds) enhance the immune system, kill microbes, and block the formation of cancer-causing compounds. In recent years garlic's broad cardiovascular benefits have also been uncovered. Garlic lowers blood pressure and discourages platelet aggregation. It also contains antioxidants that protect the arteries from free radical damage.

Dozens of studies have been conducted on garlic's ability to lower cholesterol. In 1993, researchers from New York Medical College surveyed all these studies and found that there was a 9 percent average reduction in cholesterol in study subjects taking one-half to one clove of garlic or its supplemental equivalent daily.[43] Even more important, garlic tends to improve the ratio of two types of cholesterol, lowering LDL and raising protective HDL cholesterol. Make a conscious effort to use garlic as a culinary spice—try adding it to sauces, salad dressings, and other dishes. Garlic may also be taken as a supplement. If you choose this form, look for an extract standardized to contain a total of 4,500 mcg of allicin per daily dose. This equals one average-size clove of garlic, without the odor.

Runner-Ups

There are many outstanding members of the plant kingdom, but I'm going to mention just a few more that should hold a prominent place in a heart-healthy diet. ***Dark leafy green vegetables*** contain antioxidants that safeguard LDL cholesterol, calcium and magnesium that relax the arteries, folic acid that keeps homocysteine levels in check, and essential fatty acids, which are highly therapeutic for the cardiovascular system. These foods are unappreciated by Americans, who eat spinach but are generally unfamiliar with other dark greens. Get acquainted with kale, collard and mustard greens, chicory, Swiss chard, and arugula and make them a regular part of your diet. Try to include at least one food from this class of vegetables three or four times a week.

In addition to soybeans, include ***kidney, pinto, garbanzo, black beans, and other legumes*** in your diet. Their combination of protein, minerals, and soluble fiber can't be beat. Studies have found that eating as little as four ounces (½ cup) of beans a day can lower LDL cholesterol. ***Oatmeal*** is a great source of a soluble fiber called beta glucan that lowers cholesterol. This cereal grain has also been shown in clinical studies to reduce the adverse effects of a high-fat meal on the endothelium, which I described earlier in this chapter.[44] I recommend eating a bowl of old-fashioned, slow-cooking oatmeal several times a week.

CHOOSE THE PROPER FUEL

I want to wrap up this chapter on diet with this thought. The engineering specs on every automobile include the type of fuel for optimum performance. For most cars it is regular unleaded gasoline. More expensive models require premium gasoline, some makes run on diesel, and a few bypass petroleum altogether and operate on battery power. If you put the wrong fuel in any of these vehicles, expect disaster.

While our bodies are much more forgiving of improper maintenance than a mechanical vehicle (just think what would happen if you accidentally put diesel in your gasoline-powered car), too much of the wrong fuel takes its toll over time. Consider how you've treated your body up to this point. Does it fit the design specs of the human body? Now think how much better it could function if you observed its proper care and feeding instructions.

The human body, as I hope I have made clear in these last two chapters, is clearly designed to be fueled by plant foods. Vegetables, fruits, grains, beans, legumes, nuts, and seeds contain plenty of the protein we need for growth and maintance. These same plant foods are also the source of essential fatty acids as well as a cornucopia of vitamins, minerals, unique phytonutrients, and life-sustaining, health-enhancing fiber. Add to this moderate amounts of lean protein from poultry—and as much salmon and other fatty fish as you desire—and you'll be running on premium.

CHAPTER 13

Nutritional Supplementation: Essential for Optimal Health

VITAMINS, MINERALS, AND OTHER NUTRITIONAL SUPPLEMENTS are an integral part of the Whitaker Wellness Institute's approach to treating serious disease. Rather than the prescription pad most doctors turn to when treating health problems, we have extensive nutritional protocols for dozens of medical conditions. For example, patients with arthritis are able to end their dependence on painkillers and regain mobility by supplementing with glucosamine sulfate and other compounds that nurture the joints. Diabetics can often replace drugs with vanadyl sulfate, chromium, and the herb *Gymnema sylvestre*. Prostate enlargement is treated with saw palmetto, and menopausal symptoms with black cohosh.

Heart disease is no different. When combined with a low-fat, nutrient-rich diet and a regular exercise regimen, targeted nutritional supplements can truly make a difference in both the prevention and reversal of heart disease. This is not conjecture. The effectiveness of these vitamins, minerals, herbs, amino acids, essential fatty acids, enzymes, and coenzymes has been proven in repeated studies published in top medical journals. It is also backed by the experience of the thousands of patients who have passed through the Whitaker Wellness Institute over the years.

The use of nutritional supplements has exploded over the past decade. You need only scan the covers at a magazine rack to observe the keen interest in this realm of medicine. Articles on vitamins, herbs, and other nutrients are no longer relegated to *Prevention* magazine but are covered in depth in publications aimed at women, parents, sports enthusiasts, and even pet owners. Daily newspapers and the evening news routinely cover developments in the field, and the Internet is home to tens of thousands of sites devoted to educating people about, and selling, nutritional supplements. Today more than half of all Americans take vitamin, mineral, and/or herbal supplements on a regular basis.

Yet controversy over the use of supplements lingers, and the most diehard critics come from within the medical profession. These skeptics raise a strong voice against the use of nutritional supplements, except when there is a specific deficiency such as scurvy (vitamin C), rickets (vitamin D), pellagra (niacin), or pernicious anemia (vitamin B12, brought on by inability to absorb this vitamin). They further insist that a "good diet" supplies the optimum amount of vitamins and minerals. According to Victor Herbert, M.D., one of the most vociferous opponents of nutritional supplements and most everything else in medicine that smacks of the alternative, "There is no data which has been published demonstrating that healthy people eating a well-balanced diet need any vitamin supplements."[1]

This is simply not true, as a careful look at the published research would show. The National Institutes of Health's Office of Dietary Supplements maintains a database of more than 400,000 scientific articles from 1,600 medical journals,[2] but few physicians consider it a useful investment of their time to plow through the research on nutrition. After all, this is an area of study that has never been valued highly in the medical education of budding physicians. As I mentioned before, when I was a medical student we had a few hours of lectures on the role of fat, protein, and carbohydrate in the body, and that was that. Even today, only a quarter of the medical schools in this country require coursework in nutrition. Postgraduate education in the high-tech, drug-intensive milieu of our hospitals only strengthens the belief that inexpensive nutritional supplements have little bearing on health. And once a doctor settles down to practice medicine, continuing education is most often obtained through drug company–sponsored publications and conferences. Is it any wonder that so many physicians take Dr. Herbert's blanket statement at face value?

In this chapter I will tell you why I prescribe a multivitamin and mineral supplement program to virtually all of my patients as a foundation for good health. In the next chapter, I will show you how specific vitamins, minerals, coenzymes, essential fatty acids, amino acids, and herbs protect and nurture the heart and cardiovascular system. First, let's examine how vitamins and minerals work in the body.

THE FUNCTIONS OF VITAMINS AND MINERALS

One of the primary functions of vitamins and minerals is as essential constituents of enzymes or coenzymes. Enzymes facilitate chemical reactions. They act as catalysts to join different molecules together or to split them apart, without being affected themselves. Coenzymes simply assist the action of enzymes. The body produces some complete enzymes that do their work by themselves. However, most enzymes require a vitamin or mineral in order to function properly, and a shortage of the required nutrient will prevent the enzyme from doing its job.

Zinc, for example, is a vital component of the enzyme that converts vitamin A to its active form in the eyes. Zinc deficiency is a well-known cause of night blindness. Another example is the role of vitamin C as a coenzyme in the synthesis of collagen. Vitamin C assists the enzyme that produces this structural component of our tissues, so without adequate vitamin C, collagen synthesis is impaired. Wounds heal slowly, gums may bleed, and skin bruises more easily.[3]

Other vitamins and minerals work on their own to promote metabolic reactions independent of enzymes. For instance, vitamin D works alone, much like a hormone, to regulate calcium metabolism. And some nutrients, such as vitamin B6 (pyridoxine), play multiple roles, sometimes acting as a coenzyme and at other times working in an independent fashion. But regardless of exactly how these nutrients contribute to the workings of various metabolic systems, without them the body simply cannot function as it is meant to. It is easy to see that adequate intakes of vitamins and minerals are crucial to health.

But what are adequate intakes of vitamins and minerals?

THE TROUBLE WITH THE RDAs

The Food and Nutrition Board of the National Academy of Sciences has issued guidelines for vitamin and mineral intake since 1941. The board has defined the recommended dietary allowances (RDAs) as "the levels of intake of essential nutrients considered, in the judgment of the Food and Nutrition Board, on the basis of available scientific knowledge, to be adequate to meet the known nutritional needs of practically all healthy persons."

Studies on both human volunteers and animals have been used to set the RDAs. A clinical deficiency of a nutrient is produced in a study subject, and starting with very small doses of that nutrient, researchers determine how much is needed to eliminate evidence of the deficiency. A modest surplus is tacked onto this minimum amount for good luck, and *voilà*! You have the RDA. There are several basic flaws in this method.

First, the focus is entirely on elimination of deficiencies rather than on the promotion of optimal health. A very small amount of a vitamin or mineral can eliminate evidence of gross deficiency. On the other hand, larger amounts of the same nutrient may stimulate the production of increased amounts of enzymes and affect metabolic activities that improve the body's health from just-above-borderline to excellent.

Riada A. Bayourni, M.D., and Sidney Rosalki, M.D., of St. Mary's Hospital in London experimented with red blood cells taken from well-nourished individuals in whom no vitamin deficiency was suspected. However, after they added vitamins B1, B2, and B6 to these red blood cells, there were marked increases in enzyme production by the cells. If the synthesis of this enzyme had been at the maximum level, adding these vitamins would not have increased it.

Next, the researchers supplemented the diets of the study subjects with vitamins B1, B2, and B6 for seven days and then repeated the lab test, again adding B vitamins to the red blood cells. This time, far fewer additional enzymes were produced by the cells, indicating that the seven days of supplementation had saturated the enzyme system and brought it to a peak level.[4] These findings raise an obvious question. Should the RDAs of vitamins and minerals be set at levels to stimulate peak production of enzymes and thus optimal functioning, or should we continue to aim for levels that produce enough enzymes only to eradicate symptoms of gross deficiency?

Another flaw in the way the RDAs are established is that very limited parameters are used. Blinded to the body of research suggesting broad and multifaceted actions of most nutrients, the Board of Nutrition considers only limited effects of each nutrient in determining the recommended vitamin and mineral intake. The RDAs are supposed to protect the "average healthy person" (if such a person exists) from blatant deficiency diseases, and by and large, they do. However, other, more subtle but equally important effects of these same nutrients are not taken into consideration at all, even when research clearly demonstrates that larger amounts may be required to enhance other areas of health.

Let's take vitamin C as an example. Small amounts of vitamin C (75 to 90 milligrams daily, according to the 2000 revisions of the RDAs) will prevent scurvy. But what about the research showing that men who got more than 300 milligrams daily of this nutrient from food or supplements had a 45 percent lower risk of death from cardiovascular disease than those getting less than 50 milligrams per day?[5] What about the scores of studies showing the positive effects of higher doses of vitamin C for improving immune function, lowering blood pressure, preventing kidney disease, reducing the risk of prostate cancer, and slowing the progression of arthritis? How can the Board of Nutrition, in the face of all this evidence, set as the RDA the small amount of vitamin C needed to prevent scurvy—and warn people against taking much more?

Finally, the RDAs leave little room for individual biological differences, and believe me, these differences can be vast. We are as unique on the inside as we are on the outside. There are many, many confounding factors, from body size to activity and stress levels to inherited variations. What is adequate for one person may be inadequate for the next. When you consider how many different functions vitamins and minerals serve, how many thousands of metabolic reactions they are involved in, the assumption that there are no inherent differences between individual needs defies reason.

THE GENETOTROPHIC THEORY OF DISEASE

The prevailing concept of disease in medicine today, which dates back to Louis Pasteur's nineteenth-century germ theory, is that individuals are normal until external factors such as germs or stress disrupt the equilibrium and cause disease. For instance, a virus infects normal cells, causing a cold. Until you had the cold you were clinically a well person. Everyone's constitution is supposedly strong—as strong as everyone else's—and those that break down do so because of external factors.

There is a competing theory, also dating back to the nineteenth century, which was proposed by French scientist Claude Bernard. Dr. Bernard believed that a person's internal environment, or "terrain," is a more important factor in disease than what that person is exposed to. He proposed that disease prevention strategies should focus on bolstering this internal terrain. Roger J. Williams, Ph.D., the remarkable biochemist who discovered pantothenic acid (vitamin B5), believed as Dr. Bernard did, that the internal environment was at least as important to health as the external one. Keenly aware of the enormous biochemical variations within the human species, he proposed that these underlying differences—and the wide variances in nutritional needs that they cause—are at the root of many of our health problems. In 1950, Dr. Williams advanced his genetotrophic theory of disease (*geneto* referring to genesis or origin, *trophic* referring to feeding or nutrition).[6] Simply stated, a genetotrophic disease develops because of variables in the "terrain" leading to deficiencies in certain nutrients. The amount of a particular nutrient required by one individual may be a hundred times that required by another, and unless this demand is met, that individual is weakened and made more susceptible to disease.

Let's take the theory of genetotrophic disease out of the textbook and into the laboratory. D. Lonsdale, M.D., and Raymond J. Shamberger, M.D., of the Department of Pediatrics, Cleveland Clinic, conducted a study involving 20 patients who had disorders such as depression, insomnia, irritability, chronic fatigue, nightmares, intermittent diarrhea and constipation, and recurrent abdominal or chest pains. Most doctors would have subjected these patients to a battery of tests that would have turned up nothing, and then prescribed antidepressants or other drugs and psychotherapy to treat their symptoms.

Drs. Lonsdale and Shamberger went in another direction and looked for deficiencies of thiamine (vitamin B1), which has a known role in nerve cell function and energy production. They measured the activity of transketolase, a thiamine-dependent enzyme, in the red blood cells of these patients and found it to be low in 12 of the 20 patients. Diet histories showed that many of the patients were eating a lot of junk food such as soft drinks and candy, which are essentially devoid of vitamins and minerals. The 12 patients with low transketolase activity were given a thiamine supplement ranging from 150 to 600 milligrams a day—megadoses surely, since the RDA for thiamin is only up to 1.6 milligrams. In all 12 patients symptoms disappeared over a period of several weeks, and their red blood cell transketolase reactions returned to normal.[7]

You may ask, why not get those people off all the junk instead? That would probably have helped. However, this study also found that there was no measurable difference between the dietary patterns of the 12 patients with abnormal thiamine function and the eight with normal thiamine function. It is likely that the combination of the junk food and the greater genetic need for thiamine shared by 12 of the patients produced the deficiency that was reversed by supplemental thiamine.

NUTRITIONAL SUPPLEMENTS FOR HEALTH MAINTENANCE

Deficiency diseases aside, Dr. Williams recommended that healthy people take vitamin and mineral supplements as "insurance" against possible deficiencies. This does not mean that a nutritional deficiency will definitely occur in the absence of supplementation any more than the failure to have fire insurance means that your house is going to burn down. But given the enormous potential for individual differences from person to person and the broad and varied functions of vitamins and minerals, supplementation makes sense.

I recommend that all my patients, regardless of their current state of health, take a daily nutritional supplement that contains potent doses of all the vitamins and minerals known to play beneficial roles in human health. I invariably get questions on the necessity and safety of such a program, as well as practical queries about the best types of vitamins and minerals. So before we move on to the specific nutrients I recommend for general health, let me answer some of these commonly asked questions.

I eat a good diet. Why should I take supplements?

If you truly do eat well, bravo to you. A United States Department of Agriculture survey suggests that few Americans eat even the minimum recommended daily servings of fruits and vegetables. Seventy-two percent, on the day surveyed, ate no vitamin C–rich fruits, and 41 percent ate no fruit at all. Eighty-two percent ate no broccoli, cabbage or other cruciferous vegetables, and 84 percent no fiber-rich whole grain foods.[8]

We're eating out more than ever—most often in notoriously unhealthy fast-food restaurants—and eating more prepared and convenience foods at home. Unfortunately, even if you are eating a well-balanced diet with lots of whole foods, you cannot be guaranteed that your food contains all the nutrients you would expect. Soil levels of some minerals vary from one geographic area to another, as does the mineral content of foods grown in various areas. Storage, processing, and cooking further deplete our food of water-soluble vitamins and minerals. Taking a daily vitamin and mineral supplement will fill the unforeseen nutritional "holes" in your diet.

Are natural vitamins better than synthetic?

For the most part, vitamins found in food and those synthesized in the lab are like identical twins—impossible to tell apart. The genuine vitamin, whether found in food or synthesized in a lab, is in most cases the same substance. Synthesized ascorbic acid, for example, is chemically identical to the vitamin C found in food. It is also less expensive and much easier to put into supplements. You would have to eat handfuls of nature's richest source of vitamin C, acerola cherries, to get the amount of that vitamin found in one capsule. Rose hips, another good source of vitamin C, contains only 25 milligrams of ascorbic acid per 100,000 milligrams of rose hips powder. A tablet containing 250 milligrams of vitamin C derived solely from rose hips would be the size of a basketball! You can bet that most nutritional supplements containing significant doses of vitamins are largely synthetic.

There are two exceptions: vitamin E and beta-carotene. Natural vitamin E and synthetic vitamin E are mirror images of each other: close, but no cigar. The synthetic version works to some degree, but because it doesn't "fit" exactly right, it is less effective than the natural version. In addition, synthetic vitamin E, which you can pick out by closely reading supplement labels (synthetic E is dl-alpha-tocopherol or dl-alpha-tocopheryl, while natural E is listed as d-alpha-tocopherol or d-alpha-tocopheryl, without an *l*) contains only the most dominant of the tocopherols, alpha. Natural vitamin E, which is often labeled "with mixed tocopherols," also contains beta-, delta-, gamma-, and other tocopherols. These other forms of vitamin E also play important, though less well-studied, roles in health maintenance.

In a similar manner, synthetic beta-carotene is a one-shot wonder, whereas natural beta-carotene with mixed carotenoids includes the gamut of these invaluable plant compounds, including lutein and zeaxanthin, which protect the eyes, and lycopene, which guards against cancer and heart disease. You may pay a little more for formulations with natural vitamin E and beta-carotene, but it's worth it. Current research demonstrates that the synthetic forms of other vitamins, however, are perfectly adequate.

Can vitamins and minerals be toxic?

You've likely heard that nutritional supplements can be toxic—even deadly—in large doses. I have yet to document a single fatality definitively attributed to a vitamin or mineral supplement. Prescription drugs, on the other hand, when used exactly as directed by physicians, are the third or fourth leading cause of death in the United States, killing more people than automobile accidents, breast cancer, prostate cancer, or AIDS.[9]

So what's the story on vitamin toxicity? Fat-soluble vitamins, particularly vitamin A and vitamin D, do have the potential of toxicity. By their very nature they collect in the fat cells and could build up to dangerous levels. This, however, would require taking highly excessive amounts over prolonged periods of time. If one were to overdose on fat-soluble vitamins, there would be early warning signs of toxicity, which would rapidly subside once the vitamin was discontinued. (Women of childbearing age should not take more than 10,000 international units of vitamin A, for it has been linked with increased risk of birth defects. The related nutrient, beta-carotene, is nontoxic.) Vitamins K and E are also fat soluble. However, vitamin K is rarely found in nutritional supplements (you see it most often in very small doses in formulas aimed at preventing and treating osteoporosis), and vitamin E has been shown to be safe in doses hundreds of times higher than the RDA.

Although some of the trace minerals are potentially toxic, as they may upset the balance of mineral metabolism as well as having specific toxicities, reports of adverse effects are rare. Virtually all multivitamin and mineral supplements contain trace minerals that are within prescribed and balanced levels. When taken as directed, they are perfectly safe.

The water-soluble nutrients, such as vitamin C and the B-complex vitamins, are very safe. Excesses of these substances are eliminated from the body in the urine. (Notice how yellow your urine is when you're taking vitamin supplements?) There have been reports of people taking very large doses of B6 by itself (2,000 to 5,000 milligrams a day; the RDA is around 2 milligrams) on the inaccurate assumption that this vitamin would serve as a diuretic. These individuals experienced weakness and loss of sensation as a result of damage to the peripheral nerves, primarily in the lower extremities. Symptoms abated with cessation of high B6 intake.

To sum it up, vitamin and mineral supplements taken in recommended doses (even if the recommendations are much higher than the RDAs), are not only safe but also a powerful boon to good health.

THE WHITAKER WELLNESS INSTITUTE BASIC SUPPLEMENT PROGRAM

To reiterate, I believe that everyone, regardless of their state of health, needs to take a daily multivitamin and mineral supplement. The goal is to saturate the system with a high but safe dose of all the vitamins and minerals that have been proven to be essential for human health. We aim high to make sure we meet the needs of all of our patients. As you recall from our earlier discussion of the genetotrophic theory of disease, everyone has unique, individualized requirements for various nutrients. By including in our basic formula rather high doses of the water-soluble nutrients, knowing the body will excrete what it doesn't use, and safe yet therapeutic amounts of the fat-soluble nutrients, we cover all the bases.

A comprehensive multivitamin and mineral supplement should contain free-radical-quenching antioxidants such as vitamins C, E, beta-carotene, and selenium. It should include adequate doses of the B-complex vitamins, which are essential for the health of the arteries, brain, and central nervous system. A broad range of minerals, including bone-building calcium, heart-healthy magnesium and potassium, as well as zinc, copper, chromium, and other trace minerals must be present.

All these nutrients are contained in the multivitamin and mineral formula we prescribe for everyone who visits the Whitaker Wellness Institute. Years ago I had my patients mix and match bottles of vitamins and minerals to approximate these recommended levels. Due to popular demand I formulated my own supplement, the Forward Daily Regimen, just to make things easier for my patients, and I have updated it several times over the past twenty years. Next is a list of my recommended daily intake of the most important vitamins and minerals for general health. These are the dosages found in Forward, and they are appropriate for adults, including women who are pregnant or lactating, and older adolescents. Children under the age of twelve to fourteen should stick with a good multivitamin and mineral supplement geared for kids.

Of course, there are other excellent brands of high-potency multivitamin and mineral supplements sold in health food stores, and you can always add to your favorite multi to meet my suggested levels. (Avoid one-a-day types of multivitamins. It is impossible to fit therapeutic levels of all of these vitamins and minerals in one capsule or tablet.) For optimal absorption, take your supplements in divided doses with meals.

Nutrient	Suggested Daily Intake
*Vitamin A	5,000 international units
*Beta-carotene	15,000 international units
Vitamin D	600 international units
*Vitamin E (d-alpha-tocopheryl)	800 international units
*Vitamin C	1,500 milligrams
*Folic acid	800 micrograms
Thiamine (vitamin B1)	50 milligrams
Riboflavin (vitamin B2)	50 milligrams
*Niacin (vitamin B3)	100 milligrams
*Vitamin B6 (pyridoxine)	75 milligrams
*Vitamin B12 (cyanocobalamin)	150 micrograms
Biotin	300 micrograms
Vitamin B5 (pantothenic acid)	50 milligrams
*Calcium	1,000 milligrams
Iodine	150 micrograms
*Magnesium	500 milligrams
Zinc	30 milligrams
Copper	2 milligrams
*Potassium	99 milligrams
Manganese	10 milligrams
*Chromium (picolinate or polynicotinate)	200 micrograms
*Selenium	200 micrograms
Molybdenum	125 micrograms
Silica	25 milligrams
Bioflavonoids	100 milligrams

*These nutrients are particularly important for cardiovascular health.

In summary, this is the basic nutritional supplement program we recommend for all of our patients at the Whitaker Wellness Institute. Other nutrients can be added as needed to address specific medical problems. In the next chapter we will cover the targeted nutritional supplements for reversing heart disease.

CHAPTER 14

Nutritional Supplements That Heal the Heart

NOW THAT I'VE LAID THE GROUNDWORK FOR NUTRITIONAL SUPplementation as a prerequisite for good health, let's look at other nutrients I suggest you add to your basic supplement program to prevent or reverse heart disease. As we discussed in Chapters 3 and 4, several mechanisms are at work in atherosclerosis. Elevated cholesterol is the best known risk factor, but it is certainly not the only one. The ratio of the various types of cholesterol and elevations in other blood fats such as triglycerides are important. So are abnormalities in homocysteine metabolism, inflammatory and clotting compounds, and other processes that affect the heart and arteries.

In this chapter I am going to briefly review the mechanisms that initiate or promote atherosclerosis and tell you about specific nutrients that intervene in these processes and help reverse heart disease. Let's begin with free radicals, or oxidative damage.

ANTIOXIDANTS: FRONT-LINE DEFENSE

We have talked so much about oxygen in this book and how inadequate delivery of this life-sustaining element to the heart muscle is at the root of angina and heart attacks. Many of the therapies utilized at the Whitaker Wellness Institute in one way or another increase oxygen delivery to the heart and arteries. However, there is also a dark side to oxygen. While oxygen is required for the production of energy that keeps us alive, it is also the primary source of free radicals in our bodies. Free radicals, as we touched upon in Chapter 3, are unstable molecules that damage other molecules by stealing electrons, creating a chain reaction of destruction.

Free radicals are perpetrators of heart disease for two reasons. First, they damage the arteries, setting the stage for atherosclerosis. Second, they transform LDL cholesterol into its oxidized form, which burrows into artery walls and contributes to plaque build-up. While it is important to lower your LDL cholesterol levels, you can see that it is equally important to protect LDL from oxidation.

Nature has an ingenious system to counter oxidation: antioxidants. Antioxidants give up electrons to reactive free radicals, stabilizing them and preventing them from disrupting other molecules. High levels of antioxidants in the blood have been shown to be protective against atherosclerosis, while low levels, as you might expect, are associated with increased risk of heart disease. A 2001 study published in *The Lancet* found that blood levels of vitamin C were inversely related to death from heart disease—men and women with the lowest levels of this important antioxidant were twice as likely to die of heart disease as those with the highest levels.[1] German researchers came up with similar findings for vitamin E and beta-carotene: Blood levels of these antioxidants were low in people with atherosclerosis. They concluded that measuring levels of antioxidants may be a valuable way of assessing risk of heart disease.[2]

Your body produces antioxidants, and you also get them in your diet (provided that you eat lots of fruits and vegetables). However, the best way to ensure optimal levels of these crucial nutrients is to take supplements of the major antioxidant vitamins and minerals: vitamin E, vitamin C, vitamin A, beta-carotene, and selenium. Don't underestimate the importance of this simple step. Researchers at the Centers for Disease Control and Prevention (CDC) in Atlanta, Georgia, recently concluded a seven-year study that included an astounding number of subjects—more than one million people—and compared death rates of those who took various combinations of multivitamin and mineral supplements and individual antioxidants with those who took no supplements. They found that individuals who took a multinutrient plus vitamin A, C, or E had a 15 percent lower risk of death from heart attack or stroke than people who did not take vitamins. Interestingly, people who took a multivitamin alone (most likely a one-a-day supplement with RDA doses) were not afforded protection.[3] This supports my contention, which I explained in the previous chapter, that the RDAs for important nutrients are just too low. The CDC researchers agreed with this, stating: "One explanation is that there may be a minimum dose of a single vitamin or combination of supplements necessary for risk reduction."[4]

Vitamin E Reduces the Risk of Heart Attack

Vitamin E is the most active antioxidant in the lipid or fatty portions of the body. It guards against the oxidation of LDL cholesterol by hitching onto LDL particles and neutralizing free radicals. Vitamin E is also highly protective of the endothelial lining of the arteries. This was demonstrated in a 1997 study carried out at the University of Maryland School of Medicine in Baltimore. When volunteers were fed a high-fat meal, endothelial function in the coronary arteries was dramatically suppressed for up to four hours. However, when the volunteers took 800 international units of vitamin E and 1,000 milligrams of vitamin C along with a high-fat meal, endothelium function remained completely normal.[5]

Vitamin E has other protective mechanisms. It improves cholesterol levels, lowers levels of C-reactive protein and other inflammatory markers, and has a slight blood-thinning effect, enhancing circulation and preventing abnormal blood clots. (We will elaborate on these attributes of vitamin E later in this chapter.) This broad spectrum of actions is likely why vitamin E has proven so effective in protecting against heart disease.

Some of the studies on vitamin E are truly astounding. Harvard University researchers followed 87,245 female nurses and more than 46,000 male physicians and found that the women and men taking at least 100 international units of supplemental vitamin E had a lower risk (40 percent and 37 percent, respectively) of heart attack or death from heart disease compared to those who took no vitamin E.[6, 7] In the Cambridge Heart Antioxidant Study (CHAOS), a 1996 double-blind, placebo-controlled trial that involved 2,002 patients, half of the study subjects took 400 to 800 international units of vitamin E daily, while the other half received a placebo. After an average period of 510 days, the patients taking supplemental vitamin E had 75 percent fewer heart attacks than those taking the placebo.[8]

Vitamin E also improves symptoms in patients with established cardiovascular disease. Japanese researchers found that one month of daily supplementation with 300 milligrams of vitamin E reduced angina in heart patients. They attributed this effect to the vitamin's ability to improve endothelial function, relax the arteries, and prevent spasms that reduce blood flow.[9] Patients with intermittent claudication, exercise-induced leg pain caused by atherosclerosis in the arteries of the legs, also benefit from vitamin E. According to a sixteen-year study by Swedish physician Knut Haeger, M.D., supplementation with vitamin E resulted in slow but significant improvements in pain and ability to exercise.[10]

The primary dietary sources of vitamin E are vegetable oils, nuts, and seeds. The average American obtains only 11 to 13 international units of vitamin E from such foods. To get 800 to 1,200 international units, the amount I recommend to patients with heart disease, you'd have to eat up to 2,000 almonds—which would also give you 16,000 calories and 1,300 grams of fat! As you can see, supplementating this important vitamin is crucial. Make sure you take natural vitamin E, preferably with mixed tocopherols, as discussed in the previous chapter. You can tell it's natural if it's listed on the label as d-alpha-tocopherol or d-alpha-tocopheryl.

Vitamin C Protects the Arteries

Just as vitamin E is the premier antioxidant in the lipid portions of the body, vitamin C is the most active in the aqueous, or water-based, components. Although this vitamin is best known as an immune booster and therapy for the common cold, it is also highly protective against atherosclerosis. We have known since the 1950s that guinea pigs, one of the few mammal species that, like humans, does not produce vitamin C, develop atherosclerosis when vitamin C is removed from their diet. When the vitamin is added back in, atherosclerosis is reversed.[11]

Higher intakes of vitamin C are associated with reductions in risk of death from heart disease in humans as well. In a five-year study, Dr. James E. Enstrom, associate professor at the University of California Los Angeles School of Public Health, and colleagues analyzed the vitamin C intake of 11,348 adults. They found that the men with the highest consumption from food and supplement sources (more than 300 milligrams per day) had a 45 percent lower risk of death from cardiovascular disease than men with the lowest intake (less than 50 milligrams). The degree of protection was less significant for women, but it was still an impressive 25 percent reduction.[12]

Vitamin C's dominant action against atherosclerosis is to protect the integrity of the arteries. It blocks free-radical damage to the endothelium and promotes healing of injuries that initiate atherosclerosis. It is also crucial for the production of collagen, an important structural material in the blood vessels and other tissues. Boosting the health of the arteries not only staves off atherosclerosis but also helps normalize blood pressure by making the arteries more responsive to signals to dilate and relax. In addition, vitamin C also has a role in protecting LDL cholesterol from oxidation. It is the third-string antioxidant in this particular play—if vitamin E and beta-carotene and other carotenoid stores are consumed, vitamin C comes to the rescue. Furthermore, it regenerates the oxidized vitamin E, refueling it so it can get back in the game. Other activities of this crucial antioxidant, which we will return to later include improving blood flow by inhibiting platelet aggregation, lowering lipoprotein(a), and elevating HDL cholesterol.

How much vitamin C should you take? As I mentioned earlier, all mammals produce vitamin C in their bodies—with the exception of primates (including us), guinea pigs, and Indian fruit-eating bats, which must get this nutrient from their diets.

To ascertain the optimal intake for humans, two-time Nobel Prize winner Linus Pauling, Ph.D., calculated the amount of vitamin C most mammals produce for their own use. For example, the average amount a goat manufactures is equal to about 5,000 milligrams per day in a human, based on body weight. Figuring in individual differences, Dr. Pauling estimated the optimal dose of vitamin C to range between 2,300 and 9,000 milligrams a day—and more could be required during times of illness or high stress.

It is impossible to get this amount of vitamin C from diet alone. Fewer than one in ten Americans eats the recommended daily servings of fruits and vegetables, our best dietary sources of vitamin C. Even if you eat five servings, you get only an average of 250 milligrams of vitamin C—and this doesn't take into account the fragility of this water-soluble vitamin. When cooked or even cut and left sitting, fruits and vegetables rapidly begin to lose their vitamin C content. Since you will get some vitamin C in your diet (peppers, cruciferous vegetables, greens, berries, and citrus fruits are particularly rich sources) I recommend a minimum supplemental dose of vitamin C of 1,500 milligrams. You can safely increase this to as much as 5,000 to 6,000 milligrams per day.

Although vitamin C is nontoxic, when taken in large doses it does have one fairly common side effect: loose stools. To avoid this problem, build your dose up gradually, starting with 500 milligrams per day. Every three or four days, add another 500 milligrams until you reach your target level. Should you have any gastrointestinal distress, cut back by 500 milligrams and stay at that dose.

Other Important Antioxidants

Although vitamins C and E are the most active of the antioxidants in protecting the cardiovascular system, they are by no means the only ones we recommend for our patients with heart disease. Vitamin A, beta-carotene and other carotenoids, and the mineral selenium each have powerful antioxidant and cardioprotective activities of their own. Coenzyme Q10, which we will discuss later in this chapter, is one of the most powerful antioxidants of all, and perhaps the most therapeutic for the heart.

Furthermore, it is important to understand that these vital nutrients work in concert in your body in an intricate dance of destruction and renewal. When vitamin E takes a hit from a free radical and stops the chain reaction of oxidative damage, it is oxidized and must be regenerated by another antioxidant such as vitamin C. Other antioxidants, such as glutathione, coenzyme Q10, and lipoic acid, can also perform this function, which is why I recommend taking a broad array of antioxidants.

My suggested doses include 5,000 international units of vitamin A and 15,000 international units of natural beta-carotene, preferably with mixed carotenoids. These two nutrients protect the arterial walls and inhibit the oxidation of cholesterol. Also make sure you take 200 micrograms of the trace mineral selenium, which has independent antioxidant activity and is required for the production of the antioxidant enzyme glutathione. Dietary intake of this mineral varies according to soil levels of selenium in the region where food is grown, and repeated studies have found that rates of heart disease and cancer are highest in areas in which selenium soil levels are lowest.[13] The best-absorbed form of this mineral is high-yeast selenium.

SUPPLEMENTS TO LOWER CHOLESTEROL AND TRIGLYCERIDES

Getting your cholesterol level under control is important in the management of heart disease. As you know, LDL is the main type of cholesterol we're aiming to lower, for oxidized LDL cholesterol builds up in the plaque in artery walls and is a prime player in atherosclerosis. Another is lipoprotein(a), a close relative of LDL cholesterol, which is surrounded with a strand of sticky protein that easily adheres to damaged areas in artery walls. VLDL cholesterol also has ramifications for heart disease. It carries triglycerides, and elevations in these blood fats are an independent risk factor for heart disease. HDL cholesterol, on the other hand, guards against heart disease by ushering cholesterol out of the arteries, so we want to raise levels of this protective type of cholesterol.

As we discussed in Chapter 12, dietary changes will go a long way toward lowering cholesterol and triglyceride levels while maintaining protective HDL. Cutting out saturated fat and adding more dietary fiber—particularly in the form of oatmeal, soy and other beans, and flaxseed—takes a big bite out of cholesterol. Many of our patients at the Whitaker Wellness Institute have seen remarkable drops in cholesterol by adding one-quarter cup of freshly ground flaxseed to their daily diet. (See Chapter 12 for details.) And eliminating white flour, sugar, and other high-glycemic carbohydrates from the diet is an excellent therapy for lowering triglycerides.

In addition to dietary measures, the following nutritional supplements stand out for their positive effects on blood fats.

Fish Oil Tackles Triglycerides

Fish oil is one of our most potent therapies for heart disease. In Chapter 12 I told you about the research linking consumption of fish, particularly fatty fish, with decreased risk of heart disease, and how its benefits stem from its omega-3 fatty acids. In review, these important fats cannot by produced in the body, so it is imperative that you get them from dietary or supplemental sources. Nature's most abundant sources of omega-3s are algae, fatty cold-water fish (which eat algae), and marine mammals like seals and whales (which eat fatty cold-water fish). Because these are not common foods on most of our dinner plates, many Americans are deficient in these important fatty acids.

Interest in the relationship between omega-3 fatty acids and heart disease gained momentum in the mid-1970s with the publication of revolutionary research on the dietary habits of the Greenland Eskimos. This group of people had an extremely low incidence of heart disease despite the fact that they subsisted on a diet composed of more than 70 percent fat. It was determined that the type of fat Eskimos ate, primarily from cold-water fish and marine mammals, protected them. This set off a flurry of studies, which firmly established that two types of fat found in these foods, omega-3 fatty acids known as eicosapentaenoic acid (EPA) and docosahexaenoic acid (DHA), provide this protection.

I will return to fish oil several times in this chapter, for it modulates many of the mechanisms of atherosclerosis, including inflammation, blood clotting, and platelet aggregation. For now we will concentrate on its very powerful effects on blood lipids. Although it affects both LDL cholesterol and lipoprotein(a) levels, fish oil is best at inhibiting VLDL production in the liver and reducing triglycerides. In a 2000 review of fish oil and cardiovascular disease, taking 2,000 milligrams of fish oil daily lowered VLDL, the primary carrier of triglycerides, by 25 percent in healthy people and by 40 to 50 percent in patients with high triglyceride levels. In addition, when taken over the course of several weeks, this supplement also has been shown to reduce concentrations of chylomicrons, triglyceride transporters produced in the intestine after a fatty meal, and remove the harmful remnants of these lipoproteins.[14]

While eating omega-3-rich fatty fish several times a week is highly protective against heart disease, few people do it, and experts estimate that as many as 80 percent of Americans do not get adequate essential fatty acids in their diet.[15] So in addition to eating fish, I recommend that all my patients supplement with two 1,000-milligram fish oil capsules daily (the average capsule contains 180 milligrams of EPA and 120 milligrams of DHA). I double, triple, or even quadruple this dose for patients with extremely elevated triglycerides.

Fish oil is very safe. Although diabetics are sometimes told to avoid fish oil because it raises blood sugar, this is simply not true. A 2000 review of studies involving 823 patients with type 2 diabetes found that fish oil supplementation in doses ranging from 3,000 to 18,000 milligrams per day had no negative effects on blood sugar control. Furthermore, it significantly lowered the triglyceride levels of the many patients in this group who had high triglycerides.[16]

The biggest complaint I hear from patients regarding fish oil capsules is the fishy taste that stays with them all day. Taking fish oil with meals helps with this problem, as does using a very high-quality supplement. Good fish oil has a slightly fishy taste and odor, but it isn't overwhelming—if your fish oil tastes really bad, it is probably rancid. Superior technology now exists to eliminate the problem of rancidity, and there are excellent brands on the market. (See the resource section for recommendations.)

The only other abundant source of the omega-3 fatty acids is flaxseed oil, which contains alpha-linolenic acid (ALA), the precursor to EPA and DHA. ALA must be converted in the body into EPA and DHA before it is put to use. In most healthy people, this conversion is seamless; in those who are ill, it may be compromised. The fact that fish oil contains fatty acids in a form that is immediately useful to the body makes it my preferred source of the omega-3 fatty acids for the treatment of heart disease. Flaxseed oil, however, is a reasonable substitute—and freshly ground flaxseed has benefits of its own, particularly in lowering cholesterol, as discussed in Chapter 12.

When you are taking fish oil, flaxseed oil, or any polyunsaturated oil, it is imperative that you also take potent doses of antioxidants, for these fragile oils are prone to oxidation. Vitamin E, in particular, will protect them from the ravages of free radicals.

Niacin: A Cholesterol-Lowering "Drug"

Niacin has been around a long time as a cholesterol-lowering agent. This B-complex vitamin (vitamin B3, also called nicotinic acid or nicotinate) is so good at lowering cholesterol that the drug companies have claimed it as one of their own. It is listed in the *Physicians' Desk Reference* as a therapy for high cholesterol levels. Niacin lowers not only LDL cholesterol, but also triglycerides, lipoprotein(a), and fibrinogen (more on this later)—and it raises levels of protective HDL cholesterol. In fact, this neglected nutrient has been tested against several classes of newer and more dangerous cholesterol-lowering drugs and come out on top.

In a 1994 clinical trial, niacin was compared to lovastatin (Mevacor), one of the popular statin drugs for reducing cholesterol. One hundred and thirty-six patients with elevated cholesterol were enrolled in a twenty-six-week study and randomly assigned to take either niacin or Mevacor. While the statin drug was more effective in reducing LDL cholesterol (average reduction of 32 percent compared to 23 percent for niacin), niacin raised HDL cholesterol by 33 percent versus 7 percent for the drug. Niacin also cut lipoprotein(a) by 35 percent, while Mevacor had no effect on this marker of heart disease.[17]

Many physicians are reluctant to prescribe this very effective, natural therapy because niacin, in the high doses required to lower cholesterol levels, has substantial side effects. Liver enzymes can go up, indicating chronic stress on the liver, and uric acid may rise, which can precipitate attacks of gout. Large doses may also elevate blood sugar, making it inappropriate for diabetics. Furthermore, niacin is not very well tolerated by many patients. Because it dilates the capillaries, patients often experience an uncomfortable flushing and tingling of the skin twenty to thirty minutes after niacin is taken. To get around this common side effect, some physicians recommend time-release niacin. I do not. A few studies suggest that it is even more toxic to the liver than regular niacin.

What we use at the Whitaker Wellness Institute instead is inositol hexaniacinate, a complex of niacin and inositol (a B-complex-like vitamin essential for normal liver function). It lowers cholesterol levels as well as regular niacin but with none of niacin's undesirable side effects. Studies dating back to the 1960s demonstrate that inositol hexaniacinate dropped cholesterol levels from an average of 344 to 286, with no side effects whatsoever.[18] This compound has been widely used in Europe for more than four decades not only to lower blood lipids but also to improve circulation and reduce calf pain in patients with blockages in the arteries of the legs.[19]

High-dose niacin, regardless of the form, should be taken under the supervision of a physician, and blood levels of liver enzymes and cholesterol should be monitored every three months or so. The usual starting dose of inositol hexaniacinate is 500 milligrams three times a day for the first two weeks, taken with meals. You can then increase your dose to 1,000 milligrams three times per day, if needed. The initial dose for regular niacin is 100 milligrams three times a day with meals, then very gradually increasing to a total daily dose of 1,500 to 3,000 milligrams per day. Upping the dose very, very slowly is key to avoiding adverse effects—do it over the course of four to six weeks. Stay away from time-release niacin. Diabetics and people with liver damage should avoid high-dose niacin altogether.

"Green" Solutions for Elevated Cholesterol

Several herbs have a proven ability to lower cholesterol. Garlic, which we discussed in Chapter 12, has positive effects on blood lipids, as does gugulipid, the active ingredient in *Commiphora mukul*, an herb with a time-honored history in the medicine of ancient India. However, the most promising botanicals for treating patients with elevated cholesterol are red yeast rice and policosanol.

Red yeast rice is the fermented product of red yeast (*Monascus purpureus*) cultivated on rice. In 1979, researchers discovered that this traditional Chinese remedy contained monacolin K (also called mevinolin or lovastatin), a substance that inhibits the acitivity of an enzyme involved in the production of cholesterol. Lovastatin was subsequently synthesized and made into the first of the statin cholesterol-lowering drugs, Mevacor, which I told you about in Chapter 9. Red yeast rice, like the statin drugs, lowers LDL cholesterol and triglycerides, and raises HDL (by 31 percent, 34 percent, and 20 percent, respectively, according to one study), but in a safer, gentler manner.[20] This natural supplement does not have the sledgehammer effects of the drugs—the dose of monacolin K, or lovastatin, is much lower, and red yeast rice contains other compounds such as sterols, isoflavones, and fatty acids that also have a beneficial effect on cholesterol levels.

The recommended dose of red yeast rice is 1,200–2,400 milligrams per day.

Policosanol, an extract of natural plant waxes from sugar cane and wheat germ, contains a compound called octacosanol, which Cuban scientists found to have exceptional effects on cholesterol levels. In one double-blind study, 437 patients with high cholesterol and other coronary risk factors were assigned to take either policosanol or a placebo for 24 weeks. During the first 12 weeks of the study, the policosanol group took 5 milligrams per day, then their dose was increased to 10 milligrams daily for another 12 weeks. Both doses significantly lowered LDL cholesterol (by an average of 18.5 percent while on a 5-milligram dose and 25.6 percent on a 10-milligram dose) and total cholesterol (by 13 and 17.4 percent, respectively). Furthermore, HDL cholesterol levels increased by an average of 15.5 and 28.4 percent with the two doses. It was well tolerated, and no adverse events were reported.[21]

This supplement has other benefits for the cardiovascular system. Like aspirin, it decreases the stickiness of platelets in the blood and has positive effects on the lining of the arteries and the function of the heart muscle. It also improves symptoms of intermittent claudication (pain in the legs while walking, caused by atherosclerosis of the arteries in the legs). The suggested dose is 10 mg per day, taken with the evening meal. (Some people may require as little as 5 mg or as much as 20 mg per day to notice effects.) It has no known toxicity or adverse side effects, even when taken in very high amounts.

Because both of these natural products work on the same enzyme system as statin drugs, they could theoretically also lower CoQ10 levels. Although there is no evidence to suggest that they actually do this, I would recommend that you take at least 100 mg of coenzyme Q10 daily when taking red yeast rice or policosanol, just to be safe. Do not take either of these herbs if you are taking a statin drug.

NUTRIENTS FOR NORMALIZING HOMOCYSTEINE

In Chapter 3 we discussed the very important role of homocysteine in the development of atherosclerosis. An elevated level of this toxic by-product of protein metabolism is as significant a risk factor for heart disease as smoking or a high cholesterol level. When homocysteine builds up in the blood, blood cells become sticky, and the oxidation of cholesterol is accelerated. The production of nitric oxide, a short-lived but important substance that protects the lining of the arteries and prevents the adherence of plaque, is also blocked. In short, high levels of homocysteine set the stage for atherosclerosis. Harvard researchers compared the plasma homocysteine levels of 271 participants in the ongoing Physicians' Health Study who had had heart attacks since the study's onset and found that the men with the highest homocysteine levels were three times more likely to have a heart attack than those with the lowest levels.[22]

B-Complex Vitamins Mop up Homocysteine

Nature in its infinite wisdom has a means of detoxifying homocysteine, a process called methylation, in which homocysteine is converted into the essential amino acid methionine. However, in order for the methylation process to run seamlessly, adequate amounts of folic acid and vitamin B12 are required. Vitamin B6, although not an active player in methylation, also keeps homocysteine levels in check by converting the toxin to cysteine, another harmless amino acid. The kicker here is that many of us do not get sufficient amounts of these B vitamins in our diets. This impedes methylation and allows homocysteine levels—and risk of heart disease—to rise.

Elevated homocysteine is also a player in hypertension, cancer, Alzheimer's disease, and other disorders, so I recommend that all my patients supplement with the B-complex vitamins, in the doses suggested in the previous chapter. However, if you have heart disease, you need even greater protection. For vitamin B6 I suggest a dose of 100 milligrams and for folic acid, 1,200 to 1,600 micrograms. Dosage recommendations for vitamin B12 are age-dependent. As we get older, absorption of vitamin B12 is frequently impaired due to declines in our production of gastric acid and a substance called intrinsic factor, both required for the absorption of vitamin B12. Therefore, if you are over sixty-five years of age, I recommend upping your intake with monthly B12 injections (talk to your doctor about this) or daily 1,000-microgram sublingual supplements. Vitamin B12 is quite safe, but very high intakes of vitamin B6 (500+ milligrams per day for prolonged periods) may cause nerve damage.

According to Kilmer S. McCully, M.D., the physician who laid the foundation for our understanding of homocysteine's role in heart disease, most people will be able to keep homocysteine levels under control with supplemental B vitamins. However, he feels that those at greatest risk may benefit from additional methyl donors, which, like folic acid and vitamin B12, help convert homocysteine into methionine.[23] The most common and readily available supplemental methyl donor is trimethylglycine (TMG, sometimes called betaine), which is obtained from beets. The recommended dose is 1,000 milligrams daily.

Because the B-complex vitamins work in tandem, you should always take them together. Select a multivitamin formula that contains the entire gamut of B vitamins, but make sure it has therapeutic (i.e., higher than the RDA) doses of vitamins B6, B12, and folic acid.

DAMPEN INFLAMMATION AND IMPROVE BLOOD FLOW

The revolutionary discovery over the past few years that atherosclerosis is an inflammatory disease has irrevocably altered the way scientists look at heart disease. Let's briefly review this concept. Active lesions in the arteries, especially the smaller, more dangerous vulnerable plaques, are hotbeds of inflammatory activity that can disrupt plaques and precipitate a heart attack. Blood levels of one inflammatory compound, C-reactive protein, have been shown in several studies to be the strongest single predictor of future heart attack or other coronary events. And when coupled with total cholesterol to HDL ratio, C-reactive protein blows the predictive value of all other markers of heart disease out of the water.[24]

Closely associated with inflammation is blood clotting. Whenever there is an injury to a blood vessel, a chemical messenger called thromboxane A2 rallies clotting factors to stop blood loss. Fibrinogen gathers platelets in the blood together to form a blood clot to seal the injury. After the immediate danger has passed, fibrinolysis gets under way to break down the blood clot and removed excess clots, which could lodge in a coronary artery and instigate a heart attack. When levels of thromboxane A2, fibrinogen, and other clotting factors are out of balance, the blood becomes sluggish, clotting increases, and you are at increased risk of heart attack.

Some researchers now believe that the statin drugs reduce the risk of heart attack not so much because they lower cholesterol but because they also dampen inflammation and bring down levels of C-reactive protein. Red yeast rice and policosanol, discussed earlier in this chapter for their ability to cut cholesterol levels, also appear to have positive effects on markers of inflammation and/or clotting. Likewise, the reason low-dose aspirin is such a powerful preventive therapy against heart disease is that it lowers inflammatory and clotting factors in the blood. (For more on aspirin, which I strongly recommend for patients with heart disease, please see Chapter 9.) Now I'm going to tell you about other nutritional supplements that intervene in the cycle of inflammation.

Fish Oil Steps in Again

As I mentioned earlier, the omega-3 fatty acids in fish oil work in several ways to enhance cardiovascular health, and one of the most important involves inflammation. EPA, one of the cardioprotective compounds in fish oil, is converted into anti-inflammatory prostaglandins, messenger molecules that regulate cellular activity throughout the body. One of these beneficial prostaglandins, PGE3, not only has mild anti-inflammatory effects of its own, but also inhibits the production of pro-inflammatory prostaglandins, which are produced in response to injury.

In addition, omega-3 fatty acids influence clotting factors in the blood. They curtail the production of thromboxane A2 and fibrinogen, which are involved in the formation of blood clots. They also stimulate the production of other chemical messengers that discourage platelet aggregation.[25] This combination of benefits is yet another reason not to overlook the importance of supplemental fish oil. (See page 224 for dietary recommendations.)

Vitamin E Does It All

We once again return to the therapeutic powers of vitamin E. In addition to its many other benefits, this versatile antioxidant also dampens inflammation. It has been shown in laboratory studies to dramatically reduce the production of a chemical messenger that rallies the immune system and signals the liver to make more C-reactive protein. As you may recall, levels of this inflammatory compound are highly predictive of heart disease risk.

Drs. Ishwarlal Jialal and Sridevi Devaraj of the University of Texas Southwestern Medical Center in Dallas measured levels of C-reactive protein in 47 patients with either mild or severe type 2 insulin-resistant diabetes (diabetics are at extreme risk of atherosclerosis) and compared them with those of a control group of 25 healthy volunteers. At the study's onset, C-reactive protein levels were twice as high in the patients with severe diabetes and one-third higher in those with mild diabetes, compared to the control group. The study subjects were then supplemented with 1,200 international units daily of vitamin E for three months. When they were retested at the study's conclusion, C-reactive protein levels in patients with mild diabetes had fallen to normal levels, and they had leveled out at about 33 percent above normal in patients with severe diabetes.[26]

Vitamin E is also a safe and gentle blood thinner. It blocks an enzyme involved in clot formation and inhibits platelet aggregation, thus improving blood flow. A 1999 British study found that doses as low as 75 international units of natural vitamin E daily over a two-week period ameliorated platelet aggregation.[27] Questions have been raised about the possibility of vitamin E thinning the blood too much, and some patients who are taking aspirin or prescription blood thinners such as warfarin (Coumadin) have been told that it is not safe to take vitamin E at the same time.

The truth is there has not been a lot of research in this area. One study suggests that taking vitamin E and low-dose aspirin concurrently provides better protection against heart disease than aspirin alone,[28] and a small study published in the *American Journal of Cardiology* reported the safety of taking Coumadin and vitamin E together.[29] Millions of people in this country—including a significant number of cardiologists—are taking both aspirin and vitamin E, and the Coumadin-E combo has never been an issue in all my years of clinical experience. Although I very, very rarely prescribe Coumadin, many of my patients take low-dose aspirin and vitamin E together and reap the benefits of both.

Again, my recommended dose of *natural* vitamin E for people with heart disease is 800 to 1,200 international units per day.

SUPPLEMENTS THAT STRENGTHEN THE HEART

The primary concern in this book, atherosclerotic heart disease, is more a disease of the arteries than the heart. However, the most serious and life-threatening outcome of this disease—a heart attack—involves damage to the heart itself. When the heart muscle is deprived of oxygen (a condition known as ischemia), inflammatory chemicals rush to the area, unleashing massive amounts of free radicals and causing cells to die. Even if the heart attack is not fatal, areas of the muscle are severely damaged, and a significant number of patients who have survived a heart attack or have extensive heart disease eventually develop heart failure. This condition arises when the weakened heart muscle simply cannot maintain circulation and fluid pools in the lungs and extremities. In fact, heart failure is often described as the end stage of heart disease.

The two supplements I am going to discuss next are crucial for anyone who has or is at risk of heart failure, as both are highly effective in protecting and preserving the heart muscle. Yet because these supplements have widespread cardiovascular benefits, I recommend them for all of my patients with heart disease.

Coenzyme Q10: Miracle Nutrient for the Heart

Every patient who comes to the Whitaker Wellness Institute with a diagnosis of heart disease is immediately started on coenzyme Q10. CoQ10 is involved in energy production within the mitochondria of your cells. It is the spark plug that gets things going. Because the heart is such a busy muscle, beating more than 100,000 times every day, CoQ10 is highly active in the heart. In addition to its role in energy production, CoQ10 has one other very important attribute: It is an exceptionally potent and active scavenger of lipid free radicals. It stabilizes the membranes of heart muscle cells and protects them against oxidative damage.

Supplemental CoQ10 has also been demonstrated to reduce chest pain and improve exercise tolerance in patients with chronic stable angina. It can lower blood pressure, improve performance on exercise stress testing, and smooth out arrhythmias.

These diverse actions make coenzyme Q10 a requisite therapy for all conditions affecting the cardiovascular system. Peter H. Langsjoen, M.D., a Texas cardiologist who has authored a number of studies on CoQ10, has been documenting the benefits of this supplement for more than thirty years. With CoQ10, Dr. Langsjoen is routinely able to reduce heart medications by 40 to 50 percent, and a significant proportion of his patients have become drug-free.

The bulk of the research on coenzyme Q10 has been on its use in the treatment of heart failure, which, as I mentioned above, is increasingly common in patients with long-term atherosclerotic heart disease. Heart failure is a serious and debilitating condition with an often-poor prognosis. It requires heavy-duty drug regimens or, in severe cases, heart transplant. Patients suffering with heart failure are virtually always deficient in CoQ10. The late Karl Folkers, M.D., who is considered to be the "father" of coenzyme Q10, measured CoQ10 levels of patients with heart failure and compared them to levels of a control group of healthy individuals. He found that three-quarters of the ill patients had moderate to severe CoQ10 deficiencies in the heart muscle.[30] Other studies have indicated that the severity of heart failure corresponds to the severity of deficiency.

The good news is that supplementing with CoQ10 dramatically prolongs the life of patients with heart failure. In one study, taking CoQ10 cut the average yearly death rate of patients with heart failure by 26 to 59 percent.[31] I have had dozens of patients at the Whitaker Wellness Institute with very serious heart failure whose conditions were reversed by taking large doses of coenzyme Q10. Some were even awaiting a heart transplant, and after taking CoQ10 for a few months, they got off the transplant list!

My first patient to experience the incredible benefits of

CoQ10 was Charmaine. When she came to see me she was as near death as any patient I had ever seen. The poor functioning of her heart had resulted in the collection of more than 70 pounds of excess fluid. Her legs were so swollen that the skin had split, and when she wasn't in a wheelchair, she was propped up in bed, breathless and disoriented. She was on all the standard medications for severe heart failure, and she had been told she had no more than six months to live. All I did was start her on a nutritional regimen, including large doses of coenzyme Q10. The results were immediate and miraculous. Within a few weeks she had lost all the extra fluid and was out of bed, engaging in most of her usual activities. Four years later Charmaine was taking no heart medications at all and was leading a normal, active life.

As I described in chilling detail in Chapter 9, I am convinced that one reason so many patients with coronary heart disease develop heart failure is because of the enormous popularity of the statin cholesterol-lowering drugs. While these drugs reduce the production of cholesterol in the liver, they also lower the production of coenzyme Q10—in the very group of patients who need it the most. According to one study, statin drugs lowered CoQ10 levels by 40 percent![32] The drug companies seem to know this, for one of them has patents on statin-CoQ10 combination drugs, but they haven't come out with such drugs, nor do they educate physicians or patients about this very real danger of taking statins.

CoQ10 is synthesized in the body, and it is present in our diet. (Beef, poultry, and broccoli are particularly good sources.) However, if you have heart disease, coenzyme Q10 should be high on your list of essential supplements. The dose we recommend for our heart patients is 200 to 400 milligrams per day, in divided doses. (Patients with heart failure may double this dose.) Because it is fat soluble, this supplement is much better absorbed when taken with some oil or fat. Oil-based capsules are probably the best-absorbed form, and chewable wafers that contain a little stabilized oil are also good. Take them with meals to ensure even better absorption.

L-Carnitine

L-carnitine is also involved in cellular energy production. It is critical in the transportation of fatty acids into the mitochondria, where they are burned for fuel. If coenzyme Q10 is the spark plug in this process, carnitine is the fuel pump, and a well-functioning heart requires both. Healthy heart tissues have plenty of carnitine reserves. Those with a less than adequate oxygen supply are often deficient in this essential nutrient, which may lead to angina and other symptoms of heart disease.

Several studies document supplemental carnitine's ability to reduce angina and risk of heart attack. It improves exercise endurance and may even be an effective alternative to drugs used to treat angina. In one study, 200 patients with angina brought on by exercise were treated with the usual drugs (nitroglycerin, beta-blockers, calcium channel blockers, etc.) alone, or drugs plus 2,000 milligrams daily of carnitine. After six months, the group taking carnitine had improvements in performance on exercise stress testing—including a 70 percent reduction in EKG changes indicative of inadequate oxygen delivery to the heart. They also experienced fewer arrhythmias and more significant drops in cholesterol and triglycerides than the patients who were taking only medications.[33]

Because they are both involved in energy production, l-carnitine and coenzyme Q10 work synergistically, and I recommend you take them both. The suggested dose of l-carnitine is 1,000 to 2,000 milligrams in divided doses. It is very safe, with no known side effects. Make sure the supplement you take is l-carnitine, not d-carnitine or d,l-carnitine—the *d* form interferes with natural l-carnitine.

PROTECT AND NURTURE YOUR ARTERIES

Maintaining the integrity of the coronary arteries is key in the prevention and treatment of heart disease. Vitamins C and E and other antioxidants protect these delicate structures from free radical damage. The B-complex vitamins keep down levels of homocysteine, which is particularly damaging to the endothelial cells lining the arteries. And the nutrients that curb inflammation also nurture the blood vessels in their own way.

There are two other nutritional supplements I want to tell you about that prevent and treat heart disease because of their unique effects on the arteries: magnesium and arginine.

Magnesium: Multifaceted Mineral for Heart Disease

Magnesium is a vital nutrient for your cardiovascular system. It increases the heart's supply of oxygen, retards vessel blockages, and prevents the formation of blood clots. Magnesium also has a relaxing effect on the smooth muscles of the arteries and other tissues. This makes it an invaluable therapy for muscle spasms, asthma (which involves dilation of the bronchioles), and, of course, cardiovascular disease.

Let's first look at magnesium's effects on high blood pressure which, in a nutshell, is caused by too much tension in the arteries. Population-based studies have shown that people who consume higher levels of magnesium have lower blood pressures. Geographic areas with naturally high levels of magnesium in the water enjoy lower rates of hypertension and other cardiovascular diseases. In a 1998 study, 60 patients with hypertension, ranging in age from the mid-thirties to the mid-seventies, were divided into two groups and given either magnesium supplements or a placebo for eight weeks. The two groups were then crossed over—those on magnesium were switched to the placebo, and vice versa, for another eight weeks. Blood pressures were significantly lower when the patients were taking magnesium, and the individuals with the highest blood pressure at the study's onset had the greatest reductions.[34]

Despite the findings of these and other studies, most physicians ignore the clear association between magnesium and hypertension. Instead, they prescribe drugs such as diuretics, which actually deplete your body of this precious mineral, and calcium channel blockers. Calcium channel blockers, as their name implies, prevent calcium from entering cells. This promotes relaxation of the artery walls so that blood can flow more freely, angina eases, and blood pressure falls.

Guess what? Magnesium does the same thing! In fact, it has been called "nature's calcium channel blocker" because it too restricts the entry of calcium into cells. This is how it relaxes the arteries and improves blood flow. Yet magnesium has none of the harmful side effects of these drugs, which in some studies have been shown to actually increase the risk of heart attack. (See Chapter 9 for more on these drugs.)

Another very important protective mechanism of magnesium is its ability to restore normal heart rhythm. Heart attacks turn fatal when abnormal arrhythmias develop. The heart turns from a powerfully beating muscle that moves life-sustaining blood throughout the body into a quivering, ineffective organ with erratic electrical activity. Because magnesium is involved in the firings of nerves and muscles, it helps smooth out arrhythmias. This can mean the difference between life and death for some patients with heart disease.

Although it is most commonly taken as an oral supplement, studies show that intravenous magnesium can correct even severe, life-threatening cardiac arrhythmias. When given to patients immediately after a heart attack, it can be a lifesaver. In one study of 194 acute heart attack patients who were not candidates for blood thinners, 96 patients received intravenous magnesium for forty-eight hours while 98 received a placebo. The benefits of magnesium treatment were dramatic. The in-hospital death rate for patients receiving magnesium was only a quarter that of the placebo group, and they also experienced far fewer complications.[35]

Unfortunately, the typical American diet of meat, dairy products, and processed foods has produced a near-epidemic of magnesium deficiency in this country, with most adults getting barely half the government's meager recommended daily amounts. If you have heart disease, supplementation is crucial to ensure adequate magnesium levels. The recommend dose is 1,000 milligrams of magnesium daily, balanced in a 1:2 or 1:1 ratio with calcium, which has heart benefits of its own (1,000 milligrams of magnesium to 1,000 to 2,000 milligrams of calcium).

Arginine: Artery-Protecting Amino Acid

The arteries are not passive pipes but responsive conduits that send out and pick up chemical signals, contract or relax as needed, and repair themselves. The inner lining of the arteries, the endothelium, produces a number of chemical messengers, and one of the most important is the gaseous molecule nitric oxygen (NO). NO signals the release of important hormones and acts as a neurotransmitter in the brain. It is used by the immune system to kill marauding bacteria and cancer cells. NO is even involved in the formation of erections. Most important for our discussion, it protects the cardiovascular system, helping to stave off heart disease.

As we discussed in Chapter 2, NO combats heart disease in several ways. It protects the endothelial cells, it is a potent antioxidant (more powerful than vitamin E, according to some studies), and it prevents platelets in the blood from sticking together. NO also relaxes the arteries and prevents arterial spasms that cause angina. (This is how nitroglycerin works to relieve chest pain in heart patients—it is converted to NO.)

Unfortunately, once the atherosclerotic process has taken hold, it gains a momentum of its own. Damaged arteries make less NO, and inadequate production of NO increases arterial damage. There is a way, however, to break this vicious cycle. An essential ingredient in the production of nitric oxide is the amino acid l-arginine.[36] By taking supplemental arginine you provide your remaining healthy endothelial cells with the raw material they require to boost production of NO. Arginine supplements have been shown to restore normal function in damaged arteries. A study published in *Circulation* showed that long-term arginine supplementation in patients with high cholesterol was associated with a reduction in the thickness of plaque.[37] Other studies have demonstrated improvements in exercise capacity, peripheral artery disease, and angina.

When NO was first discovered in the arteries, it was named endothelium-derived relaxing factor (EDRF) because it is such a powerful vasodilator. Released by the endothelium, it signals the smooth muscle cells of the arteries to relax, thus increasing their diameter. Therefore, NO is a primary regulator of blood pressure, and when its synthesis is inhibited, blood pressure soars. Boosting NO levels with supplemental arginine is an effective therapy for hypertension. An Italian study of patients with newly diagnosed mild hypertension demonstrated that two grams of oral arginine lowered systolic blood pressure by 20 mm Hg after only a week of supplementation.[38]

The recommended starting dose of arginine is 1 gram three times a day, although some people require double that dose (2 grams three times a day) to notice benefits. Like other amino acids, arginine is best absorbed when taken on an empty stomach, or at least in the absence of protein. If you experience stomach upset when taking it this way, try it with some carbohydrate-containing food, but eating protein at the same time may impair absorption. Consult your physician before starting arginine if you are taking Viagra, nitroglycerin or a related drug, or if any of the following currently apply to you: pregnancy, migraines, autoimmune disorders, AIDS, cirrhosis, depression, or breast cancer

Iron: One Supplement You Don't Need

If you have heart disease, there is one nutritional supplement you do not want to take, and that is iron. Iron is an essential mineral, and deficiencies are quite common in areas of the world where malnutrition is an issue, as well as among teenage girls and pregnant women in this country. However, for most Americans—and particularly those concerned about heart disease—the issue with iron is not deficiencies but excesses. Unlike other minerals, iron is not excreted from the body. Once inside, it must either be used or stored, and excesses of stored iron are very harmful. Iron accelerates the production of free radicals that bode ill for many systems in the body, including the heart and arteries. It oxidizes LDL cholesterol, and it harms the arteries, both through free radical damage and by interfering with the action of nitric oxide. High iron stores have been linked to an increased risk of heart attack.[39]

Eating lots of iron-rich red meat can cause excessive iron buildup, as can hemochromatosis, a fairly common inherited disease. An often-overlooked source of excess iron is nutritional supplements, so make sure your multivitamin and mineral supplement does not contain iron (unless, of course, you are at high risk of iron deficiency). I also recommend having periodic blood tests for ferritin levels, especially as you get older. If you are storing too much iron, there is an easy and altruistic way of getting rid of it: give blood regularly.

(although arginine fights many types of cancer, very high doses may increase breast tumor growth). While there are no firm contraindications to arginine in these conditions, I believe it is prudent to wait until further research clarifies potential interactions.

SUPPLEMENTS TO IMPROVE INSULIN RESISTANCE

As we discussed in Chapter 3, insulin resistance and heart disease all too often go hand in hand. This condition arises from an inability of the cells to properly utilize insulin—insulin knocks on the cells to let glucose in, but there is no answer. Blood sugar levels thus rise, and the pancreas churns out more and more insulin until the cells finally get the message and allow glucose to enter. Insulin resistance is associated with elevated triglycerides, lowered HDL cholesterol, and abnormalities in clotting and inflammatory factors.

If you are overweight, especially around the abdomen, and have high blood pressure or high triglycerides, it is likely that you are insulin resistant. Because heart disease and insulin resistance are so closely related, the Whitaker Wellness Institute treatment program for the two conditions is similar. (For more on insulin resistance and diabetes, read my book *Reversing Diabetes*.) Both include regular exercise, a diet very close to that detailed in this book, and a basic high-dose nutritional supplement regimen like the one described in the previous chapter. For my heart disease patients who are also diabetic or insulin resistant, however, I like to add the following supplements.

Chromium-Vanadium: One-Two Punch Against Insulin Resistance

Two of the most effective supplements for insulin resistance and type 2 diabetes are the trace minerals chromium and vanadium. Both of these minerals improve insulin resistance by increasing the cells' sensitivity to insulin—they stimulate receptors on the cells that let glucose enter.

At least fifteen controlled studies support chromium's positive effects on blood sugar and insulin levels. It affects another aspect of insulin resistance as well: Chromium facilitates weight loss and thus helps combat obesity. In addition, this mineral modestly improves blood lipid levels.[40] Chromium deficiencies are not uncommon in people with atherosclerosis. Howard A. Newman, M.D., of Ohio State University, compared angiography findings with blood chromium levels and found that patients with signs of coronary artery disease had significantly lower chromium levels than patients with intact arteries.[41] The best-absorbed forms of chromium are chromium polynicotinate and chromium picolinate, and my recommended dose is 200 to 400 micrograms per day.

Much of the research on vanadyl sulfate, the most commonly used form of the trace mineral vanadium, has involved using very high doses (100 to 150 milligrams) to treat diabetes. Several studies have demonstrated that this mineral lowers blood sugar levels in both type 1 and type 2 diabetics, sometimes quite dramatically.[42] The dose of vanadyl sulfate we recommend for our patients with insulin resistance is much less than the therapeutic dose for diabetes. Fifteen to 45 milligrams per day is adequate to help improve insulin sensitivity, and it is safe and well tolerated by most people. Minor side effects may include gastrointestinal upset.

Versatile Lipoic Acid

Lipoic acid (also called alpha lipoic acid or thioctic acid) is an antioxidant that works in both the aqueous and lipid areas of the body. It is a very small molecule and is thus able to enter virtually all tissues to neutralize free radicals. Because it is so powerful and versatile, we use lipoic acid at the Whitaker Wellness Institute for many conditions. Lipoic acid has been very well studied for its ability to lower blood sugar and to improve insulin sensitivity, and for this reason it should be of interest to heart patients who also have insulin resistance.[43] The recommended dose is a minimum of 100 to 200 milligrams per day, although patients with diabetes may take up to 600 milligrams.

REVIEW OF SUPPLEMENT RECOMMENDATIONS

As I mentioned in the previous chapter, a foundation of good health is a high-potency daily multivitamin and mineral supplement. If your multinutrient supplement does not meet my recommended levels of vitamins and minerals listed on page 246, make sure you beef them up to approximate the suggested doses. Once you have this covered, then consider adding some of the nutritional supplements for reversing heart disease discussed in this chapter. These supplements are safe and well tolerated. If you are pregnant or nursing, consult your physician before taking any of these supplements. (With the exception of fish oil, I do not routinely recommend these "extra" supplements for children.)

In this chapter's text, I grouped the various nutritional supplements according to which risk factors they address. Here, in summary, I am listing them with suggested doses and primary modes of action. (Keep in mind, however, that many supplements have multiple therapeutic benefits.)

Do not be overwhelmed by this rather lengthy list—it could have been much longer. Other herbs such as hawthorn, additional amino acids like l-lysine, and other nutrients also have a place in the treatment of heart disease. I only included what I feel to be the cream of the crop. Notice that the starred nutrients are found in most multivitamin and mineral supplements (although most likely in smaller doses). With the exception of arginine, take your supplements with food and in divided doses. At the institute we suggest taking them with breakfast and with dinner for maximum absorption, tolerance, and compliance.

Nutritional Supplement and Primary Actions	Suggested Dose
To Counter Free Radicals (Antioxidants)	
*Vitamin E	800–1,200 international units
*Vitamin C	1,500–5,000 milligrams
*Beta carotene	15,000 international units
*Vitamin A	5,000 international units
*Selenium	200 micrograms
To Lower Cholesterol and Triglycerides	
Fish oil	2,000–10,000 milligrams
Inositol hexaniacinate (niacin derivative)	500–1,000 milligrams 3 times a day
Red yeast rice	1,200–2,400 milligrams
Policosanol	10 milligrams
To Keep Homocysteine in Control	
*Folic acid	1,200–1,600 micrograms
*Vitamin B12	100–1,000 micrograms (age-dependent)
*Vitamin B6	100 milligrams
Trimethylglycine	1,000 milligrams
To Strengthen the Heart Muscle	
Coenzyme Q10	200–400 milligrams
L-carnitine	1,000–2,000 milligrams
To Protect and Relax the Arteries	
*Magnesium	1,000 milligrams (balanced with 1,000–2,000 milligrams calcium)
L-arginine	3,000 milligrams
To Improve Insulin Resistance	
*Chromium	200–400 micrograms
Vanadyl sulfate	15–45 milligrams
Lipoic acid	100–200 milligrams

*Found in most multivitamin and mineral supplements, although not always in suggested doses

CHAPTER 15

Exercise for a Healthy Heart

IMAGINE SITTING IN YOUR DOCTOR'S OFFICE. HE SAYS, "I'M GOING to write you a prescription that will help you lose weight, eliminate insomnia, reduce stress and anxiety, curb your appetite, improve your creativity, tone your muscles, enhance your self-image, increase your confidence, protect you from a heart attack and diabetes, and, regardless of how you feel now, make you feel better."

"Wonderful," you say, "but that must cost a lot."

"No, it's free except for about thirty to forty-five minutes of your time four or five days a week. It's exercise."

Virtually every patient who comes to the Whitaker Wellness Institute goes away with an exercise prescription—it is an essential part of our treatment program for all health challenges, and heart disease is no exception. A sedentary lifestyle is a well-recognized independent risk factor for heart disease. Unfortunately, according to a 2000 article, published in *The Lancet*, despite all the evidence of its benefits, cardiologists rarely prescribe exercise to their patients with heart disease.[1] Even if an exercise program is suggested, its significance is rarely stressed, and patients are given little help in implementing and sticking with an exercise regimen.

While I am not suggesting that exercise is a cure-all, it truly is a powerful therapy for the prevention and treatment of heart disease. Exercise adds years to your life and life to your years. It not only lessens the likelihood that you might have a heart attack, but if you do have one, you're more likely to live through it.

THE CASE FOR EXERCISE

Physicians have historically viewed lack of physical activity as only a minor risk factor for heart disease. Yet scores of studies clearly show an inverse relationship between physical activity and death from heart disease: The more active you are, the lower your risk. The research dates back to 1953, when Professor Jeremy Morris of the British Medical Research Council published a study comparing the death rates of the bus drivers and conductors of the London Transport Department. The paper, entitled "Coronary Heart Disease and Physical Activity at Work," reported that conductors had one-third less heart disease than drivers, and only half the number of fatal and nonfatal heart attacks. The reason? Exercise![2]

As you probably know, most buses in London are double-decker, and the conductors' job was to collect fares from each passenger. While the drivers sat all day, the conductors were constantly moving. Collecting fares on a double-decker bus required a level of exertion equivalent to climbing up and down the stairs of a two-story house a hundred times a day. Since this was the first study of its kind, Dr. Morris pointed out that the reduced death rate of the conductors could be due to other causes, but his observations opened everyone's eyes to the potential value of exercise.

Further studies quickly followed. One study revealed that among postal workers, those who delivered mail on foot had one-half the heart problems as those who sorted mail. Another showed that active railroad switchmen had only one-third the incidence of heart disease as sedentary ticket clerks. Yet another compared the rates of heart disease of farmers who did one to two hours of heavy labor every day and men engaged in less active work—farmers had an 82 percent lower risk of heart disease compared to sedentary workers.

Daniel Bruner, a doctor from Israel, had a unique opportunity to study people living on a kibbutz. This was an ideal study group, for the environment, diet, and facilities were uniform, regardless of age, sex, or occupation. The one difference among the kibbutz residents was job duties. Some did clerical work, prepared food, or took care of the children, while others worked in the fields or did carpentry and building. Dr. Bruner found that heart disease was 2.5 to 4 times greater in the sedentary workers than in the active workers. In every large study of this type, heart disease rates in active workers were considerably less than those of their sedentary counterparts.

"But, doctor," you may lament, "I'm not a postman or a bus conductor. My job requires that I sit at a desk for eight hours a day!" Activity doesn't have to be work related—and for most of us, it will not be. In 1973, twenty years after his landmark study of the bus conductors, Dr. Morris published a study of the leisure-time activities of 17,000 British civil servants. He found that those who engaged in vigorous leisure activities such as brisk walking, swimming, bicycling, or soccer for thirty minutes a day had only one-third the heart problems of those whose leisure activities were sedentary. He also found that the more vigorous the exercise, the lower the incidence of heart disease.[3]

All that matters is that you get moving. Dr. Ralph S. Paffenbarger, Jr., professor of epidemiology at Stanford University School of Medicine, rated various activities in terms of calories of energy expenditure. For instance, climbing one flight of stairs once a day expends 28 calories per week, while walking one city block per day expends 56 calories. Light sports burn 5 calories a minute, and strenuous sports 10 calories a minute. Dr. Paffenbarger then surveyed 17,000 men concerning their activities during a typical week and divided them into three groups based upon the number of calories they expended in exercise. He found that the sedentary men who burned up fewer than 500 calories a week in exercise had twice the heart attack rate as the men who expended more than 2,000 calories a week.[4] If you average thirty minutes a day briskly walking, swimming, bicycling, or jogging, you can easily meet this caloric expenditure.

If you've already had a heart attack, exercise may be even more important. In a 2000 study, published in *Circulation*, researchers enrolled more than 400 men and women who had had heart attacks and followed them for seven years. They found that the people who increased their exercise following their heart attacks were much less likely to suffer a second heart attack—they reduced their chances of a second event by 78 percent! An intriguing aspect of this study was that the physical activities weren't exceptionally vigorous. Walking, swimming, even heavy gardening offered protection.[5]

Even if you don't have heart disease, regular physical activity will improve many aspects of your health—and likely extend your life. Exercise reduces death rates from all causes, not just heart disease. Medical records of thousands of Harvard University alumni, who are part of a long-term study begun in 1962, were analyzed and compared with their exercise habits. The benefits of physical activity were striking. The men who engaged in regular physical activity experienced a significantly lower risk of death, not just from heart disease but from all causes, compared to men who were inactive.[6]

HOW EXERCISE BENEFITS THE CARDIOVASCULAR SYSTEM

By the time we reach adolescence, most of us have some degree of plaque present in our arteries. Our unhealthy diet and lifestyle begin to take their toll early in life. Regular physical activity may not entirely reverse the atherosclerotic process, but it will slow it down. Here are the primary ways in which exercise benefits the cardiovascular system and reduces the risk of heart attack.

1. *Exercise Conditions the Heart*

Regular exercise causes a sustained and measurable increase in the function of the heart. It increases the efficiency of oxygen utilization by the heart, which means that a conditioned heart can extract more oxygen from the blood than an unconditioned heart. As we age, our capacity to utilize oxygen goes down. However, regular physical exercise can give a sixty-year-old the same maximum oxygen utilization as a forty-year-old.

Like any muscle, the heart becomes stronger with regular use. The conditioned heart is able to pump more blood with each beat than the unconditioned heart. This reduces the workload of the heart and the resting heart rate drops. The average heart rate of an unconditioned heart at rest is about 75 to 85 beats per minute. After several weeks of exercise, as the heart becomes stronger and more efficient, resting heart rate may slow to 65, 60, or even lower. A decline of 20 beats per minute quickly adds up—1,200 fewer beats per hour, 28,800 fewer beats per day, and 10,512,000 fewer beats per year—and means less work for the heart.

Another advantage of a slower heartbeat is that it results in more blood flow in the coronary arteries. The heart receives blood only between beats, because the valves that allow blood to flow to the heart muscle are closed when the heart contracts to pump blood. They open only when the heart is relaxed in the resting phase of its cycle. Since the conditioned heart has a much longer rest period, more blood is able to flow to the heart muscle.

2. *Exercise Improves Blood Lipids and Thins the Blood*

Although exercise does not significantly lower total cholesterol levels, it is one of the few things that has been shown to raise levels of protective HDL cholesterol. It does this by burning up the fatty complexes that make up LDL cholesterol and replacing them with the denser HDL variety. This has a favorable effect on the arteries and protects against atherosclerosis. Exercise also clears triglycerides out of the bloodstream. In fact, regular exercise has been shown to bring triglyceride levels in the 250 to 350 mg/dl range down to normal in less than a week. As a result, blood cells are less likely to stick together and impede circulation, and the blood is thinner and more fluid.

3. *Exercise Enlarges the Coronary Arteries*

The Masai, a cattle-herding people in Africa, thrive on a high-fat diet. Wandering from grazing ground to grazing ground with their cattle, Masai men have their food supply with them on the hoof. They milk their cows and regularly bleed them, collecting the blood in a gourd, mixing it with milk, and drinking it. In spite of this high-fat concoction, they seem to have no heart disease. George Mann, M.D., of Vanderbilt University, published a study in the 1960s showing that the electrocardiograms of the Masai were normal and that heart attacks were indeed rare.[7] This study was gleefully pounced upon by the meat and dairy industries in this country as proof that meat and milk didn't cause atherosclerosis.

However, when Dr. Mann went back to Africa and performed autopsies on 50 Masai warriors who had died of various causes, he found that their arteries were as severely damaged by atherosclerosis as those of American men of the same age. The difference was that their arteries were twice the size of the average American's. He attributed this to the fact that the Masai put in ten to twenty miles a day walking with their cattle. Their arteries, enlarged by exercise, were able to deliver an adequate supply of blood and oxygen, even though they were loaded with plaque.[8]

4. *Exercise Increases Collateral Circulation*

When the coronary arteries begin to close down due to atherosclerotic blockages, the body attempts to build new arteries that travel around the blockages. These new circulatory pathways are called collaterals, and they have spared millions of men and women from a fatal heart attack. In a sense, there is a race between the progress of atherosclerosis and the development of collateral arteries: If atherosclerosis wins, you could have a heart attack. If collateralization wins, you are spared. Numerous studies have shown that exercise accelerates the development of collaterals.

5. *Exercise Reduces Blood Pressure*

Hundreds of studies clearly prove that regular exercise lowers blood pressure, which is a very significant risk factor for heart disease. Improvements in blood flow engendered by regular exercise result in lower resistance on the arteries and thus lower blood pressure. An Australian research team analyzed twenty-nine randomized controlled trials, involving 1,533 participants, of the effects of exercise on hypertension. In study subjects who had exercised, systolic blood pressure was reduced by an average of 4.7 mm Hg and diastolic blood pressure by an average 3.1 mm Hg, compared to sedentary study participants. These reductions were independent of exercise intensity—high-intensity exercise was no more effective than moderate-intensity workouts. An interesting finding of this study was that as a means of controlling blood pressure, exercising three times a week was plenty. More frequent exercise sessions yielded no additional effects.[9]

6. *Exercise Improves Insulin Resistance*

Exercise also has a profound influence on the prevention and treatment of insulin resistance, the condition in which cells become unresponsive to insulin's message to let glucose in. As we discussed in Chapter 4, insulin resistance is a very significant risk factor for heart disease. Exercise enables cells to extract glucose from the blood, even in the absence of insulin, by prompting special proteins called GLUT-4 transporters to rise to the cells' surface and let in glucose.[10] In addition to its immediate effect of lowering blood sugar, exercise also improves insulin sensitivity over the long haul. It increases the number of GLUT-4 transporters and thus the cells' ability to properly utilize insulin.

Another way in which exercise combats insulin resistance is by promoting body fat losses and increasing muscle mass. Loss of abdominal fat is particularly important in preventing and controlling insulin resistance, for it is more metabolically active than other fat stores. A 2000 study found that regular exercise lowered abdominal fat stores, which resulted in reductions in insulin levels. The authors of this study suggested that decreasing abdominal fat may lower insulin secretion and prevent or improve insulin resistance and all the conditions associated with it, including atherosclerosis, hypertension, and abnormalities in blood lipids.[11]

7. *Exercise Facilitates Weight Loss*

Excess weight is another risk factor for heart disease. If you want to lose pounds and maintain your ideal weight, of course you'll need to watch your diet. But it has been my experience over the past thirty years that it is impossible to sustain normal weight without regular exercise. Fad diets, prescription weight-loss drugs, and magic supplements that promise to melt away pounds with no changes in your lifestyle are absolute bunk. Even if you do lose a few pounds at the onset, you can expect them to come back on. For the vast majority of people, weight maintenance boils down to this: If you eat more calories than you burn, you'll gain weight, and if you burn more calories than you eat, you'll lose weight. The best way to burn more calories is to exercise. As you increase your lean muscle mass and shed excess body fat with exercise, your resting metabolism rate will increase. This means you'll burn more calories even when you are not exercising, which obviously gives a further boost to weight under control.

ADDITIONAL BENEFITS OF EXERCISE

Exercise physiologists sometimes describe the benefits derived from exercise as the "SAID" principle: specific adaptations to imposed demands. In other words, the body will respond or adapt to the repetitive forces placed upon it, becoming stronger and able to perform better the next time it is called upon to do that particular task. The bones become denser, the muscles more powerful, and the cardiovascular system more efficient at pumping blood and oxygen throughout the body. Here are a few of the additional benefits of regular physical activity.

A Mood Elevator

You may find runners to be arrogant, humble, opinionated, flexible, pushy, courteous, loud, or soft-spoken. But you won't find them to be depressed. In fact, regular physical exercise and depression are virtually incompatible, so much so that exercise is a common prescription for emotional problems. One psychiatrist I know of in the San Diego area conducts group and individual therapy sessions while walking or jogging along the beach!

John H. Greist, M.D., professor of psychiatry at the University of Wisconsin, divided depressed patients into three different groups. Eight patients received no therapy but were enrolled in a jogging program. Seven patients received behavior modification training, and nine received insight-oriented therapy. After twelve weeks the runners fared the best—six of the eight got over their depression completely, while those enrolled in behavior modification reported some improvement, and patients in the therapy group were more depressed than before they started.[12]

How could jogging succeed where therapy failed? Mood is influenced by a complex balance of neurotransmitters and other chemical messengers in the brain. Antidepressant drugs manipulate the amounts and balances of these various brain chemicals. Exercise does the same thing, only in a more natural and much safer way. It literally floods the entire system with norepinephrine, a neurohormone that energizes the brain, and endorphins, which activate the pleasure centers in the brain and promote optimism and that elusive feeling of well-being.

Walter M. Bortz II, M.D., from Stanford University School of Medicine, measured norepinephrine and endorphin levels in several well-trained athletes before, during, and after a particularly grueling race. (The winner of this 100-mile race finished in eighteen hours and thirty-five minutes!) To qualify for entry, each participant had to have completed a fifty-mile race. The norepinephrine and endorphin levels of these athletes were higher than the laboratory's normal values before the race, and they went up markedly during and after the race. They were, in fact, the highest levels ever recorded by that laboratory.[13]

No doubt about it—exercise stirs up the "feel-good" brain chemicals. And you don't need to run a hundred miles. A 2000 study of older adults with major depression demonstrated that exercising just fifteen minutes three times a week proved as effective as the prescription antidepressant Zoloft in relieving depression. Six months later, patients who had exercised were less likely to have relapsed into depression than those who had taken the drug.[14]

Better Brain Function

Exercise improves blood flow and oxygen delivery not only to the heart but throughout the body. Vigorous exercise can increase your oxygen uptake by 1,000 percent! Nowhere is this more beneficial than in the brain, for this three-pound organ utilizes 25 percent of the oxygen you take in. If the brain is deprived of oxygen for only a few minutes, brain cells die. By delivering more oxygen, glucose, and other nutrients to the brain, exercise improves alertness, memory, and other aspects of cognitive function.

Exercise's effects on mental function were demonstrated in a study conducted by researchers at the Veterans' Medical Center in Salt Lake City, Utah. They compared the cognitive function of senior citizens who were sedentary to others who exercised by briskly walking for fifty minutes three times a week. After four months, they administered tests of reaction time, visual organization, memory, and mental flexibility to the study participants. The exercisers outperformed the couch potatoes in every category.[15]

Stronger Bones

Stress on the bones stimulates the formation of new bone cells. Regardless of age, people who engage in regular weight-bearing exercise have higher bone density. The repeated stress placed on the bones when you jog, walk, climb stairs, play tennis, or lift weights breaks down bone cells, and they are replaced with stronger, newer growth. (Swimming is not a weight-bearing exercise since the body is supported by water.)

One of my colleagues, a sports medicine specialist who has trained professional athletes, told me that when the runners he treated complained of sharp pain in their lower legs he often suspected a hairline fracture. However, in many cases, doing X rays on these athletes was a waste of time. Their leg bones were so dense that he couldn't make out the microfractures. All exercisers receive this same protective benefit, with studies suggesting that regular weight-bearing exercise of any type can increase bone mass by 5 to 10 percent. However, the absolute best activity for improving bone density is weight lifting. If you are at risk for osteoporosis—this condition of thin, weak bones is particularly prevalent among older women of slight build—adding just two sessions of weight training per week to a good aerobic exercise program just might turn your condition around.

WHAT TYPE OF EXERCISE?

For most people, the word "exercise" brings to mind aerobic activities such as fast walking, jogging, swimming, tennis, squash, and cycling. These activities cause the heart to beat faster, the lungs to bring in more air, and oxygen delivery to the muscles and heart to increase. I definitely recommend aerobic exercise as a means of strengthening the cardiovascular system. Whatever form of aerobic exercise you choose—brisk walking is fine—exercise to the point that you get your heart and respiration rates up. If you feel like you aren't working hard enough, you probably aren't. (More on this below.)

A less well recognized but equally important form of exercise is weight training, also referred to as anaerobic exercise, isometrics, weight lifting, or strength training. Whatever the moniker, this type of exercise increases the tone and bulk of muscle. I cannot overstate the benefits of weight training, especially as we get older. We lose more than six pounds of lean muscle mass per decade of life after our twenties, and this loss is accelerated after age forty-five. Some of this decline is age-related. However, the primary reason our muscles shrink is that we don't use them. And only one thing restores muscle mass: weight training. (As I mentioned earlier, weight training is also crucial for maintaining bone density.)

It is never too late to begin weight training. You need to lose the idea that weight lifting is for muscle-bound, hard-bodied young men and women. The people who would benefit most from this type of exercise are older men and women who are rapidly losing muscle mass. Yet few adults of any age do regular strength training—and only 5 percent of older men and 1 percent of older women engage in this type of exercise, according to a 2000 survey by the Centers for Disease Control and Prevention.[16] This is unfortunate, for it is exactly the type of activity that experts state keeps older people independent and out of nursing homes.

I wish there were a way to begin weight training on your own. However, after years of giving patients vague recommendations to buy hand weights and do specific exercises, I am convinced that you need some instruction to get started right. It doesn't have to be with a personal trainer, although this is a very good option. A group class at your gym or some instruction from a friend experienced in weight training would be fine. Once you get the hang of lifting and understand the basics of proper technique, you can continue on your own.

Regardless of what type of exercise you engage in, each session should begin with five or ten minutes of gentle stretching and warm-up to loosen your major muscles and prevent strain and injury. Each stretch should be done slowly and held for fifteen to thirty seconds. Never force a muscle or bounce during a stretch. When the muscle is stretched too fast, it reacts by tightening slightly to protect itself from tearing. You end up with a muscle that is tighter than it was before you began the stretch! Some people enjoy forms of exercise such as yoga and tai chi, which involve gentle stretching exercises, often in conjunction with deep breathing. These activities can be very pleasant and imbue a sense of tranquility and calm that relieves stress and negative emotions. I highly endorse them but suggest you do them in addition to—not in place of—aerobic exercise and weight training.

BEFORE YOU BEGIN, GET AN EXERCISE STRESS TEST

The first thing you need to do before starting an exercise program is to see your doctor about an exercise stress test. The best way to evaluate the engine of a car is not to just look under the hood but to start it up, drive it around, and kick up the RPMs to see how it runs at higher speeds. An exercise stress test is like a road test of your heart, revealing problems that wouldn't be seen on a resting electrocardiogram (EKG). It is not uncommon for a patient to have an entirely normal resting EKG but have abnormalities when the heart beats at a higher rate during and just after exercise. Such abnormalities are often present in the absence of symptoms—which is why exercise stress testing is so valuable.

An exercise stress test can show if exercise brings on an oxygen deficit, stimulates abnormal rhythms, or results in a drop in blood pressure. It will reveal electrical abnormalities that could compromise the pumping efficiency of the heart and other changes indicative of coronary artery disease. One of the most important observations is simply how long you can exercise on the treadmill and how you feel while exercising. A trained interpreter of stress test findings can even locate blocked arteries and estimate their severity by evaluating changes in electrical activity during an exercise stress test. (For more on exercise stress testing, refer to Chapter 6.) Armed with this information, your physician can help you design an exercise program.

YOUR EXERCISE PRESCRIPTION

If you came to the Whitaker Wellness Institute, you would receive an individualized exercise prescription. It would designate the types of exercise you should engage in, as well as frequency, intensity, and duration. Conditioning the heart means building up to specific goals, then working to maintain them. We would teach you how to monitor your heart rate and heed your built-in warning system to determine your ideal level of intensity. We would also show you how to modify your program as your conditioning improved.

This is not to say you cannot create your own exercise prescription. Incorporating exercise into your daily life requires a good measure of common sense as much as anything else—key concepts are moderation and regularity. If you have heart disease, however, I cannot emphasize enough the importance of having an exercise stress test before you get started on an exercise program.

Here are the basic principles of a therapeutic exercise program for heart disease.

1. Type of Exercise: Your choice, but it must be vigorous enough to elevate your heart rate.
2. *Exercise Heart Rate: The highest heart rate that is safe for you is age-dependent. To determine yours, subtract your current age from 220. If you are sixty years old, your maximum heart rate is 160; if you are forty, it is 180. You should never allow your heart rate to go above this number. Your exercise or training heart rate should be 75 to 85 percent of the maximum. For example, if you are fifty years old, 220 − 50 = 170; 75 to 85 percent of 170 = 128 to 145. Therefore, you should aim for a pulse rate between 128 and 145 beats per minute.
3. Frequency: Generally, exercise should be done at least four times weekly and at most six times weekly. Take one or two days of rest every week.
4. Duration: You should start slowly and build up to about forty-five minutes a day, in divided sessions if necessary. New research suggests that short bursts of activity scattered throughout the day, rather than a single, prolonged exercise session, are also beneficial for the heart.[17]

A typical prescription for someone sixty years old might be as follows:

Type: Walking briskly
Frequency: 5 times weekly
Exercise heart rate: 120 beats per minute (220 − 60 = 160 × .75 = 120)
Duration: 35 minutes per session

*The best way to monitor your heart rate is to find your pulse on one of your carotid arteries, the large arteries on either side of your neck, or inside one of your wrists. Check your pulse immediately after you stop exercising (this is important), count the number of beats in six seconds, then multiply it by ten.

THE MET SYSTEM

I want to tell you about a more precise method of prescribing exercise that we use at the clinic. We base our exercise prescriptions on what is known as the MET system (MET is short for metabolic equivalent). It is useful because so many patients with heart disease or hypertension take drugs that alter or blunt the normal heart response during exercise. These patients cannot get an accurate measure of how hard they are working by measuring their pulse or heart rate. The MET system quantifies the amount of work a particular activity demands from the heart. One MET is equal to the amount of oxygen or energy expended at rest. All activities, from washing dishes to digging a ditch, can be assigned a MET value. The MET system allows you to understand exactly what activities and level of exercise are safe and therapeutic and what activities should be avoided.

The following chart gives the MET levels for selected activities. (Note: The MET values in the chart are not related to the more-familiar lists of calories burned with specific activities. This is a completely different system of evaluating the physiological demands of exercise based on the oxygen and energy requirements of the heart.)

SELECTED ACTIVITIES AND THEIR MET LEVELS

Self-Care	*MET Level*	*Housework*	*MET Level*
Lying down	1.0	Sweeping floor	2.0
Sitting	1.0	Polishing furniture	2.0
Standing, relaxed	1.0	Peeling potatoes	2.5
Eating	1.0	Scrubbing floors	3.0
Talking	1.0	Cleaning windows	3.0
Dressing and undressing	2.0	Making beds	3.0
Washing hands and face	2.0	Ironing (standing)	3.5
Strolling	2.5	Mopping	3.5
Showering	3.5	Snow shoveling	8–15
Walking downstairs	4.0		
Walking upstairs	6.0		

Physical Conditioning		*MET Level*
Walking on level ground	2 mph (1 mile in 30 minutes)	2.5
Cycling on level ground	5.5 mph (1 mile in 10.54 minutes)	3.0
Cycling on level ground	6 mph (1 mile in 10 minutes)	3.5
Walking on level ground	2.5 mph (1 mile in 24 minutes)	3.5
Walking on level ground	3 mph (1 mile in 20 minutes)	4.5
Cycling on level ground	9.7 mph (1 mile in 6.18 minutes)	5.0
Swimming (crawl)	1 foot per second	5.0
Walking on level ground	3.5 mph (1 mile in 17 minutes)	5.5
Walking on level ground	4.0 mph (1 mile in 15 minutes)	6.5
Jogging on level ground	5.0 mph (1 mile in 12 minutes)	8.0
Rope skipping	60-80 per minute	9.0
Cycling on level ground	13 mph (1 mile in 4.37 minutes)	10.0
Swimming (crawl)	2 feet per second	10.0
Running on level ground	6 mph (1 mile in 10 minutes)	10.0
Running on level ground	7.5 mph (1 mile in 8 minutes)	11.5
Running on level ground	8.5 mph (1 mile in 7 minutes)	14.0
Swimming (crawl)	2.5 feet per second	16.0

Physical Conditioning		MET Level
Running on level ground	10 mph (1 mile in 6 minutes)	16.5
Swimming (crawl)	3.0 feet per second	20.0
Running on level ground	12 mph (1 mile in 5 minutes)	20.0
Running on level ground	15 mph (¼ mile in 1 minute)	30.0
Swimming (crawl)	3.5 feet per second	30.0

Occupational	MET Level
Writing at desk	1.5
Typing	2.0
Heavy assembly work	4.0
Janitorial work	4.5
Carpentry	2–7
Home improvement (painting, plumbing)	3–8

Recreational	MET Level
Painting (sitting)	1.5
Playing piano	2.0
Driving	2.0
Fishing	2–4
Playing a musical instrument	2.5
Canoeing, rowing, and kayaking	3–8
Billiards	3.0
Sexual activity	3.5
Bowling	2–4
Golf (using golf cart)	2–3
Golf (walking, carrying bag or pulling cart)	4–7
Sailing	2–5

Recreational	MET Level
Gardening (raking, weeding)	3–6
Gardening (hoeing, digging, shoveling)	4–8
Mowing lawn (power or hand mower)	4–6
Dancing	3–7
Softball	3–6
Table tennis	3–5
Tennis	4–9
Scuba diving	5–10
Skating (roller and ice)	5–8
Horseback riding	3–8
Hiking	3–7
Backpacking	5–11
Skiing (cross-country)	6–12
Skiing (downhill)	5–8
Squash, racquetball and handball	8–12
Basketball	3–12
Football (touch)	6–10
Volleyball	3–6
Gymnastics	10.0
Handball and paddleball	8–12

We determine each patient's maximum MET capacity, or ability to perform work, based on their performance on the exercise stress test. When you first get on a treadmill, it is set at a low speed, with no incline. As the test progresses, the treadmill speeds up in programmed stages (usually every minute), requiring you to walk faster and your heart to work harder. Depending on your exercise tolerance, the treadmill may also be tilted to varying degrees, requiring you to work harder still.

Each stage on the treadmill corresponds to a designated MET level, which indicates the workload of that intensity of exercise on the heart. (In most cases, one minute on the treadmill equals one MET.) Once your maximum MET level is determined, specific exercise recommendations can then be made, corresponding to the physical limitations and clinical findings revealed by the exercise stress test. For example, if you exercised on the treadmill for ten minutes at gradually increasing intensity without symptoms or abnormalities, you maximum MET capacity would be 10. Any activity on the previous charts with a MET value of 10 or less would be within your physical ability. However, if at seven minutes into your stress test an abnormality occurred—perhaps an EKG finding indicating that your heart was not receiving adequate blood flow to sustain that level of exercise—you would be assigned an exercise program with a MET value of 5.5 to 6.5. We would not want you to work at the intensity that brought on problems. By sticking with the activities in your recommended MET range, you would be assured that you were getting the benefits of exercise without endangering yourself.

The MET system also has prognostic value. Numerous studies have shown that if your MET capacity is 10 you can rest assured that your risk of heart attack is minimal and the natural treatment program outlined in this book is the best course for you. The risk of a fatal heart attack in a person whose MET capacity is 12 or more is very low indeed. If your MET capacity is 5 or less, you should be closely monitored by your physician, and you may require more aggressive care.

A PROGRESSIVE EXERCISE REGIMEN

Once your maximum and target MET capacities have been established, you can begin a progressive exercise program based on your clinical and functional status. The three-level program outlined on the next few pages covers the needs of just about everyone. Level I is designed for patients with known cardiovascular disease, diabetics with complications, and patients with severe pulmonary disease or major neuromuscular limitations. Level II is aimed at the majority of the population—those who are generally healthy, with a few risk factors for heart disease and poor physical conditioning. Level III is for regular exercisers who are already in excellent shape. If you do not know your target MET level (and you don't plan to have the recommended exercise stress test), begin at the level that seems most compatible with your current state of health and fitness, and progress from there.

Recommendations for weight training are also included in these three exercise prescriptions, with particular emphasis on the number of repetitions of weight-lifting exercises. Regarding weight training, the emphasis in level I is endurance, in level II a combination of strength and endurance, and in level III strength and bulk. As I mentioned earlier in this chapter, I highly recommend that you first get some assistance from a personal trainer or someone else experienced in weight training. Once you understand the basics, you can work out on your own.

Start slowly. If in a burst of enthusiasm you try to make up for years of inactivity, you're going to be sore and uncomfortable the next day. Nothing dissipates resolve like exhaustion and injury. Increases in your exercise program should come gradually and comfortably. Start the program with the idea that this is something you will be doing for years to come. Looking down the long road of your life ahead, you'll be less apt to rush into things or worry about seeing immediate results.

PROGRESSIVE ONE-YEAR EXERCISE PROGRAM

Notes for levels I, II, and III exercise prescriptions:

1) Frequency of exercise should be four to five times per week. Duration of each session will vary, as indicated on the charts on p. 268. Numbers of weight-training sessions will also vary according to your level of conditioning.
2) Select activities from the charts on page 268 that are appropriate for your personal target MET level. Every four weeks the program recommendations will change as your conditioning improves. If you discontinue your exercise program for longer than two weeks, resume at one MET level below the level at which you were exercising previously.
3) Exercise recommendations are for sea level and average weather conditions. If you live in a high altitude or a humid area, begin at one level below your prescribed MET level so you don't overexert yourself.
4) Always warm up for five to ten minutes with gentle stretching and slower activity before you begin exercising. Cool down for an equal amount of time after exercise.
5) One MET assumes a 2.5 percent grade when walking outdoors or on a treadmill.
6) If no treadmill test has been done, determine your training heart rate using the formula on page 261.

LEVEL I: Beginning Rehabilitative Phase

Maximum MET capacity of 4 to 7 (based on exercise stress test); for patients with known cardiovascular disease, diabetics with complications, and patients with severe pulmonary disease or major neuromuscular limitations. Add one weight-training session per week, emphasizing endurance and aiming for two sets of 25 reps for each exercise.

TARGET HEART RATE ________ 6 SECOND PULSE __________

WEEK	METS	MPH	MIN/ MILE	WATTS BIKE	TOTAL TIME
1–4	2	1.5	34	25	20
5–8	2.5–3	1.5	30	25	30
9–12	3.5	2	27–30	40	30
13–16	3.5	2	24	40	30
17–20	3.5	2.5	24	40	45–60
21–24	4.5	2.5	20	50	30
25–28	4.5	2.5	20	50	45–60
29–32	5.5	2.5	17	75	30
33–36	5.5	2.5	17	75	45–60
37–40	5.5	3	17	75	30
41–44	6.5	3	15	100	45
45–48	6.5	4	15	100	30
49–52	6.5	4	15	100	45–60

LEVEL II: Intermediate

Maximum MET capacity of 8 to 11 (based on exercise stress test); appropriate for the majority of people who are generally healthy (perhaps with a few risk factors for heart disease) but in poor physical condition. Add two weight-training sessions per week, emphasizing strength and endurance and aiming for one set of 25 reps for each exercise with heavier weights.

TARGET HEART RATE __________ 6 SECOND PULSE __________

WEEK	METS	MPH	110 Yrd. (sec.)	440 yrd. (min:sec)	MIN/MILE	WATTS (BIKE)	DURATION
1–4	5.5	3.5	65	4:20	17	75	30
5–8	5.5	3.5	65	4:20	17	75	45
9–12	6.5	3.5	65	4:20	17	100	20
13–16	6.5	4	56	3:44	15	100	30
17–20	6.5	4	56	3:44	15	100	45
21–24	7.5	4	56	3:44	15	125	20
25–28	7.5	4	56	3:44	15	125	30
29–32	7.5	4	56	3:44	15	125	45
33–36	8.5	4.5	50	3:20	13.5	150	20
37–40	8.5	4.5	50	3:20	13.5	150	30
41–44	8.5	5	45	3:00	12	150	45
45–48	10	5	45	3:00	12	175	30
49–52	10	5	45	3:00	12	175	45

LEVEL III: Advanced

Maximum MET capacity of 12 to 18 (based on exercise stress test); for people who are already in good physical condition. Add two weight-training sessions per week, emphasizing strength and bulk, aiming for one set of 25 reps for each exercise with heaviest weights.

TARGET HEART RATE __________ 6 SECOND PULSE __________

	WALK			RUN			WALK/RUN
WEEK	Pace (mph)	Distance (yd./mi.)	Time (min:sec)	Pace (mph)	Distance (yd./mi.)	Time (min./sec.)	Reps
1–8							
Thurs-Sat	4.5	3 mi.	40:00				1
Wed-Sun	4	110 yd.	1:00	5	220	1:30	18
9–16							
Thurs-Sat	4.5	3 mi.	40:00				1
Wed-Sun	4	110 yd.	1:00	5	0	3:0	4

	WALK			RUN			WALK/RUN
WEEK	Pace (mph)	Distance (yd./mi.)	Time (min:sec)	Pace (mph)	Distance (yd./mi.)	Time (min./sec.)	Reps
17–24							
Thurs-Sat	5	3 mi.	36:00				1
Wed-Sun	4	110 yd.	1:00	6.8	220	1:06	8
25–32							
Thurs-Sat	5	3 mi.	36:00				1
Wed-Sun	4	110 yd.	1:00	6.8	220	1:06	8
33–40							
Thurs-Sat	6	3 mi.	30:00				1
Wed-Sun	4	110 yd.	1:00	7.5	440	2:00	8
41–48							
Thurs-Sat	7.5	3 mi.	24:00				1
Wed-Sun	4	110 yd.	1:00	8	880	3:16	4
49–52							
Thurs-Sat	8.5	3 mi.	21:00				1
Wed-Sun	4	110 yd.	1:00	11.2	440	2:40	8

DECIDE TO GET FIT

We live in a society that requires very little physical activity. I think this is great. Unlike those who long for a return to simpler times, I relish modern conveniences and comforts. The work-saving advances we take for granted have liberated us in many ways. We no longer have to spend the bulk of our days in tasks required for mere survival. We have time to create, express, and live like at no other time in human history. We have hot and cold running water (no need to lug water from the well), instant communication with telephones, faxes, and e-mail (no jogging into town to see so-and-so), at-home entertainment from television and VCRs (we are now spectators, seldom participants), stoves and furnaces that provide heat by simply turning a switch (when was the last time you chopped, stacked, and hauled

Can Exercise Be Dangerous for People with Heart Disease?

You've likely heard about someone who dropped dead while jogging or engaging in other exercise. With so many people dying every day from heart disease, the grim reaper is bound to select an occasional jogger. The actual risk of death during vigorous exercise, however, is quite small. At the Cooper Clinic, exercise guru Dr. Kenneth Cooper's clinic in Dallas, medical records of 2,934 men and women, ages seventeen to seventy-three, taking part in vigorous exercise programs were analyzed. Over a five-year period this group logged 374,798 hours of exercise, which included 2,726,272 kilometers of running and walking. During these five years there were only two cardiac events and no fatalities recorded. The researchers concluded that if a person exercised for thirty minutes three times a week for one year, the risk of adverse events related to the heart would be from .002 to .027 events per year for men and .005 to .05 events for women.[18]

Sudden death from cardiac causes does occur, and 6 to 17 percent of such deaths happen during or shortly after vigorous exercise. However, according to a 2000 Harvard study carried out over twelve years, regular vigorous exercise plays an important role in reducing the risk of sudden death during exercise.[19] The people who run into problems are those who sporadically barrel into high-intensity activities rather than following a regular and frequent exercise schedule. When you consider all the exercise studies that show a decreased risk of heart attack with regular exercise, even in people with diagnosed heart disease, it is easy to see that not exercising is much more dangerous than exercising. Exercise regularly and moderately—none of this weekend warrior stuff—and you can do so with confidence that you are engaging in a life-sustaining activity.

wood?), and automobiles or buses for transportation (how many pairs of walking shoes do you wear out each year?).

It is important that we spend some of the leisure time these labor-saving innovations have given us in physical activity. Getting fit begins with a decision to start exercising. I can arm you with all the information you'll need to set up an exercise program. Only you can make the decision to exercise.

HOW TO STICK WITH IT

The jogging paths and gyms of the country are paved with good intentions. I can't tell you how many patients have shared similar stories about exercise. They know how good exercise is for them, so they start a program and do very well—for three or four days. Exercise is difficult, no question about it. All creatures—dogs, cats, humans, even birds—exercise only out of necessity. If an animal is fed well and not required to work for his food, he will spend the whole day lying in the sun. Humans are no different. Our natural bent is toward relaxation.

Starting an exercise program is fairly easy. Sticking with one will require willpower and resolve, especially in the beginning, until regular activity becomes just another part of your daily life. Here are some guidelines for success I've shared with or learned from patients at the Whitaker Wellness Institute to help make exercise a habit.

First, make a commitment to exercise. Once you've decided on the types of activities you want to do, schedule your exercise sessions just as you would plan business meetings or social affairs. Get out your calendar or planner—or make copies of the form on page 273—and write down the date, the type and duration of the exercise you plan to do, and what time you plan to do it. Be very specific. For example, on Monday, you may take a forty-five-minute walk before breakfast. On Tuesday, you've scheduled an

Exercise Log Week of ___/___/___ to ___/___/___

Day of Week	Activity	Exercise Time	Done!	How I Feel
Monday			☐	
Tuesday			☐	
Wednesday			☐	
Thursday			☐	
Friday			☐	
Saturday			☐	
Sunday				
Comments:				

FIGURE 11: Exercise Log

appointment with a trainer at the gym over your lunch hour. On Wednesday, you walk again in the morning. Thursday takes you back to the gym, this time after work at 5:00. Friday, no exercise. Saturday is the day you meet a friend for tennis at 10:00. Sunday, another day of rest.

Once your weekly schedule is in place, all that remains is that you follow through. Post your exercise calendar or schedule on the fridge or in another prominent place as a reminder of your commitment. After you complete each exercise session, check it off. This may sound like a lot of work, but I know from my own personal experience as well as that of countless patients that it really does help you stay on the straight and narrow.

Utilize strategies that will enable you to stick with your program. A devoted runner once said to me that the hardest part of running was putting on the shoes. Here are some proven ways of keeping on track:

- Make your exercise social. Arrange to meet with people of comparable physical fitness on a regular basis. This obligates you to go out and exercise and it works much more successfully than relying on your own willpower. An added bonus is that this regular social activity cultivates friendships. For a period of about sixteen months, I regularly met two friends at 6:00 A.M. for a five-and-a-half-mile run. Many a morning I would have stayed in bed if I had not made a commitment to meet my friends, and they admitted to the same. We met four to six days a week, and our miles mounted up. When I moved out of the neighborhood they gave me a going-away T-shirt, which I wore with pride. Printed on the shirt was I RAN 1,645.5 MILES WITH TIP AND MIKE. Had it not been for Tip and Mike, I would have slept away at least half of those miles.
- Join an exercise class or sports club. Aerobics classes are great because they are scheduled at specific times. Tennis,

racquetball, and squash programs have challenge ladders that require you to play regularly and compete against people of similar ability. Cycling clubs sponsor weekly group rides, and running clubs organize regular jogs. Merely signing up for such activities forces you to work them into your schedule. If you join a group or class, particularly if you pay for it, you are likely to attend. As you get in condition and start feeling better, you'll begin to look forward to your activities and your new active and energetic friends. Soon it becomes a regular part of your life, and you're on your way to reaping the benefits of exercise.

- Make exercise a part of your commute. If you can walk or ride a bike to work (and freshen up when you arrive), do it. This is without question the best way to be consistent. After all, you have to go to work and get back home. Once I had a routine where I drove my car, with bicycle strapped on a rack on top, for five miles of my fifteen-mile commute. I then parked the car, jumped on my bike, and pedaled the remaining ten miles. At the end of the day it was ten miles back to the car, or I didn't get home! This also added up to substantial savings on gas over time. The "gas mileage" of a bicycle, computed as calories of energy, is about 912 miles to the gallon.
- Join a sports team or competition. Over the years I have played on football teams, basketball teams, and tennis teams. I have run marathons and ten-kilometer races, golfed in tournaments, and cycled in races. One of my most recent competitions was a body-building contest. My wife, Connie, and I decided to enter the Body-for-LIFE Challenge sponsored by a company that makes sports supplements. No, we didn't win, nor were we expecting to. We entered because we had been slacking off a bit on exercise and wanted the structure this program offered. Because we were in a contest, we didn't miss a scheduled day of exercise

during the twelve-week program. Check out your community center or health club. You'll find a wide variety of team sports for all ages. Also look for runs/walks or golf and tennis tournaments sponsored by nonprofit organizations. One event or another is going on every weekend in many areas.

- Take a vacation built around exercise. Several years ago I had a bee in my bonnet to ride a bike across the country. I signed up with a company that organizes such rides and spent ten weeks pedaling down the back roads of America from Washington State to Washington, D.C. We traversed the Cascade Mountains, rode through Yellowstone, enjoyed the flat farmland of the northern plains, skirted the Great Lakes, rode through the Amish country of Pennsylvania, and ended up dipping our wheels in the Potomac River. The cross-country bike tour was a great stimulus to exercise not only during the trip itself, but in the months leading up to it. Believe me, you wouldn't want to be staring at the Cascade Mountains the first week out on the road without a lot of training under your belt. I'm glad I did that trip, but I would never do it again—ten weeks is a heck of a long time. Much more fun was a weeklong bike trip I organized for subscribers of my monthly newsletter *Health & Healing*. Thirty-four of us cycled along the C&O Canal in Virginia, West Virginia, and Maryland during a glorious week in autumn. We rode only an average of twenty-five or thirty miles a day (compared to the frequent 100-mile days during the cross-country trip), and we stopped to enjoy the fall foliage, visit Civil War battle sites, and enjoy one another's company. As you can tell, I like cycling, but the options are many. How about hiking through one of our national parks, trekking the Appalachian Trail, or touring the California wine country on foot? Use your imagination or get hooked up with a company that plans such events. Again, it isn't just the exercise during the trip, but the preparations you must make in order to enjoy your exercise vacation.

In summary, whatever activity you choose, the important thing is to stick with it. I've seen hundreds of patients blossom here at the institute with the group walks and the scheduled exercise classes, only to fade when they get home. Consistency is absolutely essential, and the only way to stay on track is to schedule exercise into your day with a commitment stronger than just good intentions. If you start a program and falter, don't give up. That particular program and structure probably were not right for you. Persevere until you find some formula that works. Your health depends on it.

CHAPTER 16

Stress, Emotions, and Your Heart

DURING THE 1991 PERSIAN GULF WAR, THERE WERE MORE CASES of sudden cardiac death among frightened Israeli citizens than there were there were deaths caused by SCUD missiles.[1] In 1996, on the day of a crucial soccer match between the Netherlands and France, heart attack deaths jumped by 50 percent among Dutch men when the Netherlands lost to France and were shut out of the European championship.

Doctors often counsel their patients with heart disease about the potential risks of sudden physical exertion. They administer treadmill stress tests to precisely measure this risk, and instruct their patients in how to exercise safely. Yet few doctors warn their patients about the dangers of emotional stress. They don't give their patients an "emotional stress test" to see how well they handle the psychological rigors of daily life. And they seldom offer suggestions for minimizing the effects of stress. Yet emotional stressors do more than just upset our mental equilibrium—they alter the functioning of the heart as well.

In fact, some studies suggest that emotional stress can be a significant risk factor for heart attack. Researchers at Harvard Medical School quantified this risk by interviewing 849 patients who had suffered a recent heart attack and found that 18 percent of them reported experiencing emotional stress prior to their heart attack.[2] What is it about emotional stress that is so . . . well, stressful? To understand how stress damages the heart and cardiovascular system, let's look at a common stress-inducing scenario of modern life: driving on the freeway.

THE STRESS RESPONSE

Whether you're a driver consumed by road rage, a highway patrol officer in hot pursuit, or a mild-mannered commuter just trying to stay out of harm's way, your body is likely responding the same way to the stress of driving at high speeds on a busy freeway. Whenever you encounter something that elicits anger, fear, or excitement, your sympathetic nervous system—the part that is not under your conscious control—shifts into high gear. In less time than it takes for you to read this sentence, messages travel from your brain to your adrenal glands, triggering the release of epinephrine and norepinephrine. You feel a surge of energy. Your senses sharpen. Your breathing quickens. Your mind becomes focused and alert. Your heart beats more rapidly and pumps more forcefully, producing up to five times its normal output. Your blood vessels constrict to raise your blood pressure. Your liver converts glycogen into glucose, which floods your bloodstream with a source of quick energy. At the same time, blood is shunted away from your digestive tract and other nonessential organs to your heart, brain, and skeletal muscles—all without any thought on your part.

The sympathetic nervous system's "fight-or-flight" response was designed to help you evade predators or duke it out with an enemy—in other words, to respond to a physical threat requiring some type of action. Few of us are faced with such threats on a daily basis. What we are subjected to is an almost constant onslaught of minor psychological stresses. Unfortunately, the body doesn't differentiate between physical danger and psychological stress—both produce the same response, the same surge of epinephrine and norepinephrine.

These hormones cause your heart to beat faster and pump harder, increasing its demand for oxygen. They constrict your arteries and raise your blood pressure. Any time you increase the force with which a fluid moves through a system, turbulence increases. Over time, the chronic increase in blood pressure that accompanies repeated stress damages the endothelial lining of the arteries, causing injuries that may lead to atherosclerosis. Platelets in the blood also become stickier as the body prepares itself to staunch a potential wound, and this raises the risk of heart attack.

THE CORTISOL CONNECTION

The story doesn't end with epinephrine and norepinephrine. These rapid and short-acting hormones are assisted by the slower and longer-acting hormone cortisol. Cortisol, which is also secreted by your adrenal glands, helps you deal with the physical demands of prolonged stress. At the same time this hormone is gearing you up for survival, it suppresses functions of the body that have to do with growth, maintenance, and reproduction. This makes sense when you're facing a physical threat to your very existence. But it can be disastrous to your health if you're under chronic stress.

One of the main functions of cortisol is to ensure that you have a steady supply of energy. It does this in several ways, and unfortunately, each and every one of these things is bad news for your cardiovascular system. First, cortisol helps your body convert fats and proteins into glucose. (Elevated blood glucose damages the arteries.) Second, it helps mobilize fatty acids from adipose or fatty tissues. (Excess fat in the blood hampers blood flow.) Third, it makes your cells less sensitive to insulin, so that glucose remains in your blood and more insulin is secreted. (This is the essence of insulin resistance, a very significant risk factor for heart disease.)

Can elevated cortisol levels contribute to a heart attack? It's quite possible. In the absence of chronic stress, cortisol levels follow a natural rhythm, peaking in the morning after you arise and reaching their lowest level in the evening just before and shortly after you fall asleep. Blood pressure follows a similar pattern. Research has shown that heart attacks are most likely to occur in the morning, when both cortisol and blood pressure levels are at their highest. In fact, the single most likely time for a heart attack to occur is on a Monday morning—the most stressful morning of the week for many of us.

IS YOUR JOB MAKING YOU SICK?

For working adults, our occupations are likely to be the greatest source of stress in our lives. After all, we spend more time with our coworkers than we do with our families. Studies show that workers reporting high job-related stress are more likely to develop high blood pressure and atherosclerosis than those with less stress. The most stressful occupational characteristic is not excessive work demands but the feeling that you lack control of your job. A five-year study of British government workers at all grades of employment showed that those who had little control over their job duties were almost twice as likely to suffer a heart attack as workers who had a great deal of job control.[3]

Strife in the home is also likely to increase the risk of heart disease, especially among women. In a long-term study of 292 women who had been hospitalized for a heart attack or unstable angina, those who reported severe marital stress had almost a 300 percent greater risk of heart attack than women who reported little to no marital stress.[4]

CAN YOUR PERSONALITY MAKE YOU SICK?

You're probably familiar with the label "type A personality." You may even know someone—a family member or coworker, or perhaps even yourself—who fits the profile. This term was coined by two cardiologists, Meyer Friedman, M.D., and Ray Rosenman, M.D., in the early 1960s to describe a set of traits they saw time and time again in their patients with heart disease. These patients were intensely competitive, overachieving, impatient, and hostile. Drs. Friedman and Rosenman wondered if these personality traits made their patients especially vulnerable to heart disease. To find out, they did a study. They selected 3,400 healthy men, gave them a personality test to determine their type, and then observed whether having a type A personality increased the risk of heart disease. Sure enough, they saw a pattern: Men with a type A personality had twice the risk of heart disease as men who did not.[5]

Although the "type A" label slowly fell out of favor, since subsequent studies failed to replicate this study, one aspect of this personality did prove to be an important predictor of heart disease: hostility. In study after study, whether researchers looked at American lawyers, twins in Finland, employees of a utility company, or middle-aged doctors, they reached a similar conclusion. Having a high degree of hostility increased the likelihood of heart disease and death.

So what exactly is hostility, and why is it so damaging to the heart? Though hostility can include many things—a cynical outlook, an explosive temper, mistrust of others—perhaps it's best described as a tendency to respond to neutral situations as if they were stressful (i.e., threatening). Minor incidents or meaningless events are interpreted as personal attacks, and a veritable arsenal of violent feelings, thoughts, and behaviors are triggered. Clenched muscles, a red face, and angry gestures are visible and dramatic signs of hostility. But chronically elevated levels of stress hormones, hypertension, and atherosclerosis are the more insidious markers of hostility at work.

ANGER AND ANXIETY CAN BE DEADLY

While having a hostile or angry personality can exert tremendous wear and tear on the heart and blood vessels over time, an episode of acute anger can trigger an immediate heart attack or sudden cardiac death. Researchers at Harvard Medical School determined that the risk of heart attack increased by 230 percent in the two-hour period following an episode of anger.[6] In fact, simply recalling an angry episode can cause the heart to beat erratically and the arteries to constrict in people with heart disease, reducing blood flow and bringing on the pain of angina.

It's no accident that anger, anxiety, and angina come from the same Greek root, a word meaning "to strangle." Anger and anxiety—fight and flight—are two sides of the same coin. Both emotions cause an identical surge of hormones and produce a similar alteration of cardiovascular function and blood flow. Clinical studies have shown that like bouts of anger, panic attacks restrict blood flow to the heart and result in chest pain in patients who have heart disease. And like anger, the experience of acute anxiety or fear can even trigger a heart attack or sudden cardiac death.

On January 17, 1994, the day that the Los Angeles area was hit by a major earthquake, the number of heart attacks was 250 percent higher than on the same day in the three preceding years. What's more, compared to the six days prior to the earthquake, the incidence of sudden cardiac death increased by over 500 percent on the day of the earthquake.[7] Interestingly, the incidence of sudden cardiac death the week after the earthquake was significantly lower than average, suggesting that people who were at risk of death from heart disease during that week died earlier as a result of the emotional stress of the earthquake.

There is also research suggesting that chronic obsessive worrying damages the heart. In a twenty-year study of 1,400 men who had no history of heart disease at the study's onset, those who reported high levels of obsessive thoughts or anxiety were almost three times as likely to die from heart disease as men who rated their level of obsessiveness as low.[8]

DEPRESSION: THE DEADLY DISEASE

Anger and anxiety are obviously stressful emotions, and their damaging effects on the cardiovascular system are easy to comprehend. What about depression? To many people, depression represents a lack of emotion rather than an excess. Yet people who are depressed tend to secrete much higher levels of the stress hormone cortisol. They also have a dramatically higher risk of heart attack and heart-related death. In a twelve-year study of almost 3,000 adults who had no history of coronary artery disease, those who were depressed or hopeless at the onset of the study were one and a half times more likely to develop fatal heart disease.[9] Likewise, of the nearly 3,000 elderly men and women with no evidence of heart disease enrolled in another study, those who had major symptoms of depression were 300 percent more likely to die from heart disease within four years than individuals who were not depressed.[10]

Depression can be especially deadly for people who already have heart disease. The first study to demonstrate that depression increased the risk of death among those with preexisting heart disease was published in the *Journal of the American Medical Association* in 1993. In this Canadian study of 222 adults hospitalized for a heart attack, depression following the heart attack quadrupled their risk of dying in the next six months.[11] And the effects of depression on mortality persisted. A follow-up study showed that after eighteen months, the relative risk of death associated with depression was 660 percent.[12]

YOU CAN LEARN TO MANAGE STRESS

If there is any theme running through this chapter, it is the importance of control to our peace of mind. Lack of control, or perceived lack of control, underlies the hair-trigger responses of the hostile personality, the obsessive worry of the anxiety-ridden adult, and the hopelessness and despair of the person afflicted with depression. Certainly there is much in life that we cannot control. But not everyone feels chronic anger or anxiety or depression in the face of all this uncertainty. What is it that separates healthy copers from those who are not?

A big part of it is attitude. Healthy copers tend to focus on the aspects of their lives that they can control rather than obsessing on the areas that they cannot. After all, while unpredictability is a part of life, there is much that is under your control. For example, you make choices every day about what and when to eat, whether to smoke or drink, which TV shows to watch (or whether to pull the plug altogether), how much (or how little) exercise to get, and on and on. Each one of these things is small, but the net effect of making many small, healthy choices can be a dramatic reduction in the amount of stress you experience.

The rest of this chapter is devoted to exploring the lifestyle changes, relaxation techniques, and other strategies that I recommend to my patients with heart disease to help them cope with stress. Some of the techniques described here may seem simple, even simplistic. But taken together they can have powerful effects on your ability to weather the emotional storms of daily life.

Eat Right for Less Stress

Many people turn to junk food—candy bars, cookies, and the like—as a way of dealing with stress or escaping from unpleasant emotions. Bad idea. Eating high-glycemic, refined carbohydrates literally stresses your body's blood sugar control mechanisms, causing dramatic fluctuations that can leave you feeling irritable and moody. For less stress, follow my dietary recommendations in Chapter 12, emphasizing vegetables and fruits, along with lean protein from fish, skinless poultry, nonfat dairy, and beans and legumes.

Avoid the Caffeine Rush

Drinking coffee all day long is as stressful as driving home in rush hour traffic—and its effects can last up to six hours! Caffeine stimulates your adrenal glands to churn out stress hormones that cause your muscles to tense, your blood sugar to rise, and your pulse and respiration to quicken. No one should drink more than one or two cups of coffee in the morning, but if you are chronically anxious, angry, or depressed, I would suggest avoiding it altogether. Drink green tea instead—it has only one-third the caffeine of coffee and has numerous proven health benefits to boot. (For more on caffeine, see Chapter 12.)

Exercise Your Emotions

Healthy copers may have as many stresses in their life as the next person, but they also take care to find outlets for their frustration. I'm not talking about punching a pillow. Research has shown that this type of "venting" actually increases anger rather than decreasing it. I am talking about having activities that are meaningful or simply enjoyable. If you're stuck in a job that offers few rewards and little control, a hobby or activity you enjoy can be a lifesaver. Lately, I've been trying to master the game of golf. The combination of physical effort, mental concentration, and simply being outdoors clears away any pent-up stress I've been carrying around.

I also make it a point to work out in the gym or play squash several times a week. As we discussed in the previous chapter, vigorous exercise stimulates the production of endorphins, your body's "feel-good" neurotransmitters. Instead of sitting down and turning on the evening news when you get home, make a practice of putting on a pair of comfortable shoes and taking a walk around the block. Simply reserving some time for yourself to do a hobby, sport, or whatever activity you choose—and honoring that commitment—will help keep stress at bay.

Maintain Social Support

While relationships can certainly be a source of stress, they may be as important for your health and well-being as eating the right foods and exercising. A number of studies have shown that people who live alone or have few significant relationships have an increased risk of developing heart disease or dying, and that close relationships are an important protective factor for those who already have heart disease. In one study, heart disease patients who were unmarried or had no significant confidant in their lives had a 300 percent increase in mortality compared to those who had a spouse or close friend to turn to for support.[13]

One great way to reach out and connect with others is through volunteering. Hospitals, nursing homes, schools, churches, homeless shelters, soup kitchens, libraries, museums: These are all possibilities for you to develop stronger ties with your community and make new friends.

Consider Getting a Pet

Anyone who has ever held a kitten or hugged a puppy knows that pets can be good for the soul. But research suggests that they also may be good for the heart. In a study of stockbrokers diagnosed with high blood pressure, those who were given a pet for six months along with a prescription antihypertensive drug showed a smaller rise in blood pressure in response to stress than those who received only the prescription drug. Other studies have shown that pet owners have lower triglyceride and cholesterol levels than non-owners, and are treated less frequently for hypertension.

In one of the earliest examinations of the effects of pet ownership on patients with heart disease, researchers looked at the mortality rate among 96 patients who had been admitted to a coronary care unit for heart attack or angina. During the year following hospitalization, the mortality rate among those who didn't own pets was 22 percent higher than that of pet owners.

Take Back Your Breath

A stressful encounter literally takes your breath away. The moment before your boss dumps a pile of work on your desk, you might be breathing calmly and evenly. But as soon as you look at the clock and realize you don't have enough time to complete the task, stress hormones kick in and your breathing changes, going from slow and deep to rapid and shallow. Your body is preparing for action, and your breath is quickening in anticipation.

An easy way to interrupt the stress response—and one that you can do anytime and anywhere—is to consciously slow your breathing. Inhale slowly, hold the breath for a few seconds, then exhale slowly. Try it: *Inhale*, two, three, four. *Hold*, two, three, four. *Exhale*, two, three, four. Repeat this three or four times. Once your breath normalizes, your body will follow. It may not "hear" you right away, but if you continue to breathe slowly and deeply, your brain and body will get the message and calm down. Instead of churning out more stress chemicals and setting you up for chronic stress, your body will learn a much healthier *relaxation response*. Your heart rate will slow, your blood pressure will drop, and less easily measured signs of stress will also abate.

For many people, combining slow, deep breathing with the

mental repetition of a word is easier than focusing on the breath itself. Choose a word that you find soothing and mentally repeat it with each inhalation and exhalation. The silent repetition of a word pulls your attention away from the alarm bells going off in your body and frantic thoughts running through your mind. You pass from the hyperalertness of stress to the alertness of focused attention to a state of relaxation and peacefulness.

Tune into Relaxing Music

One of the easiest ways of reducing stress is listening to music. In a study of patients who had suffered a recent heart attack, those who listened to music for twenty minutes in a quiet, restful environment experienced an immediate and significant reduction in respiration and heart rate, as well as oxygen demands of the heart. Their anxiety level dropped significantly as well and remained lower for an hour after the music was ended.[14] I'm a big believer in the therapeutic power of music and often play classical music in the office while I'm working. The type of music you choose depends on your personal tastes, but I guarantee that you can find some kind of music to foster peace and relaxation.

Soothe Stress with Ginseng

Winding down with alcohol after a hectic day or reenergizing in the afternoon with caffeine are common but unhealthy ways to deal with the fatigue and overstimulation of chronic stress. A far healthier choice is to make use of herbs known as adaptogens, which improve the body's ability to adapt to a broad range of physical and biochemical stressors and can help you feel more energetic and alert as well.

Panax ginseng (also known as Korean or Chinese ginseng) is such an herb. It has been used in Oriental medicine for thousands of years, and scientific studies have shown this herb enhances stamina, facilitates concentration, and improves overall well-being. The source of ginseng's adaptogenic properties are phytochemicals called ginsenosides, which help balance the glands that are involved in the stress response. Panax's first cousin, Siberian ginseng, also increases resistance to stress, plus it has a calming effect on the central nervous system.

The recommended dose of Panax ginseng is 75 to 150 milligrams (standardized to contain 7 percent ginsenosides). For Siberian ginseng, the recommended dose is 150 to 300 milligrams (standardized for 0.8 percent eleutherosides). Ginseng should be used cyclically, taken daily for two months, then off for at least two weeks. This cycle may be repeated as often as required. Although some experts warn that high doses of ginseng may cause elevated blood pressure in some people, my review of the medical literature on ginseng reveals no evidence of this. If chronic stress is a concern of yours, I recommend giving ginseng a try. Monitor your blood pressure the first two or three weeks of the trial period and never exceed the recommended dose. If you observe an increase in your blood pressure while taking ginseng, discontinue it at once.

Ease Anxiety with Kava

Kava, which comes from the root of a plant native to the South Pacific Islands, has been in use as a safe, natural anxiety remedy for over 3,000 years. The active constituents of this herb, kavalactones, reduce anxiety and induce a state of calm by acting directly on the brain's limbic system, which is the seat of your emotions. There have been more than 800 studies of the benefits of kava as an anti-anxiety agent, most of them done in Europe. In a recent double-blind study, 101 patients with chronic anxiety were randomly given daily doses of kava or a placebo. After eight weeks, patients taking kava noted improvements in mood and general well-being and experienced a significant reduction in nervousness, heart palpitations, chest pains, and dizziness when compared to the placebo group.[15]

If you are overly anxious, nervous, and edgy, give kava a try.

Look for a kava extract standardized to contain 30 percent kavalactones, and take 150 mg one to six times daily with meals, as needed. (Take the lowest dose that works for you; do not exceed the maximum recommended dose.) Kava should be taken for a maximum of three months, followed by a rest of two to four weeks. This cycle may be repeated as needed. It should not be taken in combination with alcohol, tranquilizers, or other drugs that act on the central nervous system, or by people with Parkinson's disease.

Lift Depression with Natural Agents

About 20 percent of patients become seriously depressed after a heart attack. Unfortunately, some antidepressants also increase the risk of heart attack. In a four-year study, published in the *American Journal of Medicine*, members of a health plan who took tricyclic antidepressants had a 220 percent higher risk of suffering a heart attack than members who took other types of antidepressants or control subjects who were not taking any prescription antidepressants.[16]

For mild to moderate depression, the herb St. John's wort (*Hypericum perforatum*) is an extremely safe and effective therapy, as effective as prescription antidepressants, according to some studies. A 1996 analysis of twenty-three clinical trials on St. John's wort involving 1,757 patients demonstrated that the herb was three times as effective as placebo in relieving the symptoms of depression. Even more important, in the eight of these studies that compared St. John's wort to a drug, the herb worked as well as the antidepressant—but with far fewer side effects and much less toxicity.

The recommended dose of St. John's wort is 300 milligrams twice a day of an herbal extract standardized to contain 0.3 percent hypericin. If you are taking a prescription drug for depression, ask your doctor about St. John's wort before starting it. St. John's wort increases the metabolism of certain drugs, thereby lessening their therapeutic effects. Drugs thus affected include: warfarin (Coumadin), digoxin (Lanoxin), theophylline (Theo-dur), triptin migraine drugs, oral contraceptives, and several types of antidepressants. Also be aware that when taken in large doses for prolonged periods, this herb may cause sun sensitivity in fair-skinned people.

Another safe and effective natural antidepressant is S-adenosyl-methionine (SAMe). Almost three-quarters of the depressed patients who try this supplement notice improvements, and unlike St. John's wort, which may take weeks before effects are noted, SAMe perks up mood within days. This amino acid derivative increases the production and activity of neurotransmitters in the brain by facilitating the methylation process (the same detoxification process we talked about in Chapter 3, which keeps homocysteine levels in check). Clinical trials involving more than 1,300 patients have examined the effects of supplemental SAMe on depression. A 1994 review of these studies confirmed its efficacy and showed it to be as effective as some prescription antidepressants.

SAMe is nontoxic, and the only reported side effects are headaches, stomach upset, and diarrhea with high doses. The recommended dose is 200 milligrams twice a day, between meals (at least thirty minutes before eating and no less than two hours after eating).

In conclusion, don't let your negative emotions get the best of you and your health. Practice some of the stress-reduction techniques described in this chapter, or others that work for you. This will not only reduce your risk of heart disease but improve every aspect of your life.

CHAPTER 17

Hormones and Heart Disease

HORMONES EXERT POWERFUL EFFECTS ON THE HUMAN BODY. Although they are present only in minute concentrations (1 molecule for every 50 billion molecules of blood) hormones orchestrate processes as diverse as conception, childbirth, sleep, and aging. These chemical messengers are produced from cholesterol, amino acids, and proteins in the glands of the endocrine system. Secreted into the bloodstream and carried to receptor sites throughout the body, they have widespread effects on virtually every organ system, including the cardiovascular system.

Dozens of hormones have been identified, and many of them act upon the heart and blood vessels. We discussed the pervasive influence of cortisol, epinephrine, norepinephrine, and other stress hormones in the previous chapter. In this chapter we will limit our discussion to the six hormones that not only have broad effects on the heart and arteries, but can also be used in supplemental form to help reverse heart disease.

DHEA: DEFENDER AGAINST DISEASE

Dehydroepiandrosterone (DHEA) is a steroid hormone produced in the adrenal glands from cholesterol. Although it is secreted in greater amounts than any of the other steroid hormones, for many years it was felt to have little use other than as a precursor to more important hormones such as testosterone and estrogen. We now know that DHEA has important independent functions. There is a direct relationship between DHEA levels and the incidence of many diseases, including diabetes, insulin resistance, Alzheimer's disease, and heart disease. Lower levels of this hormone are to be expected in older people. DHEA production peaks around age twenty, then begins to fall—a seventy-year-old's level is only 10 percent that of a twenty-year-old. However, there are also significant differences in DHEA levels among people of similar age, depending on their state of health.

A low blood level of DHEA is a specific and independent marker of heart disease in men.[1] In a 2001 study, researchers at the New England Research Institutes in Watertown, Massachusetts, measured DHEA and DHEA-sulfate (the most common blood marker for DHEA) in 1,709 men, ages forty to seventy, then followed them for nine years. They found that men with the lowest levels of DHEA and DHEA-sulfate were the most likely to develop heart disease over the study period. Furthermore, a low DHEA level was predictive of heart disease independently of age, obesity, diabetes, hypertension, smoking, blood lipids, alcohol intake, and physical activity.[2]

DHEA protects the heart and arteries in several ways. It influences enzymes that affect blood lipids and helps keep cholesterol and triglyceride levels in check. This hormone also inhibits platelet aggregation and normalizes blood-clotting factors.[3] Another positive influence of DHEA is its ability to increase insulin sensitivity. You will recall from our discussion in Chapter 4 that insulin resistance and the cluster of conditions known as syndrome X are significant risk factors for heart disease. There is a close inverse relationship between insulin resistance and DHEA: High insulin levels are almost always accompanied by lower DHEA levels.[4] One reason for this may be because of the link between insulin and cortisol. As you saw in the previous chapter, when levels of the stress hormone cortisol remain high, they unleash a cascade of negative actions—including a dampening of DHEA production.

I order a DHEA-sulfate blood test for most of my patients over the age of forty, and if it is low, as it often is, I recommend supplementing with DHEA. This is particularly important for patients who have or are at risk of heart disease. Although the cardioprotective effects of DHEA have been seen to a greater degree in men than in women, I suggest that both sexes supplement with this hormone. It has so many proven benefits that physiological replacement (bringing levels into the average range for a young adult) can only be beneficial. Furthermore, DHEA has a well-documented "side effect": People taking it report that they just feel better.

DHEA is available over the counter, but make sure you purchase only pharmaceutical-grade DHEA. The normal starting doses are 25 milligrams per day for women and 50 milligrams for men. Have your DHEA-sulfate blood level tested prior to taking it and again after three months, and adjust your dose if needed. DHEA is safe and has few side effects. Because this hormone is readily converted in women's bodies to testosterone, excessive amounts may cause oily skin, acne, or slight facial hair growth. These will disappear if you cut back on your dose. I do not recommend that DHEA be taken by individuals with a history of prostate, breast, or other hormone-sensitive cancers. It may exacerbate the condition by elevating hormone levels.

THYROID DEFICIENCIES ARE COMMONLY OVERLOOKED

The thyroid, a small gland located just below the voice box, secretes hormones that regulate metabolism. Hyperthyroidism, secretion of excessively high levels of thyroid hormones, is a serious condition marked by rapid heartbeat. It is usually treated by radioactive iodine, which destroys portions of the gland, or with surgical removal. Much more common, however, is hypothyroidism, or secretion of too little thyroid hormone. An underactive thyroid results in fatigue, weight gain, dry skin, cold hands and feet, hair loss, memory problems, constipation, and menstrual irregularities. Less well recognized, however, are hypothyroidism's adverse effects on the cardiovascular system.

Marlene was told by her doctor that her high cholesterol (373) and triglycerides (429) were "inherited." Because she always seemed tired and had put on some weight, she asked whether low thyroid, which she had read about in my monthly newsletter, might be a factor. Her doctor didn't think so and wrote her a prescription for a cholesterol-lowering drug. Convinced that her thyroid was at the root of her symptoms, Marlene consulted a new doctor, who agreed that it could be a factor. He started her on low-dose natural thyroid, along with other natural lipid-lowering agents such as niacin and garlic, and took her off the drug. After just one year on this program, her "inherited" cholesterol had dropped to 198 and her triglycerides to 64!

Hypothyroidism is unequivocally associated with blood lipid abnormalities. In addition to raising total cholesterol, it lowers protective HDL cholesterol. But it contributes to an increased risk of heart attack in other ways as well. According to a 2000 article, published in the journal *Thyroid*, hypothyroidism may also cause impairments in the function of the heart that show up primarily with exercise. These include endothelial dysfunction, constriction of the blood vessels, and changes in heart rate. And in patients who have had bypass or angioplasty, hypothyroidism is accompanied by a trend toward higher rates of angina and restenosis of the arteries.[5]

Hypothyroidism is much more common than you might suspect. According to the American Association of Clinical Endocrinologists (AACE), about one in eight women from thirty-five to sixty-five years of age has low thyroid function, as does one in five over sixty-five. (Although men are not immune to this condition, its incidence is about seven times greater in women.) If you are a woman over the age of fifty, you may think symptoms such as fatigue, mood swings, and forgetfulness are the consequences of menopause. But many of the symptoms of hypothyroidism mimic those of menopause. As a result, this condition frequently goes undiagnosed in this group of women.

The AACE estimates that half of the 13 million Americans who have thyroid disorders don't know it. Therefore, the routine blood tests I perform on my patients almost always include screening for thyroid activity. The gold standard for the diagnosis of hypothyroidism is the thyrotropin test, a highly sensitive test that measures blood levels of thyroid stimulating hormone (TSH). This pituitary hormone acts like an on/off switch, regulating the production and secretion of thyroid hormones. When thyroid function is low, levels of TSH are abnormally high. Other tests measure free or total T4 (thyroxine) and T3 (triiodothyronine), hormones produced by the thyroid gland. While these tests will help your doctor monitor your condition, normal levels of these hormones don't always rule out hypothyroidism. Always insist on the more sensitive TSH test.

If you suspect low thyroid function in spite of normal blood levels, here's a test you can perform at home. Since the thyroid gland controls all metabolic processes, you can get a pretty good idea of the health of your thyroid gland by measuring your underarm basal (resting) temperature. This is easier with a basal thermometer you can find in your drugstore, but a regular thermometer will do. To perform the test, shake the thermometer down at night and keep it at your bedside. First thing in the morning, while you're still in bed and before you move around, put it under your armpit for exactly ten minutes. Record the temperature and repeat this process for four days to get an average temperature reading. Women who are still menstruating should note that only temperatures taken on the first through fourth day of the cycle are accurate. Normal readings are between 97.8 and 98.2. Temperatures consistently lower than 97.8 degrees suggest inadequate thyroid production.

Thyroid replacement therapy usually returns thyroid activity to normal and thus reduces risk of heart disease. While the best-selling brand is Synthroid, I never prescribe this synthetic hormone to my patients with low thyroid function. Synthroid contains only T4, and T4 is not the only hormone produced by the thyroid gland. This is why I recommend Armour Thyroid or another form of natural desiccated porcine (pork) thyroid, which contains all the active elements of the thyroid gland. Natural thyroid has been around much longer than Synthroid and possesses a long history of safety and effectiveness. If you have hypothyroidism, I urge you to go natural. Your body will know the difference. See the resource section for sources of natural thyroid.

TESTOSTERONE AND THE MALE HEART

You probably know that testosterone is the hormone that gives men big muscles, a deep voice, a beard, and a randy sex drive. But you might not be aware that it also affects the heart. This effect was long believed to be adverse. After all, men have much higher rates of heart disease than women, until menopause, anyway. And testosterone levels are one major difference between men and women. Research over the past few years, however, suggests that testosterone actually inhibits atherosclerosis.

A research team from Columbia University's College of Physicians and Surgeons in New York City followed 55 men with chest pain or other signs of atherosclerotic heart disease. They discovered that based on comparisons of their angiograms, the men with low levels of testosterone were much more likely to have significant atherosclerosis than men with higher testosterone levels. The researchers concluded that low testosterone levels may be a risk factor for coronary artery disease.[6]

Other studies have documented the relationship between testosterone and specific risk factors for heart disease. Decreased levels of this hormone corresponded with elevations in triglycerides and lipoprotein(a), and with reductions in HDL cholesterol.[7] Testosterone appears to help maintain arterial responsiveness to signals to dilate or contract and to improve blood flow in men with existing heart disease.[8] One study, an arm of the ongoing Massachusetts Male Aging Study, has found that low testosterone levels play a role in the development of insulin resistance and type 2 diabetes, both risk factors for atherosclerosis.[9]

A very interesting study, published in *Circulation* in 2000, reported on supplemental testosterone as a therapy for angina. Forty-six men, average age sixty-two, who had chest pain related to heart disease plus low-normal testosterone levels were divided into two groups and given either testosterone patches or dummy patches to wear for fourteen weeks. At the study's conclusion, the men using the testosterone patches had astounding improvements. They were able to increase their time on the exercise stress test before experiencing angina by 37 percent, compared to the 15 percent increase in the placebo group. Study participants also reported improvements in their social functioning and mental and emotional health.[10]

At the Whitaker Wellness Institute, we frequently prescribe testosterone for our older male patients if blood tests show that their levels are below those of a young adult. However, if you ask your own physician about testosterone, you may get a blank stare. Although therapeutic use of this hormone is becoming more popular, it is still, in my opinion, vastly underused. This makes no sense. Men's testosterone levels decline with age, just as women's estrogen and progesterone levels do. Women are almost always offered the option of hormone replacement; men rarely are. It's time the medical profession embraces this safe, inexpensive therapy for heart disease, flagging libido and energy, loss of muscle mass, and other age-related conditions associated with declining testosterone levels.

Testosterone is available in several different modes of delivery: lozenges, injections, and topical ointments rubbed into the skin. (Never use oral testosterone, for it may be toxic to the liver.) It can be ordered from compounding pharmacists, who prepare prescriptions for a fraction of the cost of AndroGel and testosterone patches. Although repeated studies show that supplemental testosterone does not cause prostate cancer, it should not be used by men who have prostate cancer, as it could fuel cancer cell growth.

ESTROGEN AND THE FEMALE HEART

No hormone has fallen in and out of favor more often than estrogen. It protects against heart disease, it increases risk of heart disease; it causes breast cancer, it doesn't cause breast cancer. Many of my female patients tell me they are confused and frustrated. Should they use estrogen replacement therapy or shouldn't they? Let's review the studies on this hormone that relate to heart disease, then we'll briefly touch on some of the other issues surrounding estrogen.

Rates of heart disease and death from heart attack, while very low in menstruating women, jump dramatically in postmenopausal women. Because this coincides with declining levels of estrogen, researchers have sought to explain this relationship and to explore the benefits of hormone replacement therapy. Estrogen replacement has positive effects on blood lipids. Cholesterol and other blood fat levels often shoot up after menopause, while lipid profiles improve with estrogen replacement: LDL cholesterol and lipoprotein(a) come down, and protective HDL cholesterol gets a boost. Estrogen deficiencies have adverse effects on the arteries, making them less responsive and reducing their ability to relax, and supplemental estrogen also ameliorates this risk factor. In addition, estrogen replacement improves insulin sensitivity, increases the availability of nitric oxide, and has antioxidant properties. It even appears to enhance the growth of new blood vessels that improve blood supply to the heart. This is not to say that supplemental estrogen improves every marker for heart disease, for it raises harmful homocysteine, triglycerides, and C-reactive protein.

However, the sum total of these effects would be an expected reduction in the risk of heart disease. Early studies bore this out. A 1991 review of more than thirty epidemiological studies showed that estrogen replacement therapy conferred a 35 to 50 percent reduction in the risk of heart disease.[11] And the first controlled clinical trial on hormone replacement therapy and heart disease, the 1995 Postmenopausal Estrogen/Progestin Intervention (PEPI), also supported its cardiovascular benefits. In this double-blind placebo-controlled trial, 875 postmenopausal women were assigned to conjugated estrogen (the most popular type of estrogen replacement), progestin (synthetic progesterone), various combinations of estrogen and progestin, or a placebo. After three years researchers noted improvements in blood lipid levels in the women taking hormones: significantly lower total cholesterol and LDL and increases in HDL. (Triglycerides, however, went up.) The most favorable response was in the women taking estrogen alone—their increases in beneficial HDL cholesterol equaled a 25 percent reduction in risk of heart disease.[12]

However, more recent studies have challenged the idea that hormone replacement protects against cardiovascular disease. A 1997 review of twenty-two smaller studies suggested that rather than protecting against heart disease, hormone replacement therapy increased the risk of coronary events.[13] The largest randomized placebo-controlled trial on this subject came up with similar findings.

The Heart and Estrogen Replacement Study (HERS), published in 1998, involved 2,763 postmenopausal women with established coronary artery disease. They were divided into two groups, given either conjugated estrogen and progestin or a placebo, and followed for more than four years. As in the PEPI trial, blood lipid levels improved in the women taking hormones. However, this did not reduce the risk of sudden cardiac death or other coronary events such as heart attack. In fact, during the first year of hormone replacement therapy, there was an increased risk of such events. (This trend began to taper off in the second year, and by year three, hormone replacement actually reduced the incidence of adverse events.) There were other negative findings as well: a 40 percent increase in the risk of gallbladder disease and a 33 percent increase in the risk of nonfatal blood clots in women taking hormones. The study's conclusion was that hormone replacement therapy should not be recommended for women with heart disease because of increased risk during the first year of therapy. It appeared to be safe after that initial year, so the study's recommendation was that women who were already on the therapy need not stop, for they would likely receive benefits.[14]

The failure of estrogen to improve the course of existing atherosclerosis has been demonstrated in subsequent studies, including the 2000 Estrogen Replacement and Atherosclerosis (ERA) trial[15] and the ongoing Women's Health Initiative. In the latter study, which is an examination of the effects of hormone replacement therapy in 27,000 healthy postmenopausal women, participants were told in April 2000 of an increase in early cardiac events affecting about 1 percent of the women. The study was not stopped, however, because the period of maximum risk had passed.[16]

All this negative evidence was sufficient for the American

Heart Association and the American College of Cardiology to change their tune regarding hormone replacement therapy. They now recommend against starting women on hormone replacement therapy solely to prevent heart attack and stroke.[17] Furthermore, the FDA requires label warnings on estrogen-progestin combination products: "Women with a history of coronary artery disease may have an increased risk of serious cardiac events during the first year of treatment with estrogen/progestin treatment."[18]

Before we throw the baby out with the bathwater, remember that an increased risk of heart attacks and deaths occurred only during the first year of use, and only in women with existing disease. Much of the problem, in my opinion (and that of the FDA, judging by the above label warning), lies with the type of hormone replacement used in virtually all of these studies—progestin (an unnatural imitation of progesterone that we will cover in the next section) and Premarin, an estrogen drug derived from the urine of pregnant mares.

Estrogen isn't one hormone but a group of hormones with similar properties. The three major forms produced in a woman's body are: 1) estradiol, the most active form of estrogen, which is secreted by the ovaries and the strongest of the group; 2) estrone, secreted by the adrenal glands and also produced in the fat cells; and 3) estriol, the weakest but safest of the three. It would make sense to prescribe natural, human-identical versions of these safe and effective forms of estrogen rather than a drug derived from the urine of pregnant mares, and, in fact, this is what we do at the Whitaker Wellness Institute.

The estrogen preparation we prescribe for our patients is called bi-estrogen. It is 80 percent estriol, the weakest but safest form of estrogen, and 20 percent estradiol, the dominant estrogen in the body, which facilitates the effectiveness of estriol. I cannot say for certain that this human-identical estrogen formulation is safer than the conjugated horse estrogens, for there have been no head-to-head studies. However, I can say that it is natural to the human body, and it has some protective effects that the stronger estrogens do not. For example, while estrone (which is in Premarin) stimulates proliferation of breast cells and may contribute to cancer, estriol has been shown to protect against estrogen-stimulated breast cell replication.

Other benefits of supplemental estrogen include prevention and treatment of osteoporosis, relief of menopausal symptoms, and memory enhancement. It has been demonstrated to reduce the risk of peripheral artery disease (caused by atherosclerosis and poor circulation in the extremities)[19] and to be useful in the treatment of heart failure.[20] Documented negatives include increased risk of gallbladder disease, endometrial cancer (when estrogen is used without progesterone), and, with very long-term use, ovarian cancer.

Less clear is the risk of breast cancer. Some studies have demonstrated an increased risk, while others have failed to show any such correlation. If there is an increased risk—and it cannot be ruled out—it appears to be small, and it is most likely to occur with extended use. And once again it's a question of what kinds of hormones you are using.

Given the many pluses and minuses associated with hormone replacement therapy, each woman must make a personal decision based on a consideration of a broad range of factors, including her own health status and risk factors. At the clinic we discuss with each woman her personal history, risk factors, and preferences, tell her the pros and cons not only of hormone replacement therapy in general but of the various types of estrogen and progesterone, then leave the decision up to her. After weighing all the factors, our patients often choose to begin therapy, and most of them are very satisfied once they get started.

Bi-estrogen must be formulated by a compounding pharmacist, who mixes the ingredients together to our specifications. (No large drug company makes bi-estrogen—it is a patent/profit issue.) Like all estrogen preparations, it requires a prescription.

You will need to work with a doctor to tailor your hormone replacement to meet your needs, for dosages vary from woman to woman and, as with any hormone replacement program, you may experience minor side effects until the proper dosage is achieved.

Our usual starting dose for postmenopausal women is 1.25 to 2.5 mg bi-estrogen. Most of our patients use bi-estrogen and natural progesterone together. Some use progesterone alone, and a very few use only estrogen (only women who no longer have a uterus). For a list of compounding pharmacies and physicians experienced with natural hormone replacement therapy, refer to the resource section.

PROGESTERONE, NOT PROGESTIN

Progesterone has taken a bad rap over the past couple of years. Several large studies of the effects of hormone replacement therapy on the cardiovascular system pointed to worse outcomes once progesterone was added to a regimen of estrogen supplementation. However, a few astute researchers are finally getting around to realizing what alternative docs have known for years: The "progesterone" used in all of these studies is not really progesterone at all but synthetic compounds called progestins. The most popular of the progestins in this country is Provera (medroxyprogesterone), a chemical derivative of progesterone with a similar but not identical molecular structure. Synthetic progestins have a host of adverse side effects in a woman's body from irritability and insomnia to breast tenderness and fluid retention to blood clots and cardiac arrest. Furthermore, these drugs can lower a woman's innate production of progesterone, which may further exacerbate hormone imbalances.

Now let's compare this to natural progesterone. Unlike Provera, which can cause fetal abnormalities if taken during pregnancy, natural progesterone is produced in abundance during pregnancy, and is in fact crucial to the survival of a fetus. It is often given to women having trouble conceiving. Do you think fertility doctors would give a woman trying to conceive Provera or another progestin? Not on your life. Yet millions of women are given prescriptions for this side-effect-riddled chemical.

While I'll be the first to agree that progestins should not be used by women with heart disease—or any women, for that matter—natural progesterone is another story. French researchers tackled this subject in a 2000 article in *Steroids*. They reported that while progestins do indeed have adverse effects on blood fats, natural progesterone has no negative effect on lipids. Furthermore, while natural progesterone does not reverse the beneficial effects of estrogen, the addition of progestin to an estrogen regimen has been shown to inhibit endothelial function, reducing the ability of the arteries to dilate by as much as 50 percent. This suggests that at worst, natural progesterone has a neutral effect on the cardiovascular system, while progestin has decidedly negative consequences.[21]

Another example of the difference between natural progesterone and progestins was demonstrated in an Italian study. Researchers treated 18 postmenopausal women with estradiol (the strongest form of estrogen) for four weeks. They then added natural progesterone, administered as a vaginal gel. After a two-week clearing-out period on estradiol alone, the patients were crossed over to progestin plus estradiol. During each phase of this study the women underwent exercise stress testing to see how long they could exercise before exhibiting signs of compromised blood flow to the heart. While taking estrogen alone, the women's exercise time on the stress test increased, compared to their baseline tests. On the estradiol/natural progesterone therapy, exercise time further improved. However, when the women were taking estradiol and a progestin, performance on the treadmill—and thus heart function—were compromised.[22]

A woman who has not had a hysterectomy should never take

estrogen by itself. It should always be balanced with natural, human-identical progesterone. The form we use at the institute is micronized oral progesterone suspended in an oil base for maximum stability and absorption. Another option is a cream or gel that you rub on your inner arms, thighs or shoulders, or vagina. Both of these forms deliver a measurable dose of progesterone that predictably raises blood levels of the hormone. I prefer oral natural progesterone because I feel that the dose can be better controlled. It requires a doctor's prescription. The topical skin preparations are available over the counter. Whichever route you go, I suggest you have blood tests of your progesterone levels to establish your appropriate dose.

HUMAN GROWTH HORMONE: PERHAPS THE MOST POWERFUL HORMONE OF ALL

Human growth hormone is secreted by the pituitary gland in large concentrations during the tremendous growth spurts of childhood and adolescence. After age twenty its production falls off by as much as 14 percent per decade. By the time we reach age sixty-five, levels are often negligible. Supplemental growth hormone has been around for years as the only treatment for children of extremely short stature caused by a deficiency in growth hormone. Its therapeutic value for adults first became apparent in 1990, with the publication in the *New England Journal of Medicine* of an extraordinary study by Daniel Rudman, M.D. In this study, six months of growth hormone administration to 21 men, ages sixty-one to eighty-one, resulted in improvements in lean muscle mass, bone density, and skin thickness that were equivalent to turning back the clock ten to twenty years.[23]

Interest in growth hormone took off like a rocket. Over the past decade we have seen positive studies on this hormone's benefits in the treatment of slow-healing wounds, brain injuries, immune dysfunction, osteoporosis, muscle wasting, and heart disease. It has been demonstrated to increase exercise tolerance, raise beneficial HDL cholesterol, and normalize blood pressure. However, the dominant effect of growth hormone on the cardiovascular system is on the heart muscle itself, making it an excellent therapy for heart failure. This condition is characterized by a weakening of the heart, which loses its ability to contract efficiently enough to pump blood throughout the body. As a result, fluids collect in the lungs and pool in the extremities. Growth hormone administration dramatically improves cardiac function in a majority of patients. Brazilian physicians reported on a patient with such severe heart failure that he was awaiting a heart transplant. He began treatment with growth hormone and over the next few months, his ejection fraction (a measurement of the heart's efficiency) climbed, his ability to exercise increased, and he was taken off the transplant list.[24]

To determine if your growth hormone levels are low, get a blood test for insulin-like growth factor-1 (IGF-1). Growth hormone is released in pulses, most significantly during sleep and heavy exercise. It travels to the liver, where it is quickly converted into IGF-1. By measuring this longer-lived compound, you can get an accurate prediction of your growth hormone level. If yours falls below 300 ng/ml, you may be a candidate for therapy, for premature atherosclerosis is common in growth-hormone-deficient adults.

Growth hormone is administered by injection with a small needle; patients inject themselves several times a week at home. Although the therapy isn't cheap, you get a lot of bang for your buck with growth hormone. In addition to the injected form, there are a number of over-the-counter products billed as growth hormone precursors, or secretagogues, which claim to stimulate the body's natural production of growth hormone. I don't recommend them at this time. The bulk of the research is on the injected hormone, and although I have seen evidence that some of these pills, powders, and sprays do raise IGF-1 levels, whether they are as effective a therapy as the hormone itself remains to be seen. Future research will tell.

Unlike the nutritional supplements we covered in Chapter 14, with the exception of DHEA and natural progesterone creams, these hormones require a prescription, and they all call for periodic monitoring to make sure your levels are in the therapeutic range. If you feel you would be a candidate for any of these hormones, bring it up with your doctor and draw his or her attention to the studies mentioned in this chapter and referenced in the back of the book. For listings of physicians familiar with natural hormone replacement therapy and compounding pharmacies that fulfill such prescriptions, see the resource section.

CHAPTER 18

EECP, Chelation, and Hyperbaric Oxygen: Big Guns Against Heart Disease

When Richard came to see me, he was in bad shape. Although he had had two bypass surgeries, the grafts had closed up and his angina had returned with a vengeance. Simply walking across the street from his parked car to my office was almost too much for him. Furthermore, his cardiologist told him that because of extensive scar tissue in his chest cavity from the previous surgeries, he was not a surgical candidate. He was deteriorating rapidly and had very few options, so he came to the Whitaker Wellness Institute as a last resort. Richard was already eating a good diet and taking an excellent nutritional supplement program. Extensive exercise was out of the question because of his chronic and severe angina.

I knew Richard needed something dramatic, so I started him on EECP. (I'll explain this therapy in detail below.) After only a handful of treatments Richard began to feel better. He was able to tolerate exercise better, and he had fewer bouts of chest pain. After the full treatment course, much to his delight, his chest pain was gone. He had a repeat PET scan, which showed substantial improvement in blood flow to his heart muscle. Richard was able to return to most of his previous activities and began enjoying life again. Over the next few years, Richard returned to the clinic periodically for a repeat course of EECP. The last time I saw him he told me he had moved to New Zealand and purchased a ranch. He was feeling great and having no problems keeping up the required manual labor.

Many of the patients with heart disease who come to the Whitaker Wellness Institute have been told that they need bypass surgery or angioplasty. They are seeking a second opinion because they hope to avoid such a drastic approach to their heart disease. Some, like Richard, come because their doctors have given them no hope at all. We start all these patients on the diet, exercise, and nutritional supplement program detailed in this book, and most of them do very well. They return home, persevere through the early weeks when breaking old habits makes for some challenging times, then settle into a way of life that works for them. Over time, their symptoms improve and their heart disease recedes. Sometimes, however, this isn't enough. A patient who is having severe and unrelenting chest pain or is able to walk only half a block before resting is in need of a more immediate fix. It isn't that lifestyle therapies won't work for these patients. As I hope I have made clear in this book, they can and they do. However, these people need more intense therapy, and they need it now.

This is why I have over the years incorporated three additional very powerful therapies into my practice. These therapies are examples of everything that is good about medicine. Unlike bypass surgery and angioplasty, they are noninvasive and involve no hospitalization, sedation, cutting, or other trauma to the body. Unlike drugs, they are nontoxic and there is no potential of harmful side effects. They are safe, relatively inexpensive, and are administered in a physician's office, not a hospital. Best of all, they work. Let's begin with the therapy that for patients with heart disease is the closest thing going to a natural bypass.

EECP: A NATURAL BYPASS

Enhanced external counterpulsation (EECP), the therapy Richard used to reverse his heart disease, has been around for more than forty-five years. It was developed at Harvard University by Harry Soroff, M.D., as a treatment for angina. Dr. Soroff figured that since angina was caused by insufficient blood flow and oxygen delivery to the heart, anything that would facilitate blood flow might relieve angina. He designed a mechanical system that literally squeezed blood out of the lower extremities and up toward the heart. It eased angina and improved circulation so much that it was quickly embraced as a therapy for heart disease and all manner of circulatory disorders—in China and other Asian countries, that is. In this country, it was inexplicably ignored.

Interest in EECP has surfaced in the past decade, however, and its benefits for the heart are supported by dozens of studies in the United States. One of them, published in the *American Journal of Cardiology*, followed 18 patients whose angina had returned following bypass surgery despite treatment with medications to help control their symptoms. Each of these patients underwent a course of EECP, receiving treatment five times a week. At the study's conclusion, 16 of the 18 patients reported complete relief from angina, while the other 2 reported less dramatic improvement. Follow-up thallium stress testing showed a complete resumption of blood flow to previously obstructed areas of the heart in 67 percent of the patients, partial resumption in 11 percent, and no change in 22 percent.[1]

Another study involved 12 patients who had significant angina—an average of 3.9 episodes a day with an average intensity of 2.9 out of 4. After completing a course of EECP, the angina episodes were reduced to an average of 0.1 per day with an intensity of only 1.7 out of 4. This means that they went from an average of almost four angina attacks a day to one every ten days.

And all these patients reported improvements in energy level, ability to work, and sense of well-being.[2]

In a 1999 placebo-controlled study, researchers at seven university medical centers, including Yale, Columbia, and Harvard, enlisted 139 patients with serious heart disease. Sixty-five percent of the patients had multivessel disease, more than half had already had at least one heart attack, and 62 percent had undergone bypass and/or angioplasty. All were having chronic and severe angina and taking multiple medications. They were divided into two groups and received either 35 EECP or sham (placebo) treatments. At the study's completion, patients in the placebo group showed little improvement. Those undergoing EECP, however, had a decrease in the number of weekly angina attacks, from 3.9 to 2.4, and required less nitroglycerin to curb their pain, from 2.6 to 1.2 doses per week. As in previous studies, they also reported an increase in exercise duration and marked improvements in their energy level and how they felt overall.[3]

EECP Provides Long-Term Benefits

The best part about EECP is that it is very effective in relieving chest pain not only during and just after treatment but for months and years afterward. Here's why. EECP stimulates the production of collateral circulation, the blood vessels we discussed earlier that grow around arterial blockages. It is the equivalent of a surgery-free bypass. In no time at all, new vessels are opened, supplying adequate oxygen and nutrient-rich blood to the heart muscle and alleviating anginal pain.

The actual therapy is somewhat difficult to describe. You lie on a flat surface and what looks like a wet suit is strapped around your lower extremities, from the ankles to just below the waist. You are then hooked up to an EKG machine that monitors your heartbeat, and in synchrony with each beat of your heart, the contraption contracts. This forces blood up the extremities and through the veins toward the heart, increasing blood flow not only to the heart but also to the brain, kidneys, eyes, and other organs. One treatment session lasts about an hour. Patients chat, listen to music, watch television, or read. Aside from the squeezing sensation, there is no discomfort. The recommended course is thirty-five one-hour treatments, taken once or twice a day. In three or four weeks, far less time than it would take to recover from bypass surgery, chest pain and other symptoms of heart disease are often eliminated.

You may wonder how long EECP's benefits last. In the multicenter study reported above, 40 patients who had undergone EECP were reexamined one year after the conclusion of their treatment course. Seventy percent continued to show improvement.[4] Most patients note benefits long after the treatment is finished. One man whose heart disease was so severe that he had been given his last rites underwent EECP because he had no other options. Five years after treatment, he remained pain-free and fully active. Furthermore, if pain does return after a number of months or years, you can safely undergo another course.

EECP is gaining popularity in this country. Although I was one of the first physicians to utilize it, its benefits are so dramatic and well documented that even Medicare reimburses for its use in patients with angina. If you've been told you have no options other than bypass surgery, get thee to an EECP center. I also recommend you check EECP out if you are afflicted with any condition involving the circulatory system, such as peripheral vascular disease, stroke, Parkinson's disease, erectile dysfunction, blindness due to retinal artery occlusion, or sudden deafness. Even though most of the American research on this therapy has been on its effects on heart disease, EECP has been studied and is widely used abroad for the treatment of these other disorders.

EDTA CHELATION: A TRIED-AND-TRUE THERAPY FOR HEART DISEASE

Ethylenediaminetetraacetic acid (EDTA) is a synthetic protein that has an affinity for minerals. When it is slowly infused into the bloodstream, it latches on to minerals such as iron, copper, lead, and cadmium, forming a tight chemical bond. It then passes through the kidneys and out of the body in the urine, taking these minerals with it. Although most of these minerals are required for optimal health (lead is an exception), when they build up in the body, friend turns to foe and they speed up the oxidation process. Removing excesses of these minerals through chelation retards free radical damage to the arteries and slows down atherosclerosis.

Chelation tackles atherosclerosis from other angles as well. It chelates excess calcium from the arterial walls, making them more responsive and better able to dilate, thus improving blood flow and general circulation. It also has blood-thinning effects and discourages the formation of potentially harmful blood clots that could initiate a heart attack. Furthermore, it is a powerful antioxidant in and of itself. Given the diverse ways in which chelation protects the cardiovascular system, you would think that this therapy would be embraced by the medical community. Unfortunately, this has not happened.

Chelation Has a Rocky History

While chelation therapy has long been recognized as the most effective therapy available for heavy metal poisoning, its benefits for the cardiovascular system were discovered largely by accident in the 1950s. When men suffering from lead poisoning from painting World War II battleships underwent EDTA chelation to remove this toxic metal from their bodies, physicians noticed that those who had heart disease were having remarkable improvements not only in their symptoms of lead poisoning but also in their chest pain and other signs of atherosclerosis.

This discovery was met with enthusiasm, and further usage confirmed the original discoveries. Chelation was well on its way to becoming an accepted treatment for heart disease until 1963, when prominent Philadelphia physician Lawrence Meltzer, M.D., published an article in the *American Journal of Cardiology* that questioned its effectiveness. He assessed the long-term effects of a single course of chelation treatment in 38 patients with severe heart disease. After three months of treatment, 66 percent of the patients noted reductions in angina, and 40 percent had improvements on their electrocardiogram. After four years, although 12 of the patients had died, 15 of them continued to experience the benefits delivered by EDTA. Based on this study, Dr. Meltzer concluded that EDTA chelation therapy was ineffective.

As I review this study today I am baffled by Dr. Meltzer's conclusion, for it is not consistent with the data in his own article. The reported annual death rate in these study subjects of 8 percent was superior to the overall death rate from severe heart disease at that time. Heart disease was a much more virulent disease in the 1960s than it is now, and these patients were quite ill to begin with. Numerous experts have estimated that the yearly death rate in comparable patients would have been between 10 and 15 percent. Rather than recognizing the obvious benefits from this early study, Dr. Meltzer illogically stated that chelation therapy is "not a useful tool in the treatment of coronary disease at the present time."[5]

Over the next few years chelation therapy lost favor as invasive procedures and powerful drugs grew in popularity. Fortunately, chelation never went away. A handful of physicians persisted in using the therapy and continued to report its substantial benefits, and close to a million patients have undergone this therapy for cardiovascular disease.

Its Benefits Are Proven

Several studies have confirmed the benefits of chelation. A 1993 analysis reviewed forty published studies and another thirty unpublished studies involving a total of 25,000 patients. All but one, a Danish study, had positive results, and 87 percent of patients overall demonstrated improvements in vascular disease.[6] Of course, the negative Danish study has probably received the most attention. But an interesting aside is that just before this study was done, Danish physicians offered chelation to seriously ill patients who were awaiting bypass surgery or amputation of an extremity. Of the 92 patients who underwent chelation, 82 canceled their surgery![7]

While studies provide compelling statistics, I have been even more impressed by the effects of chelation that I have witnessed in my own patients. John came to see me with severe chest pain and a recommendation from his physician to undergo repeat bypass surgery. His memories of his triple bypass ten years earlier were anything but pleasant, so he was looking for alternative ways to relieve his debilitating chest pain. I put him on our lifestyle program, along with a course of EDTA chelation therapy. He began to improve almost immediately. After only six treatments his pain was dramatically reduced, and after eighteen sessions he had virtually no symptoms. When John first began therapy, I asked him what he would be doing if he were well. He told me that he wanted to travel. Six months after his treatment at the Whitaker Wellness Institute, John climbed the stairs of the Statue of Liberty without any pain. A year later he was in Siena, Italy, climbing the thirty stories of stairs of the Siena Tower—and he had to stop only twice to catch his breath.

Sixty-one-year-old Richard was hospitalized with severe chest pain and told that if he didn't have bypass surgery he would die. Richard signed himself out of the hospital against medical advice and came to the institute for chelation. A year and a half later, he was pain-free and taking no heart medications. Thomas, sixty-four, had a calcified heart valve, numerous blockages in his coronary arteries, and an 80 percent blockage in one of his carotid arteries. He was told he was a "walking time bomb" and that bypass surgery, replacement of his heart valve, and carotid endarterectomy (surgical reaming out of the artery in his neck) were his only options. He said no thanks, and took his chances with lifestyle changes and chelation. A year later his heart valve was functioning normally, his carotid blockage had receded to only 15 percent, he was taking no drugs, and he felt great. Robert had severe blockages in two of his coronary arteries and was given a "death sentence" unless he had surgery. He chose to go on a heart-healthy diet, do regular exercise, and start chelation therapy. Two years later he was off all drugs, had no angina, and was jogging four miles a day.

My favorite patient story regarding chelation isn't about coronary artery disease, but it is an amazing testimony to the power of this therapy. J.J. was a fifty-three-year-old high school teacher with a long history of diabetes. He was plagued with recurring open, ulcerated sores on his feet that just wouldn't heal in spite of massive doses of antibiotics. He was finally told that his only option was amputation. On the day J.J. was to have surgery, he called his substitute teacher. This teacher had heard of chelation therapy and my clinic and suggested that J.J. check us out. He left the hospital against his physician's advice and came to the Whitaker Wellness Institute. We started him on a comprehensive treatment program, which included an immediate course of chelation. Today J.J. is walking around on his own two legs, teaching, coaching, and living life to its fullest.

Chelation is administered in a physician's office, usually once or twice a week. You sit in a recliner and an IV is inserted into a vein in your arm. Then you sit back and relax, sleep, read, or chat with others undergoing the same treatment while EDTA slowly circulates through the miles of blood vessels in your body. Each treatment takes about three hours, and a complete course is between twenty and thirty treatments. Patients with a chronic condition often continue with ongoing maintenance treatments once a month. Although the initial IV needle insertion may be uncomfortable, the procedure itself is painless and completely safe. I recommend EDTA chelation therapy for patients with hypertension, atherosclerosis, angina, and circulatory disorders such as intermittent claudication, peripheral artery disease, and diabetic complications of the lower extremities.

SATURATE YOUR CELLS WITH HYPERBARIC OXYGEN

Food, water, and oxygen are the three requisites for life, but our most immediate need is for oxygen. If your cells are deprived of this life-sustaining element for even short periods of time, they will die. Cut off blood and oxygen supply to the brain (the essence of a stroke) and neurons begin to die within minutes. Block its delivery to the heart, and you have the coup de grâce in heart disease. Virtually all of the therapies we have discussed in this book directly or indirectly improve oxygen delivery to the heart and arteries. Now I want to tell you about hyperbaric oxygen therapy, a treatment we utilize at the Whitaker Wellness Institute that literally floods the body with oxygen—including areas affected by severe atherosclerosis.

Hyperbaric (meaning above normal pressure) oxygen therapy is a way of delivering massive amounts of oxygen to oxygen-starved tissues. The best way to explain how it works is to visualize a Coke. Open the can and there is a pop as built-up gas (carbon dioxide) is released. Pour it into a glass and it immediately fizzes up as gas bubbles escape from the liquid. After a time, the bubbling stops and the drink becomes flat because at normal atmospheric pressure, gases will not dissolve in liquids—they simply escape into the atmosphere. To get the fizzy effects of carbonation, these soft drinks must be bottled under pressure.

This is essentially how hyperbaric oxygen therapy works. While at normal atmospheric pressure oxygen is carried only on the hemoglobin in your red blood cells, in a pressurized environment oxygen dissolves in all of your body's fluids and is transported to all tissues, even those with a poor or absent blood supply. As you breathe oxygen in a hyperbaric oxygen chamber, your cells are flooded with many times their normal amount of oxygen. Believe it or not, inside a hyperbaric chamber a patient's heart could actually be stopped with no ill effects—oxygen would enter and sustain the cells even if there were no blood flow. In fact, before the invention of the heart-lung machine, some of the very early open-heart surgeries were performed in hyperbaric oxygen chambers.

Oxygen Under Pressure

Hyperbaric oxygen therapy is administered in a specially designed chamber. After you are comfortably situated in the chamber, pressure is slowly increased to 1.4 to 3 times normal atmospheric pressure. You'll probably notice increased pressure in your ears, similar to what you feel when a plane takes off or lands, but there is no other discomfort. Then you breathe 100 percent oxygen through a small mask while relaxing or listening to music. A typical treatment session lasts forty-five minutes to two hours, and at its completion pressure is slowly returned to normal. Sessions are repeated from five to forty times, depending on the condition being treated.

The effects of this massive infusion of oxygen are remarkable. For patients who have just suffered a heart attack, hyperbaric oxygen can be lifesaving. It lessens damage to the heart muscle by providing dying cells with oxygen and minimizing fluid accumulation that leads to cell death. It also enhances the effects of clot-busting drugs administered right after a heart attack. A group of physicians at the Long Beach Memorial Medical Center in Long Beach, California, studied 46 patients who were admitted to the hospital with an acute heart attack. All of the patients were treated with a clot-dissolving drug, tissue plasminogen activator (TPA), but 24 of them also received two hours of hyperbaric oxygen therapy.

Those who received hyperbaric oxygen reported relief from angina after an average of 271 minutes from the time they first noted symptoms, and most noted relief within ten minutes of entering the chamber. The patients who were treated with the drug alone did not experience pain relief until 671 minutes post–heart attack. These physicians also reported that the therapy hastened the recovery of normal electrical activity in the heart, which as we discussed in Part I becomes erratic during a heart attack. EKGs of the oxygen-treated patients calmed down in an average of 188 minutes, compared to 374 minutes for those treated only with drugs. There was also evidence that the heart muscle cells of the patients who received hyperbaric oxygen were actually being saved. Furthermore, the ejection fraction, which indicates the pumping efficiency of the heart, was better in the hyperbaric group.[8]

Hyperbaric oxygen therapy is also useful in less dire circumstances. It relieves angina, smoothes out arrhythmias, and improves circulation. It also stimulates angiogenesis, the growth of collaterals. The high pressure inside a hyperbaric oxygen chamber causes the arteries to constrict, which is harmless, since oxygen is suffusing the cells. Once you leave the chamber, your body compensates for this theoretical reduction in blood flow by growing new blood vessels. As you go in and out, in and out of the chamber, more and more new blood vessels spring up around blocked arteries.

Hyperbaric oxygen-induced angiogenesis is particularly evident in the small vessels of the brain, making it a remarkable therapy for strokes, which can afflict patients with hypertension and heart disease. Stroke patients can often avoid paralysis, speech difficulties, and other impairment if hyperbaric oxygen therapy is administered immediately after the stroke. Jackie, an active seventy-six-year-old, came to our clinic for hyperbaric oxygen therapy after suffering a stroke during an angioplasty. She hobbled into the office for her first treatment, using a walker and aided by her son and daughter-in-law. Two weeks and eight treatments later, she carried her walker over the threshold, and now she's out dancing three nights a week.

It even helps months or years after a stroke. Vic, a seventy-one-year-old who had two strokes in the summer of 1999, left the hospital in a wheelchair with severe speech, vision, and hearing deficits. After one month in a rehabilitation center, he was sent home. His wife was advised that there was no hope of improvement and it was suggested that she put him in a nursing home. Instead, after reading about hyperbaric oxygen therapy, she brought her husband to the clinic for treatment some six months after his initial stroke. Vic returned for a second course of treatment a few months later, and the last time we saw him, he was walking at least a mile a day and was back to his former activities.

More than 30,000 scientific studies have been published on hyperbaric oxygen therapy over the past seven decades. It has proven useful in the treatment of almost 200 medical conditions, ranging from chronic fatigue and fibromyalgia to multiple sclerosis and Lyme disease. Its benefits in facilitating wound healing are legendary. Oxygen not only encourages new tissue growth but also dramatically curtails infection, since oxygen kills many types of bacteria. Many patients with deadly poisonous spider bites or flesh-eating bacteria, who would otherwise have lost limbs if not their lives, have been saved by this therapy.

While hyperbaric oxygen has been heartily embraced by physicians in many countries, there are fewer than 350 hyperbaric chambers in the United States, and most of them are in hospitals that restrict use to only fourteen Medicare-approved applications, such as treating decompression illness (the bends), serious skin and bone infections, carbon monoxide poisoning, skin grafts, gangrene, and peripheral artery disease. This is unfortunate. In my opinion, this safe therapy should be standard emergency room treatment right after a heart attack. Furthermore, it should be available to the millions of patients with other conditions who would fare much better than with the drugs and surgical procedures they are currently receiving.

IF THESE THERAPIES ARE SO GOOD, WHY DON'T MORE DOCTORS RECOMMEND THEM?

This a question that has haunted me since I was a young resident, first learning about effective therapies that were not taught in medical school. The answer isn't that there's a lack of research supporting these "alternative" therapies. The efficacy of every therapy discussed in this book has been confirmed in scientific studies. In fact, most of them have more supporting research than many of the surgical procedures commonly used for heart disease—some of which, as we discussed in Part II, are not only unproven but actually "disproven."

Nor can the resistance to these therapies be explained by concerns about safety—surgical procedures and prescription drugs kill more than a hundred thousand Americans every year and harm millions more. And the risks of bypass surgery are, for most patients, greater than their risk of dying from heart disease while being treated with more conservative therapies.

In my opinion, this leaves only one explanation for the bias against alternative therapies: the threat that these therapies pose to the status quo. If these therapies were to gain a foothold in medicine, guess what they would replace? The multibillion-dollar hospital-based cardiology wards and surgical suites, and entire classes of best-selling pharmaceuticals. There is just too much invested in the heart disease industry as it now exists.

I sense that the resistance against alternatives in medicine is gradually changing, but like most revolutions in the history of humanity, it is changing from the ground up. More and more people like you are learning about the remarkable benefits of these and other unique, safe, and noninvasive therapies. You are coming to realize the dangers and irrationality of the old approach to the treatment of heart disease. You realize that doctors are not demigods but rather people with the same foibles and weaknesses as everyone else. You are taking charge of your own health like never before.

I suspect that managed care will hasten this process. The financial incentive of managed care is to cut costs by withholding expensive treatments. The effectiveness and easy implementation of therapies like those discussed in this and previous chapters—which cost a fraction of the expense of bypass, angioplasty, and lifelong drug regimens—should make them mighty attractive. We will likely see more and better coverage for EECP, chelation, hyperbaric oxygen, nutritional supplements, and lifestyle change programs, at the expense of drugs and surgery.

PART IV

The Dietary Program for Reversing Heart Disease

CHAPTER 19

How to Approach the Dietary Program

BECAUSE OF THE IMPORTANCE THAT FOOD HAS IN OUR LIVES, WE are devoting an entire section of this book to the diet for reversing heart disease. Food is much more than the fuel that keeps us going—it is a big part of our lives. We don't eat things because they're good for us but because they taste good, and what tastes good to us is what we have grown up with. Offer a bowl of menudo, a soup made with intestines, to natives of Mexico, and their mouths will water. Explain its contents to someone who has never had it before and you're likely to get a polite "No, thank you." The same goes for haggis, the Scottish delicacy made of a sheep's stomach, and the Korean favorite, kimchee, a spicy, smelly, fermented cabbage dish. Food also has layer upon layer of emotional meaning. A bowl of grits takes me right back to my mother's kitchen in Atlanta. Birthday cakes, fried chicken on Sunday, grandmother's turkey dressing, your family's special Christmas dessert: We love these foods because we associate them with good times in our lives.

This program requires changes in your eating habits. I know this isn't easy, and at first glance it may seem impossible—this is a normal reaction to any kind of change, dietary or not. One thing that will make it easier is to always keep your eye on your goal: better health. You are obviously a highly motivated individual or you wouldn't be reading this book. Having read Chapters 11 and 12, you now understand the reasoning behind this diet—how it can improve your health and actually reverse many of the risk factors for heart disease—and your resolve should be firmer than ever. As you become familiar with the principles of this dietary program and make it part of your life, you will find that eating healthfully becomes easier and easier. I'll go so far as to predict that one of these days this new way of eating will become so ingrained that you will lose your cravings for the unhealthy foods you left behind. Your best motivation, however, will be noticeable improvements in your health and how well you feel.

RECIPE FOR SUCCESS

I do not underestimate the efforts required to adopt and adjust to this dietary regimen. The entire thrust of this program is a clarion call to change the habits that make us sick, and changing eating habits is more difficult than changing any other habitual behavior. There are two philosophies on how to approach this program. One is to ease into it: Reduce red meat consumption from five nights a week to two, cut desserts back from every evening to two or three times a week, switch to low-fat varieties of cheese, and gradually add more and more of the recommended foods.

Another philosophy is to just jump into the program. Go cold turkey. Clean out your cupboards, restock your fridge, and make an abrupt about-face. This means following the program to the letter—no compromises. In my opinion, the latter approach is the best. Think of it like this. How many alcoholics do you know who control their habit by drinking moderately? How many smokers are able simply to cut back on the cigarettes they smoke? The best way to control these addictions is simply to stop. Dietary changes require the same degree of discipline.

This is the approach we take with the patients who spend a week with us at the Whitaker Wellness Institute. The clinic program of diet, exercise, and nutritional supplementation outlined in this book is designed to produce results—and produce them quickly, so patients can see changes before they return home. They are often astonished that improvements in cholesterol, triglycerides, blood pressure, weight, energy, pain, and sense of well-being come about so rapidly. After all, most of them have been battling heart disease for years and have already tried many conventional therapies. One of my favorite things about the weeklong clinic program is watching the transformation of frightened, debilitated patients into enthusiastic and motivated proponents of the regimen.

For one week our patients eat nothing but the heart-healthy foods and dishes described in this section. Of course, for them it's easier because someone else does the shopping and cooking. However, at the same time, our nutritionist and professional chef are teaching them how to shop, cook, eat in restaurants, and stick with this program after they return home. Because it takes about twenty-one days to change a habit, we encourage our patients to strictly adhere to the program for a minimum of two more weeks. This is a crucial period, for they must integrate their new lifestyle into the real world. We have found that if people are extremely vigilant during this time—for a total of three weeks—they are much more likely to stay on track over the long run. After this period, the new lifestyle starts to become second nature, and improvements in health accelerate. Once they've experienced how well they feel on their new regimen, they are less likely to go back to their old habits.

People who successfully implement this program generally go through three phases. The first phase is one of negativity—you may be discouraged and feel it will be impossible to make all these changes. The food is different from what you're used to. If you are a diehard meat-and-potato eater, you may have never considered eating anything besides meat or chicken as a main dish. It gets easier during the second phase, as you learn the tricks of the trade. What was once foreign and strange becomes familiar, shopping is easier, and the uncomfortable disruption of your old routines is replaced by the pleasure of instituting new ones. During this time you will invariably notice improvements in your health. You will likely be taking less medication, your blood pressure and weight will drop, and you will have more energy.

In stage three, your new diet will become old hat. Your taste buds will grow to enjoy the taste of "real" food, not doctored up with sugar, fats, and salt. Expect to get off track on occasion—after all, you're only human—but when you do, it will only remind you of how far you have come, how much you have changed. You will know you've arrived when this dietary program is not a "diet" but simply the way you eat. I remember when I first started this program years ago, one of my favorite snacks was air-popped popcorn we made at home. At the movies one night I bought some popcorn—the regular salted, buttered kind—and it just about knocked my socks off. I wondered how I ever tolerated so much fat and salt!

Of the thousands of patients who have completed this program at the institute, without exception those who enjoy the most success and get the most pleasure out of their new regimen choose not to look upon it as an exercise in deprivation but rather as an opportunity to improve their health and enhance their lives. Their continuing good health becomes a mission, a hobby, an avocation, and a labor of love.

REVIEW OF DIET PRINCIPLES

Before we go on, let's recap the general guidelines of the diet for reversing heart disease. To revisit these principles in detail, go back to Chapter 12.

Make Plant Foods the Basis of Your Diet

The healthiest foods for humans are vegetables, fruits, beans, and whole grains. They are excellent sources of the nutritional components that fight heart disease: fiber, carbohydrates, vitamins, minerals, and phytonutrients. The best plant foods are those that are in their natural state, and if they are organic, so much the better. Vegetables, fruits, beans, legumes, and whole grains should make up about 60 percent of your total caloric intake.

Processed and refined plant foods, particularly refined grains and sugars, are another story. Products made with sugar and white flour, such as white bread, crackers, pastries, and cookies, as well as cold cereals, rice cakes, and other snack foods have a high glycemic index rating. (So do starchy root vegetables like white potatoes and turnips, and tropical fruits like pineapple and ripe bananas. However, because they are whole foods they aren't as problematic as processed foods.) These foods cause too rapid an elevation in blood sugar and insulin. This is particularly harmful for diabetics but is also of concern for the many patients with heart disease who are insulin resistant. Regular consumption of these foods may cause elevated triglycerides, low HDL cholesterol, abdominal weight gain, hypertension, and other manifestations of insulin resistance, or syndrome X. Because of the very close association between insulin resistance and heart disease, I recommend that all patients with heart disease avoid or seriously restrict their consumption of these foods.

Eat Only Healthy Fats

Saturated fat from animal foods elevates cholesterol. Trans fatty acids in fried foods and hydrogenated oils raise total cholesterol *and* lower protective HDL. Excess fat in the bloodstream impedes blood flow and interferes with a number of metabolic processes. Monounsaturated olive oil, on the other hand, improves circulation and lowers blood pressure, while omega-3 fatty acids in fish and flaxseed oils are a blessing to the cardiovascular system. Polyunsaturated oils from sunflower seeds, almonds, and other nuts and seeds are also good—provided that they are cold-pressed and unprocessed (which most brands are not). The point is, there are good fats and there are bad fats, and if you have heart disease, you need to learn the difference.

My general recommendation is that about 20 percent of your daily calories should come from healthy fats. Enjoy raw nuts, avocados, olive oil, and fatty fish, but be vigilant about avoiding saturated and processed trans fats. The best cooking oil is olive oil, for it can better tolerate heat without breaking down into unhealthy by-products as polyunsaturated fats do. (Canola oil is a distant second because of the extensive processing required to extract this monounsaturated oil.). Polyunsaturated flaxseed and other cold-pressed vegetable oils are good for salad dressings, but they are fragile and should never be heated.

To coat the nonstick skillets, baking pans, and griddles you will be using to prepare your food, use an olive oil cooking spray such as Pam, or purchase a kitchen sprayer and fill it with extra-virgin olive oil. If you feel you need something to spread on bread, check out the low-fat margarines that are free of trans fatty acids or boast beneficial plant sterols. (Read labels very carefully, for most margarines contain harmful trans fats.) Butter (preferably organic) on very special occasions is acceptable, but do not take this as license to use it regularly. When cooking try Butter Buds Brand Natural Butter Flavored Mix or a similar product to get that good old butter flavor.

Eat Enough Protein—But Not Too Much

Don't obsess about protein. Eat a healthy diet and you'll get plenty of this essential nutrient. You don't have to pork out on meat and eggs either. As we discussed in Chapter 12, soy and other beans, legumes, nuts, and seeds are very good sources of protein, as are fish and skinless poultry. Replace ground beef with ground turkey breast. If possible, purchase organically fed free-range poultry and eggs. Even though you will pay a little more for them, you'll likely find that your total food bill will be lower with this way of eating, since you're cutting out red meat and convenience foods. Your daily protein intake should be about 20 percent of total calories.

Don't Overeat

We eat too much. The average American's idea of a normal serving of meat, for example, is eight ounces—and a 16-ounce steak is not considered unusual. Restaurants serve gigantic portions on oversized plates. Fast food joints specialize in 48-ounce beverages and "super-sizes" of everything. It's no wonder we're so heavy.

This program does not require that you count calories or grams of fat. I know from experience that this drives people nuts. You will, however, need to monitor your portions, and the guidelines below will help you learn to eyeball appropriate serving sizes without having to compute calories and the like. (The "typical" serving size in reference charts and on food labels for meat, poultry, and fish is just four ounces.) If you're still hungry, eat more of the recommended foods. Nobody gets fat eating vegetables, beans, and fruit. Eating slowly will also help you eat less. It takes about twenty minutes for the signal of fullness to reach your brain, so if you're gobbling down your food in half that time, you're likely to overeat.

RECOMMENDED DAILY INTAKE AND PORTION SIZES

Carbohydrates (60 percent of total calories)

- Vegetables: 5 to 8 servings; limit starchy vegetables (white potatoes, turnips, corn) to two to three times a week. 1 serving = 1 cup raw (the size of a tennis ball) or ¾ cup cooked vegetables. If you find you're still hungry, eat more from this food group.

- Fruit: 3 to 4 servings; go easy on dried fruits and tropical fruits. 1 serving = 1 medium whole fruit or ¾ cup sliced fruit.
- Starches and grains: 3 to 4 servings from the bread, cereal, pasta, and grain categories. Pasta is fine, but prepared foods made from refined grains and flour (cold cereals, most breads and snack foods) promote insulin resistance. 1 serving = 1 slice of bread, ½ bagel, or ¾ cup cooked cereal, pasta, or grain. Try to not exceed this number of servings.

Protein (20 percent of total calories)

- 3 to 4 servings of lean protein
- Fish or poultry: 1 serving = 4 ounces (about the size of a deck of cards)
- Beans: 1 serving = ¾ cup cooked beans
- Soy products: 1 serving = 4 ounces tofu, 1 cup soy milk, ½ cup soy protein
- Raw nuts and seeds: 1 serving = 2 tablespoons nuts, seeds, or nut butter
- Dairy: 1 serving = 1 cup nonfat cottage cheese or yogurt
- Eggs: 1 serving = 1 whole egg, 2 egg whites, or ¼ cup Eggbeaters or another frozen egg product

Fat (20 percent of total calories)

- Eat only natural, unprocessed fats. Trim meat, skin poultry, and go easy on whole-fat dairy. Limit oil intake to 2 to 3 tablespoons of olive or flaxseed oil (with occasional use of other cold-pressed oils). Strictly avoid fried foods and those made with hydrogenated oils (including margarine, regular peanut butter, store-bought pastries and baked goods, and deep-fried foods).

SHOP SMART

Shop in the produce section, spend time among the dried beans and grains, visit the frozen vegetables—and quickly breeze through the prepared, canned, and boxed food. Get familiar with a local health food store. It is the only place you will find some of the healthful oils and sweeteners I recommend. And get into the habit of reading labels. Although most of the foods you will be purchasing will be fresh, you will use some boxed, canned, and frozen foods. Before you purchase them, scrutinize their labels carefully.

Pay attention to sugar in its various guises: corn syrup, fructose, fruit juice solids, maltose, etc. You will be astounded by how much sugar is in some products. Also focus on sodium content and aim for less than 1,000 mg a day. (As we discussed in Chapter 10, sodium-potassium balance is the real key. If you eat lots of potassium-rich plant foods, you can get by with more sodium.) And carefully check labels for fat. Avoid anything with saturated fat or hydrogenated or partially hydrogenated oils. As long as you are eating the right types of fat (most processed foods contain unhealthy fats), you don't need to be so fanatical about precise amounts.

A final bit of advice. Never go to the grocery store when you're really hungry. Things you wouldn't normally buy—convenience foods, desserts, even candy bars—somehow manage to sneak into your shopping cart. Once when I was shopping, the smells wafting from the bakery enticed me to buy a couple of loaves of French bread that had just come out of the oven. By the time I got home, one of them was half gone!

Deciphering Food Labels

- Sugar content is listed in grams. To turn this into something more tangible, use this quick conversion: 4 grams equal 1 teaspoon of sugar. A can of regular Coke contains 39 grams of sugar (in the form of high fructose corn syrup)—almost 10 teaspoons. An eight-ounce container of fat-free fruit yogurt has 28 grams, or 7 teaspoons.
- To determine the percentage of fat, do a quick ratio of fat calories to total calories. A one-ounce serving of cheddar cheese contains 85 fat calories and 110 total calories: 85/110 = 77 percent fat. (You can either divide 85 by 110 or eyeball it to realize that it's pretty darn high.) Furthermore, the label notes that two-thirds of the fat is saturated fat. A serving of reduced-fat crackers, which has 40 fat calories out of 140 total calories, is almost 29 percent fat. Since most of it is partially hydrogenated vegetable oil shortening, this is a product you'd want to stay away from, reduced fat or not.
- If you want to figure out the percent of protein in a given product, multiply each gram of protein by 4 to get protein calories. That same serving of cheddar cheese contains 7 grams or 28 calories from protein and so is 26 percent protein. (7 grams x 4 protein calories per gram = 28 protein calories/110 total calories = 26 percent). The crackers have 3 grams or 12 protein calories per 140 total calories and are thus 8.5 percent protein.

DINING OUT

This program in no way means that you have to give up dining in restaurants. I realize how many meals are eaten in restaurants these days—I eat out pretty often myself. It is possible to stay on track in restaurants and still enjoy yourself. It goes without saying that some restaurants are easier than others. All-you-can-eat salad bars are perfect. Just make sure you don't slather your vegetables with high-fat dressings—put them on the side and use judiciously. Also go easy on mixed salads such as potato salad and coleslaw, since they are loaded with unhealthy oils and mayonnaise. A piece of bread or a few crackers with your meal are fine, but you really need to get out of the habit of eating a lot of bread. As I have repeatedly pointed out, many people who have heart disease also have insulin resistance, and these fast-burning carbohydrates can do a number on your blood sugar and insulin levels.

When you are ordering from a menu, it is perfectly acceptable to request modifications and to even order things that are not on the menu. The golden rule is to be very precise when you order and to make sure the waiter understands you. Be polite but specific, and most waiters will be more than willing to work with you. If you happen to get a waiter with an attitude, ask to speak to the manager.

Good choices are fish, chicken breast, vegetables, and pasta, but make sure you specify how you want them prepared—baked or broiled rather than breaded and fried. "On the side" will become your mantra. Salads with dressing on the side. Fish broiled without butter, with the sauce on the side. Of course, you could order these things without the sauces and dressings altogether, but what the heck, you're in a nice restaurant. Enjoy the extra flavor by dipping your fork into the sauce or dressing, then stab a bite of fish, salad, or whatever, and eat it. Enough of the sauce/dressing will cling to the fork that you'll get a hint of flavor, but you will eat only a small portion of what you would eat if the food were drowned in the sauce.

As a rule, better restaurants are more amenable to your requests and desires than lower-priced ones. It seems like the lower you go on the price scale, the less likely you are to be able to get low-fat, healthy food. You can still eat in fast-food joints, but stick to salads with dressing on the side and grilled chicken. If you find that certain "blacklisted" foods are just too tempting for you—pizza or hamburgers might be your hot buttons—simply stay away from those types of restaurants.

SNACKING

Any diet program that does not include snacks is on shaky footing. When we're really hungry, we want something to eat, and we want it fast. If you don't have healthful options, you'll go for whatever is handy. Give these tasty, easy-to-fix snacks a try.

- Leftovers
- A piece of fruit
- Raw vegetables and dip (choose your favorite from the salad dressing recipes in this book or purchase fat-free dips)
- Apple slices with raw nut butter (1 tablespoon nut butter per apple)
- Raw nuts and seeds: almonds, sunflower seeds, pumpkin seeds, etc. (2 tablespoons total)
- Nonfat cottage cheese, plain or with fruit (¾ cup cottage cheese, ½ cup fruit)
- Crackers and avocado (4 small rye or whole-wheat crackers and ¼ avocado)
- Smoothie (see recipe on page 359)
- Soybeans, raw in pod (Edamame) (½ cup)
- Nonfat yogurt, plain, with added fruit and sweetened with stevia (¾ cup yogurt, ¼ to ½ cup fruit, 3+ drops stevia, to taste)
- Half a sandwich (choose from sandwich recipes in Chapter 21, pp. 380–381)
- Whole wheat tortilla with salsa
- *Whitaker Wellness Health & Nutrition Bar

*See the resource section.

STAYING ON TRACK

Staying on the straight and narrow can be challenging. There will be many, many times when you will be confronted with less than perfect food choices. Consider all the picnics, wedding receptions, office parties, birthday parties, potluck suppers, and family gatherings in your future. Life is built around socializing, and socializing is built around eating. When you are unable to obtain your ideal foods, you'll just have to choose the next best thing—or in some cases, the lesser of two evils.

We've talked about potential pitfalls of eating in restaurants, but the truth is most accidents (falling off the program) happen at home. That stash of cookies you have "for the kids" slowly disappears. You cook your traditional high-fat lasagna because your family loves it. Unless you have a will of steel, don't keep things in the house that you don't want to eat. (This is especially true of snack foods.) And make the effort to learn how to modify that lasagna recipe and make it healthier. Your family loves you enough to support your efforts to improve your health.

In the next chapter we will talk about getting started on the diet for reversing heart disease: shopping for staples, modifying recipes, and cooking basics. Then in Chapter 21 I will provide you with kitchen-tested recipes from the Whitaker Wellness Institute that will make this transition an ease and a delight.

CHAPTER 20

Getting Started

IN THIS CHAPTER, WE ARE GOING TO SHOW YOU HOW TO TRANSform your kitchen and meals into something that would do a health spa proud. We will teach you how to follow the general dietary guidelines, what to keep on hand for quick meals and snacks, and how to convert your favorite recipes into similar but healthier versions. This information should serve only as a starting point to help you get over the initial hump. I have no doubt that by following these guidelines you will be able to develop your own recipes, favorite dishes, and shortcuts. However, these simple hints may spare you from a lot of frustration in the beginning.

SHOPPING GUIDE

You can do most of your shopping in your local grocery store, but I strongly recommend that you get acquainted with a health food store. My family does most of our shopping in such a store. We prefer organic fruits and vegetables, and we love the bins full of beans, nuts, and grains. If you don't have access to a good health food store, don't worry—you will get by fine at the grocery store. If you cannot find something, it never hurts to ask your grocer to stock it. I have provided in the resource section mail order sources for hard-to-find items.

Here are some of the food items you will be using frequently. You don't have to buy everything listed here, particularly the perishables, but it is a smart idea to keep a good stock of staples on hand. There likely will be a few things on this list you aren't familiar with, so I have included brief explanations.

Beans and Grains

- Barley
- *Beans: garbanzo, white, red, navy, pink, black, black-eyed peas, pinto (your favorites)
- Brown rice (not white)
- Bulghur (cracked wheat)
- Lentils
- Split peas
- Whole wheat flour (stone-ground preferred)

*Dried beans you cook are best, but frozen or canned beans are also fine. Make sure you rinse canned beans well to remove excess sodium and added sugars.

Breads

- Pita bread (sprouted-grain or whole wheat preferred)
- Rye bread, 100 percent
- Ry-Krisps and 100 percent whole wheat, low-fat crackers
- *Sprouted grain bread
- Tortillas (whole wheat preferred)
- Whole wheat bread (stone-ground best)

*Sprouted-grain breads have the best glycemic rating. Next best are breads made from stone-ground whole grains. Store bread in the freezer.

Cereals

- *Bran flakes, 100 percent
- Multigrain hot cereal
- Oatmeal, long-cooking (not quick oats)

*Most cold cereals, even though they are low in fat, have a very high glycemic index. A bowl every once in a while is acceptable, but hot cereals are much better. Oatmeal, because of its cholesterol-lowering fiber, is excellent.

Dairy/Eggs/Poultry/Fish/Meat Substitutes

- Cheese, low-fat (use in moderation; keep grated Parmesan on hand)
- Chicken breasts, skinless (big bags of boned, individually frozen breasts are handiest)
- Cottage cheese, nonfat
- Eggs, preferably from organically fed hens; Eggbeaters or other egg-white products (avoid egg substitutes)
- Fish, your choice (fatty fish such as salmon, tuna, sardines, anchovies, mackerel, and trout are best; others are fine, including shellfish, shrimp, and lobster)
- Ground turkey or chicken breast (This is the lowest-fat ground meat you will find. Regular ground chicken or turkey contains fatty skin.)
- Milk, nonfat and soy milk, low-fat
- Soy meat substitutes (Look in the freezer section of your grocery or health food store for low-fat, low-sodium soy "meats": burgers, bacon, lunch meats, and ground beef. They are surprisingly delicious.)
- Tofu (firm or extra-firm is easiest to work with)
- Turkey
- Yogurt, plain, nonfat

Condiments/Cooking Ingredients

- *Arrowroot (a thickening agent) or cornstarch
- Baking powder (aluminum-free)
- Baking soda
- *Brown rice syrup (low-glycemic sweetener; nice drizzled over cereal, pancakes, or desserts)
- Butter Buds

- *Cardia Salt (a healthy salt substitute that contains half the sodium of salt, along with potassium, magnesium, and the amino acid lysine; see resource section to order)
- Cornstarch
- *Flaxseed oil (store in refrigerator)
- Herbs and spices (your choice)
- Ketchup (low-sugar)
- Mustard
- NuSalt or NoSalt (potassium chloride salt substitutes that contain 500 milligrams of potassium per 1/8 teaspoon and no sodium—good idea if you have hypertension)
- Olive oil, extra-virgin
- *Stevia (herbal sweetener available in powder or liquid; good sweetener for beverages, yogurt, and cereal, and can be used in baking with some modifications)
- Tapioca
- Vanilla extract
- *Vegetable seasoning (made from dehydrated vegetables and grains; contains less than 250 milligrams per teaspoon of sodium compared to 2,000 milligrams in a teaspoon of salt)
- Vinegar (balsamic and apple cider are best)
- Whole wheat flour (stone-ground preferable)
- *Xylitol (a healthy, low-glycemic sweetener derived from birch trees; looks and tastes like granulated sugar and may be used in baking)
- Yeast

*You may find these items only in health food stores. Also see the resource section for mail order sources.

Fruits

- Applesauce, unsweetened
- Apricots, dried (other dried fruits have a very high glycemic rating)

- Fresh fruits (your choice; remember that ripe bananas and tropical fruits have the highest glycemic rating)
- Frozen fruits packed without sugar (berries, cherries, peaches, etc.)

Nuts and Seeds

- Raw nuts and seeds, all types
- Raw nut butters (almond is particularly nice)

Pastas

- All pastas (with the exception of prepared pastas stuffed with high-fat meat or cheese)

Vegetables

- Fresh vegetables (The only vegetables you should use in moderation, because of their high glycemic rating, are starchy root vegetables such as white potatoes, turnips, carrots, and corn.)
- Frozen vegetables (without sauces or excess salt)
- Canned vegetables (a very distant third—rinse well to remove sodium)

SUBSTITUTIONS AND RECIPE MODIFICATIONS

Do not throw away your favorite cookbooks, no matter how unhealthy the recipes may seem. Almost all recipes, except those that require lots of red meat, can be adapted to your new program. You can substitute unacceptable ingredients with some of the suggestions below—or leave them out altogether.

HEALTHY SUBSTITUTIONS

Ingredient	Use Instead	Recipes and guidelines
Bacon	Fat-free bacon bits	Available at your health food store
Broth	Homemade	Make low-sodium broth by boiling chicken and fish bones, vegetables, and herbs.
	Vegetable seasoning	You'll find lower-sodium vegetable seasonings in health food stores.
Butter	Butter Buds	Mix in water for liquid or sprinkle on food. Use in baked goods and over vegetables.
	Olive oil	For dipping bread, like the Italians do
	Ground nuts and seeds	May be used in baking instead of butter. Grind and measure as you would butter.
Cheese	Reduced-fat varieties	A little cheese for flavor is fine; a lot is not. Grated Parmesan really perks up food.
Chocolate	Carob powder	Use like semisweet chocolate in baking.
Cream	Nonfat evaporated milk	Makes a nice thickener in sauces.
	Nonfat yogurt or cottage cheese	Blended and thinned with a little milk, these are also good in sauces.
Flour	Whole wheat flour	Stone-ground is best. Try whole wheat pastry flour for a lighter result.
Mayonnaise	Nonfat varieties	Or see recipe for olive-oil mayo on page 376.
Ground beef	Ground turkey or chicken	Breast is leanest; most ground poultry has added skin.
	Soy protein granules	This is a great way to get soy protein in your diet. Good in spaghetti, tacos, etc.
	Cooked beans	Your chili won't miss the beef if you add extra beans.
Milk	Nonfat, soy, or rice milk	Soy milk contains heart-healthy components.

Ingredient	Use Instead	Recipes and guidelines
Oil	Olive oil	Best for cooking
	Cold-pressed vegetable oils	Fine for salad dressings, but never heat. Store in fridge or freezer.
	Olive-oil pan spray	To coat or grease skillets and baking dishes.
Peanut butter	Natural, nonhydrogenated	Avoid the usual grocery store brands of peanut butter
	Raw nut butters	Sold in health food stores; store in fridge
Pie crust	Grapenuts crust	See recipe on page 410; or make crustless pies or quiches
Salt	Salt substitutes	Use vegetable seasoning (best in soups and cooked dishes), NuSalt or NoSalt (potassium chloride), or Cardia Salt.
	Herbs	Perk up food with extra herbs.
Soy sauce	Low-sodium	Note that even low-sodium soy sauce has a lot of sodium; dilute with water.
	Bragg's Amino Acids	Lower sodium, soylike flavor; available in health food stores.
Sour cream	Nonfat sour cream	Use in equal amounts or substitute nonfat yogurt.
Sugar	*Stevia	This herbal sweetener, sold in health food stores, is best in drinks and cereals.
	*Brown Rice Syrup	Drizzle this syrup over pancakes, fruit, and desserts.
	*Xylitol	Looks and tastes like sugar.
Whipped cream	"Whipped Dream"	Blend ¾ cup nonfat milk, 1 cup nonfat cottage cheese, and 1 teaspoon vanilla.

*All three of these sweeteners can be used in baking, but modifications must be made. For more information, see the recipes in the next chapter, and the resource section.

COOKING BASICS

Part of successful cooking is having a few essential items in the kitchen. The most important is nonstick cookware. This healthier approach to cooking involves using far less fat than you might be used to, and if you're sautéing vegetables or cooking eggs in aluminum, stainless steel, or cast-iron skillets, you're asking for trouble. In addition to a couple of nonstick skillets of varying size, a nonstick cookie sheet is also recommended. No other specialized equipment is necessary, although several of our recipes do call for a blender or food processor.

If you cook regularly and enjoy spending time in the kitchen, you will have no problem with this program once you get the knack of it. In fact, making these changes likely will inspire you and bring out your creativity. As with anything new, you will have successes and failures as you go along, but I suspect that you will have a lot of fun with this. You will quickly adapt and even improve upon the suggested recipes in this book. If you are an inexperienced cook, then any kind of food preparation is going to be a challenge at first. However, the recipes in this book are no more difficult to prepare than those in any other cookbook, and in many cases, they are easier. So let's get started.

CHAPTER 21

Recipes for Reversing Heart Disease

CONTENTS

ONE WEEK OF MENUS

	BREAKFAST	LUNCH	DINNER
Monday	Hot Whole Grain Cereal* with nonfat milk/soy milk Apple Yogurt with stevia	Taco Salad* Guacamole* and Salsa* Whole wheat tortilla Sliced oranges	Tasty Trout* with Lemon Sauce* Greens and Spuds* Cucumber Salad* Berry Delicious*
Tuesday	Poached eggs (2) Sprouted-grain toast Grapefruit	Vegetable Soup* Rye crackers with almond butter Carrot and celery sticks	Marinated Chicken Breasts* Mock Mashed Potatoes* Mushroom Gravy* Spinach-Mushroom Salad* Apple Crisp*
Wednesday	Oatmeal with nonfat milk/soy milk Fruit Salad with Yogurt and Nuts*	Tuna Melt* Coleslaw* Cherries	Spinach Lasagna* Green salad Garlic bread*
Thursday	Mexican Egg Scramble* Whole wheat tortilla Fresh strawberries	Hummus Sandwich* Tabouli* Tangerine	Oriental Chicken Salad* Miso Soup* Dessert Fruit Salad*

	BREAKFAST	LUNCH	DINNER
Friday	Apple Pancakes* Applesauce Yogurt with stevia	Split Pea Soup* Egg Salad* Rye crackers Blueberries	Pasta Putanesca* Salad Caprese* Bread Sticks* Fresh Fruit Ice Cream*
Saturday	Veggie Omelet* Sprouted-grain bagel Grapes	Curried Chicken-Rice Salad* Whole wheat pita bread Tangerine	Teriyaki Chicken* Barley Pilaf* Marinated Broccoli* Poached Fruit*
Sunday	Whole Wheat Waffles* Berry Syrup* Cottage cheese	Turkey Chili* Tomato slices Pear	Broiled Salmon Steaks* Curried Quinoa* Green salad Baked Apples*

*Recipe included in this chapter

BREAKFASTS

Breakfast Tips

- Start out with a piece of fruit, which is preferable over juice. Fruit juices are a very concentrated form of sugar and have a high glycemic rating. Whole fruit also contains an abundance of heart-healthy fiber that juice lacks.
- Contrary to popular belief, you can eat eggs—up to seven a week. (If you have diabetes, you should limit yourself to two or three per week.) You may have as many egg whites as you wish. The healthiest ways to fix eggs are poached and soft boiled. Also try some of our egg (and scrambled tofu) recipes.
- Go easy on breakfast breads, for most have a very high glycemic rating. Doughnuts and pastries are no-nos because of their high content of unhealthy hydrogenated fats and trans fatty acids. Look for sprouted-grain bread and bagels or stone-ground whole wheat bread.
- Rather than the usual French toast, pancakes, and waffles made with white flour, try our recipes. Top them with brown rice syrup or the Berry Syrup recipe we have included.
- While hot cereals made from whole grains are excellent, most cold cereals have a very high glycemic index. The best of the cold cereals are those made from bran. Try some of the following cereal recipes.
- For extra fiber, protein, and heart-healthy omega-3 fatty acids, grind one-fourth cup of flaxseed and sprinkle it on cereal.

Swiss-Style Meusli

1 cup uncooked regular oatmeal (slow-cooking)
¼ cup chopped or slivered almonds
1 cup shredded apple
1 tablespoon raw sunflower seeds
1 tablespoon raw sesame seeds

Mix ingredients together. Serve with nonfat milk or soy milk.

Serves 2

Granola

½ cup oatmeal (not cooked)
¼ cup rye flakes
¼ cup barley flakes
¼ cup freshly ground flaxseed
1 tablespoon sesame seeds
1 tablespoon raw almonds (or other nuts)
1 tablespoon raw pumpkin seeds
2 tablespoons brown rice syrup

Mix all ingredients. Serve with soy milk or nonfat milk. Add chopped fruit if desired.

Serves 2

Hot Whole-Grain Cereal

1 cup whole grains*
2–3 cups water (as directed)
*Oatmeal, barley, wheat kernels, buckwheat groats, teff, multigrain cereal, quinoa (a South American native that contains very high-quality protein), or other whole grains

Bring water to a boil, add grain, cover, and cook until done. Cooking times will vary, depending on grain. Follow package directions.

Serves 2

Hot cereal variations: To cooked hot grains, add one of the following:

Brown rice syrup and cinnamon
Chopped dried apricots
Almond extract, ⅛–¼ teaspoon plus ¼ cup chopped almonds
Chopped fruit, ½ cup, your choice
Carob powder, 1 tablespoon, plus stevia or other sweetener, to taste

Overnight Wheat Berry Cereal

⅔ cup wheat berries
2 cups boiling water
A wide-mouthed thermos

Here's a unique way to make hot cereal. It works with other grains as well. The evening before, place boiling water and wheat berries in a wide-mouthed thermos. Close thermos and allow it to sit overnight. The cereal will be ready to eat in the morning. Serve with soy milk or nonfat milk, and flavor with cinnamon, xylitol, or stevia.

Serves 2

French Toast

1 whole egg
1 egg white
2 tablespoons soy milk or nonfat milk
½ teaspoon vanilla
½ teaspoon cinnamon
4 slices sprouted-grain bread

Blend first five ingredients. Dip bread into egg mixture. Brown both sides in hot skillet or on griddle, lightly sprayed with olive oil spray. Serve with brown rice syrup or Berry Syrup.

Serves 2

Apple Pancakes

¾ cup whole wheat flour
1 teaspoon cinnamon
1 teaspoon baking soda
¾ cup water
1 tablespoon olive oil
½ large apple, grated
2 egg whites, stiffly beaten
2 drops stevia

Blend dry ingredients well, then stir in water, oil, stevia, and apple until well blended. Fold in egg whites. Using ¼-cup measuring cup, pour onto hot griddle sprayed with olive oil. Serve with unsweetened applesauce, brown rice syrup, or Berry Syrup.

Serves 2

Whole Wheat Waffles

1 cup water
1 tablespoon olive oil
1 egg white
1 teaspoon baking powder
½ cup unsweetened applesauce
½ teaspoon vanilla
1½ cups whole wheat flour

Put all the ingredients into a blender or food processor, except for the flour. Blend. While the blender or food processor is running, add the flour a little at a time. Cook on a medium-hot waffle iron, sprayed with a pan spray. These waffles are naturally sweet and crunchy. If you do desire additional sweetening, use a little brown rice syrup, unsweetened applesauce, or fruit sweetened with xylitol or stevia.

Serves 2

Berry Syrup

1 cup mashed fresh or frozen blueberries or strawberries
2 teaspoons tapioca granules
½ cup water
2–6 drops stevia (to taste)

Combine all ingredients and bring to a boil over medium heat in a saucepan. Stir constantly until thickened, about five minutes. Serve warm over French toast, pancakes, or waffles.

Serves 2

Cinnamon Toast

2 slices sprouted-grain bread
2 teaspoons brown rice syrup
½ teaspoon cinnamon

Toast bread under broiler. Turn over and drizzle 1 teaspoon of brown rice syrup over each slice, then sprinkle lightly with cinnamon. Place under broiler for another minute or so.

Serves 2

Italian Scrambled Eggs

½ yellow onion, chopped
1 zucchini, sliced and quartered
4 ounces fresh mushrooms, sliced
½ green pepper, chopped
1 teaspoon olive oil
¼ teaspoon salt
¼ teaspoon pepper
1 tablespoon minced fresh basil (or ½ teaspoon dried), to taste
2 eggs (or 4 egg whites)

In a nonstick skillet, sauté the onion, zucchini, mushrooms, and green pepper in the olive oil over medium heat. Add the seasonings. Beat the eggs or egg whites with a fork and pour onto skillet, stirring frequently to keep it from sticking. Cook until the eggs are set but still moist.

Serves 2

Veggie Omelet

½ cup chopped mushrooms
½ cup chopped onion
1½ teaspoons olive oil (divided use)
4 egg whites and 2 whole eggs
4 teaspoons water
Dash pepper
¼ teaspoon salt (or salt substitute to taste)

Sauté vegetables in ½ teaspoon olive oil until tender-crisp and set aside. Mix eggs with water, pepper, and salt or salt substitute and beat lightly. Heat small nonstick skillet over medium heat. Coat bottom of pan with ½ teaspoon olive oil. Pour in half of egg mixture. Gently shake pan and lift edges of omelet as eggs cook, tilting pan to let uncooked eggs underneath. Slide from pan, add half of vegetables, fold, and serve. Repeat with remaining egg mixture.

Makes 2 omelets

Mexican Egg Scramble

1 small onion, chopped
½ green pepper, chopped
1 teaspoon olive oil
4 egg whites and 2 whole eggs
1 tablespoon water
¼ teaspoon pepper
¼ teaspoon salt (or salt substitute to taste)
3 tablespoons salsa

Brown onion and green pepper in olive oil in a medium skillet over medium-high heat for about five minutes. Lightly beat eggs, egg whites, water, pepper, and salt or salt substitute. Pour into skillet over onion and peppers and continue to cook, stirring, until eggs are set. Serve with salsa.

Serves 2

Tofu Scramble with Spinach

1 cup chopped onion
1 teaspoon olive oil
½ container firm tofu
1 teaspoon onion powder
1 cup fresh spinach, cleaned and chopped
2 tablespoons grated Parmesan cheese

Give this recipe a try—it isn't as weird as it sounds. Sauté onion in olive oil until tender. Crumble tofu and add to onion, sprinkle with onion powder, and blend well. Continue cooking for 2 to 3 minutes. Add spinach and stir just until spinach is wilted. Sprinkle on cheese, cover 1 to 2 minutes until cheese melts.

Options: Spinach may be replaced with ½ cup sautéed green pepper, zucchini, mushrooms, or a mixture of your favorites.

Serves 2

Fruit Salad with Yogurt and Nuts

1 apple cut into chunks
1 pear cut into chunks
2 tablespoons raw sunflower seeds
2 tablespoons raw almonds
2 tablespoons raw pumpkin seeds
1 cup plain nonfat yogurt

Mix fruit, seeds, and nuts. Stir into yogurt.

Serves 2

Smoothie

1 apple (or other fruit)
1 cup berries (or other fruit)
¼ cup flaxseed, freshly ground
2 scoops protein powder
½ cup nonfat yogurt (optional)
1 cup soy milk (or water)
1 cup ice

Mix all ingredients in blender and blend until smooth. Adjust soy milk and ice to obtain desired thickness. This is a delightful, well-balanced, and nutritious breakfast that you can eat on the run. The variations are endless. Use your imagination and the fruits in season for a rich supply of nutrients.

Serves 2

SOUPS

- Make soup in volume—double or triple the recipe if it makes only a few servings. Then enjoy the leftovers or freeze individual-sized servings for quick meals later.
- Most soup recipes call for a lot of salt. Canned stock or bouillon cubes are also loaded with sodium. Try using the vegetable seasoning I told you about in the previous chapter as your soup base—it is tasty and has a fraction of the sodium of other soup bases.
- Soups are a good way to clean out the fridge and make use of odds and ends in your vegetable bin. Also, throw some canned beans in every batch (rinse beans to remove sodium) for additional protein and fiber.
- When making bean soups from dried beans, soak the beans overnight, then pour off the soaking water, rinse, cover, and bring to a boil. Discard that water too, cover again, then cook as usual. This will get rid of some of the sugars in the beans that cause gas.

Vegetable Soup

5 cups water
½ cauliflower head, diced
1 cup peas, fresh or frozen
1 carrot, scrubbed and sliced
1 small yellow onion, diced
¼ small head of cabbage, chopped (approximately 1 cup)
⅛ teaspoon pepper
2 tablespoons vegetable seasoning (or more to taste)

Start the water boiling as you prepare the vegetables. Add the vegetables to the pot one by one as they are ready, along with the seasonings. Cover the pot, and cook for 20 minutes, until vegetables are tender.

Serves 4

Miso Soup

3 cups water
1 tablespoon vegetable seasoning
½ cup onion, thinly sliced
½ cup firm tofu, cut into ¼-inch cubes
3 tablespoons miso paste
1 tablespoon chopped green onion

Miso is a Japanese staple made of fermented rice or soybeans and is sold in health food stores and Asian markets. It is strong-flavored and very nutritious. It also contains a lot of sodium, so if you are salt sensitive, eliminate vegetable seasoning and cut miso paste back to 2 tablespoons.

Heat water and vegetable seasoning in medium saucepan, add onion, and simmer for 5 minutes. Add tofu and simmer 1 to 2 minutes longer. Mix miso with 2 tablespoons of the broth and add back to soup. Garnish with green onions and serve.

Serves 2

Lentil Soup

4 cups water
1 tablespoon vegetable seasoning
¾ cup lentils
1 sliced carrot
1 teaspoon onion powder
¼ cup chopped parsley

Rinse lentils under running water. Simmer all the ingredients about 30–40 minutes, or until the lentils are tender.

Serves 2

Split Pea Soup

1 cup uncooked split peas
5 cups water
¼ cup salsa
1 cup chopped onion
2 tablespoons vegetable seasoning
1 tablespoon tomato paste

Rinse peas under running water. Put all ingredients together in a pot. Bring to a boil, then simmer until the peas are tender, at least 1 hour. Watch carefully and add more water if needed.

Serves 3

Quick Multi-Bean Soup

5 cups water
½ cup cooked garbanzo beans
½ cup cooked baby lima beans
½ cup cooked black-eyed peas
1 medium zucchini, sliced
1 cup chopped celery
2 cups chopped cabbage
2 tablespoons tomato paste
1 tablespoon vegetable seasoning

Put all ingredients in a large pot. Bring to a boil and cook for 20 minutes.

Serves 4

Turkey Chili

1 pound ground turkey breast
1 medium onion, chopped
1 green pepper, chopped
1 teaspoon olive oil
2 cups water
1 16-ounce can tomatoes, chopped
1 16-ounce can kidney beans, rinsed
2 tablespoons tomato puree
2 tablespoons vegetable seasoning
½ teaspoon red chilis (or to taste—very hot)
1–2 tablespoons chili powder (to taste)
2 chopped green onions

Sauté the ground turkey, onion, and green pepper in olive oil in a large pot over medium heat. Add the remaining ingredients to the pot and simmer until flavors are thoroughly blended, at least one hour. Add more water as needed. Garnish with green onions.

Serves 6

Minestrone

¾ cup sliced carrot
¾ cup sliced celery
¼ cup chopped onion
¾ cup green beans
1 cup sliced zucchini
1 quart water
1½ cups tomato puree
¾ cup cooked kidney beans
2½ tablespoons chopped parsley
2½ tablespoons chopped green onion
1 teaspoon basil
4 tablespoons vegetable seasoning
½ cup macaroni
4 teaspoons grated Parmesan cheese

Put all ingredients, except for the macaroni and the cheese, in a large pot. Bring to a boil and simmer for 20 minutes. Add macaroni and simmer for another 15 minutes. Garnish each bowl with a teaspoon of parmesan.

Serves 4

Cream of Vegetable Soup

Basic Cream Soup
2 medium chopped carrots
2 medium chopped onions
1 small chopped green pepper
3 chopped zucchini
3 stalks chopped celery
½ cup chopped parsley
1 teaspoon onion powder
1 tablespoon vegetable seasoning or salt substitute
½ tablespoon pepper
2 cups nonfat milk

Cover vegetables with water and simmer until tender. Drain, then puree in blender or food processor with milk and seasonings. Return to pan and heat to serving temperature. Add more milk to obtain desired thickness.

Serves 3 to 4

Variations

Add to vegetables before cooking:

Spinach: 1 package thawed frozen spinach or 1 pound chopped fresh spinach, cleaned and stemmed, and 1 clove minced or pressed garlic

Mushroom: 2 cups chopped mushrooms and ½ teaspoon thyme

Pea: 1½ cups fresh or thawed frozen peas, ½ teaspoon marjoram, and ½ teaspoon thyme

Tomato: 1 cup tomato puree and 1 clove minced or pressed garlic

SALADS AND SALAD DRESSINGS

- Every lunch and dinner, no matter how informal, should be accompanied by a salad, or at least some raw vegetables. Several of the salads listed below make great main dishes. You can also add chunks of cooked chicken or fish to any salad and turn it into a main dish.
- Salads give you a chance to pack in lots of nutrients. Go for variety: romaine, spinach, arugula. Remember, the darker the leafy greens, the more nutritious. Always throw in other raw veggies, such as onions, celery, and tomatoes.
- For added fiber and nutrition, toss a handful of cooked beans or ¼ cup freshly ground flaxseed in your salads.
- The best salad dressings are those you make yourself with olive oil or flaxseed oil. Try the recipes below.

Chef's Salad

1 head romaine, butter, red or green leaf lettuce
1 grated carrot
2 chopped large tomatoes
2 ounces alfalfa sprouts
½ cup thawed frozen peas
2 hard-boiled eggs, chopped
½ pound cooked chicken breast, cubed
¼ cup raw hulled sunflower seeds

Wash and tear lettuce into a large bowl. Add remaining ingredients. Toss well with your favorite dressing from the recipes on pages 375–378.

Serves 3

Curried Chicken-Rice Salad

1 teaspoon curry powder
½ cup fat-free mayonnaise (or homemade, page 376)
2 cups cooked, chilled brown rice
1 pound cooked chicken breast, cubed
½ cup slivered almonds
½ cup finely chopped celery
2 green onions, chopped
2 tablespoons parsley, chopped
Fresh crisp greens

Mix curry powder in mayonnaise. Place all other ingredients in a bowl, except for the greens, and toss lightly with mayonnaise. Serve on a bed of fresh crisp greens.

Serves 4

Salad Caprese

2 large tomatoes, sliced
¼ small sweet onion (optional), thinly sliced
2 thin slices mozzarella cheese
8 large fresh basil leaves
2 teaspoons olive oil

Arrange the tomato, onion, cheese slices and basil on individual salad plates. Sprinkle one teaspoon olive oil over each plate.

Serves 2

Cucumber Salad

¼ cup vinegar
4 ounces plain nonfat yogurt
1 teaspoon dill
¼ teaspoon black pepper
1 large cucumber, peeled and sliced very thin
1 small, thinly sliced onion

Mix first four ingredients. Marinate the cucumber and onion slices in the dressing for several hours or overnight.

Serves 2

Spinach-Mushroom Salad

1 large bunch spinach, stemmed
4 ounces mushrooms, sliced
½ hard-boiled egg, chopped
¼ small onion, chopped

Combine and serve with an olive oil and vinegar dressing (page 375).

Serves 2 to 3

Coleslaw

2 chopped green onions
½ head shredded cabbage (or mix purple with green)
¼ teaspoon garlic powder
1 tablespoon celery seed
1 teaspoon mustard
1 large shredded carrot
1 chopped green pepper
1 cup plain nonfat yogurt
½ cup fat-free Italian salad dressing (or homemade)

Combine all dressing ingredients. Mix with cabbage and onions and refrigerate overnight.

Serves 4

Bean Salad

1 cup cooked kidney beans
1 cup cooked green beans
1 cup cooked garbanzo beans
1 small chopped onion
½ chopped green pepper
5 tablespoons vinegar
3 tablespoons olive oil
¼ teaspoon onion powder
¼ teaspoon garlic powder
⅛ teaspoon black pepper
4 lettuce leaves

Combine all the ingredients except the lettuce in a bowl with a tight-sealing lid. Allow to marinate for at least an hour, gently shaking the bowl several times to mix the seasonings with the beans. Serve on lettuce leaves.

Serves 4

Tuna-Macaroni Salad

1 cup uncooked macaroni
1 tablespoon flaxseed or olive oil
2 tablespoons vinegar
1 teaspoon prepared mustard
½ teaspoon salt (or salt substitute to taste)
1 cup cooked peas
4 tablespoons chopped pimentos (optional)
2 hard-boiled eggs, chopped
2 tablespoons minced sweet or dill pickles
1 6-ounce can water-packed tuna, drained
Lettuce

Cook the macaroni according to the package directions. Drain, rinse, and immediately toss with the oil to prevent sticking. Mix the next three ingredients and toss with the macaroni. Add the remaining ingredients except the lettuce, tossing lightly. Serve on lettuce.

Serves 3

Oriental Chicken Salad

1 large chicken breast, cooked, thinly sliced into 1-inch pieces and chilled
1 head lettuce (romaine preferred), coarsely chopped
½ bunch green onions, chopped
1 cup fresh bean sprouts
¼ cup sesame seeds

Combine salad ingredients. Toss with Sesame Dressing (recipe on page 375). Sprinkle with sesame seeds.

Serves 2

Taco Salad

½ pound ground turkey or chicken breast
1 teaspoon olive oil
1½ teaspoons chili powder (divided use)
½ teaspoon salt (or salt substitute to taste)
3 cups lettuce (romaine preferred) torn into bite-size pieces
¼ cup onion, thinly sliced
1 tomato, coarsely chopped
¼ cup black olives, sliced
½ cup kidney beans
4 tablespoons fat-free, sugar-free ranch dressing
1 ounce cheese, low-fat, grated
Guacamole
Tortillas

Brown ground turkey in olive oil in medium skillet over medium-high heat, adding 1 teaspoon chili powder and salt or salt substitute. Drain and set aside. Combine salad ingredients in large bowl. Mix ranch dressing with ½ teaspoon chili powder and toss with salad, along with meat mixture. Top with cheese. Serve with Guacamole (see next recipe) and tortillas.

Serves 2 to 3

Guacamole

1 ripe avocado
½ small tomato, chopped
1 green onion, thinly sliced
Juice of ½ lemon
¼ teaspoon salt (or salt substitute to taste)
1 tablespoon salsa
Whole wheat tortillas
Salsa

Mash avocado with fork in small bowl. Add remaining ingredients. Serve with whole wheat tortillas and extra salsa.

Serves 2

Greek Salad

3 cups lettuce (romaine preferred) torn into bite-size pieces
½ cucumber, sliced
¼ cup onion, thinly sliced
1 tomato, coarsely chopped
¼ cup black olives, sliced
1 tablespoon crumbled feta cheese
1 tablespoon olive oil
2 tablespoons vinegar
1 clove garlic, minced
¼ teaspoon salt (or salt substitute to taste)
¼ teaspoon black pepper

Combine salad ingredients in large bowl. Mix last five dressing ingredients in small bowl, then toss with salad.

Serves 2

Marinated Broccoli

1 cup broccoli spears, coarsely chopped
2 tablespoons onion, chopped
1 tablespoon olive oil
1 tablespoon vinegar
¼ teaspoon salt (or salt substitute to taste)
⅛ teaspoon pepper

Mix oil and vinegar with salt and pepper. Combine broccoli and onions in small bowl, toss with dressing. Let marinate for one hour before serving.

Serves 2

Tabouli

2 cups boiling water
1 cup bulghur
2 tablespoons olive oil
4 tablespoons lemon juice
½ teaspoon salt (or salt substitute to taste)
⅛ teaspoon ground pepper
1 cup fresh parsley, chopped
2 large tomatoes, chopped
1 cucumber, chopped
½ onion, chopped

Pour boiling water over bulghur, stir, and let stand for 30 minutes. Drain in a strainer, squeezing out excess moisture. Place in a large bowl. Mix the olive oil, lemon juice, salt or salt substitute and pepper and stir into bulghur. Add chopped parsley and vegetables and mix well. Chill at least two hours before serving.

Serves 4

Roasted Vegetables in Mustard Vinaigrette

1 eggplant, thinly sliced
2 small zucchini, sliced
½ pound mushrooms, sliced
1 teaspoon olive oil
¼ cup vinegar
¼ cup olive oil
2 tablespoons mustard powder
2 tablespoons celery seed
Salt to taste
Pinch of pepper
Lettuce leaves

Brush vegetables with 1 teaspoon olive oil, then roast under broiler, three or four minutes, on both sides. Let cool. Mix the vinegar, oil, mustard powder, celery seed, salt, and pepper. Top with a spoonful of dressing.

Serves 4

Apple Salad

1 cored and cubed red apple (peeling optional)
1 cored and cubed green apple (peeling optional)
1 cored and cubed yellow apple (peeling optional)
¼ cup chopped almonds
2–3 tablespoons lightly toasted sesame seeds

Combine all ingredients and serve with Fruit Salad Dressing (see recipe page 413).

Serves 3

Salad Dressings

Basic Oil and Vinegar Dressing

2 tablespoons olive oil or flaxseed oil
2–3 tablespoons vinegar (balsamic is nice)
1 clove garlic, minced
¼ teaspoon seasoned salt (or salt substitute to taste)
Pinch black pepper

Mix all ingredients together.

Serves 2–3

Sesame Dressing

1 tablespoon olive oil
1 tablespoon sesame oil
2 tablespoons lemon juice
1 clove garlic, minced
¼ teaspoon seasoned salt (or salt substitute to taste)
Pinch black pepper

Mix all ingredients together. This is an excellent dressing for Asian salads such as Oriental Chicken Salad.

Serves 2–3

Homemade Mayonnaise

1 egg
½ teaspoon salt (or salt substitute to taste)
½ teaspoon mustard powder
2 tablespoons cider vinegar
1 cup virgin olive oil

Combine egg, salt or salt substitute, mustard powder, and vinegar in blender or food processor with ¼ cup olive oil. Blend on low and while blending, slowly but steadily pour in remaining oil. This recipe has as much fat as any mayonnaise, but it is made with healthy virgin olive oil and has no additives.

Makes 1¼ cups

Yogurt-Chive Dressing

1 cup plain nonfat yogurt
½ teaspoon salt (or salt substitute to taste)
2 finely chopped scallions
6 tablespoons chives
2 tablespoons vinegar
½ teaspoon pepper
½ teaspoon onion powder

Mix all ingredients together.

Makes 1½ cups

Spicy Dressing

¾ cup water
¾ teaspoon mustard powder
½ cup cider vinegar
2¼ teaspoons garlic powder
¾ teaspoon paprika
3–4 drops stevia
¼ teaspoon cornstarch
¼ teaspoon ground black pepper
1½ teaspoons crushed oregano

Combine all ingredients in a small saucepan. Bring to a boil. Cook, stirring until thickened, about 2 minutes. Pour into a small bowl. Chill, and mix well before using.

Makes about 1¼ cups

Tangy Thousand Island Dressing

1 cup plain nonfat yogurt
¼ cup tomato paste
⅛ teaspoon pepper
1 teaspoon mustard powder
½ teaspoon onion powder
3 tablespoons chopped dill pickle
½ teaspoon horseradish

Combine the ingredients and chill before serving.

Makes about 1½ cups

Creamy Artichoke Dressing

1 cup canned water-packed artichoke hearts, drained
½ teaspoon onion powder
1 teaspoon fat-free cottage cheese
⅔ cup buttermilk
1½ teaspoons vinegar
1 teaspoon diced green onion
¼ teaspoon basil

Blend all ingredients until the dressing is smooth. Chill well before serving.

Makes about 2 cups

SANDWICHES

- Make your sandwiches on sprouted-grain bread if possible, for it not only has the lowest glycemic index rating of all breads but it is high in fiber, quality protein, and other nutrients. Whole wheat bread, preferably stone-ground, is also acceptable, as are whole wheat pita and rye bread made from 100 percent rye flour. Some of the spreads are also very good on whole wheat or rye crackers. And try some of the bread recipes in the bread section below.
- Use mustard liberally but only fat-free or homemade mayonnaise. Pile lettuce, onions, tomatoes, and other vegetables on your sandwiches.
- Check the fat and sodium content of lunch meats. As a rule, labels on these products are not a pretty sight. Low-fat cheese, or a very thin slice of your favorite regular cheese, on occasion is fine. Use your best judgment when eating these foods that are high in saturated fats.
- Love peanut butter? Because peanuts are roasted, even the health food store brands are less than ideal. If you are going to indulge, make sure the word "hydrogenated" does not appear on the label. The best nut butters are raw, organic almond, sesame, and other nut/seed butters. Eat with a minimal amount of jam or jelly.
- Check your health food store for vegetarian hot dogs and hamburgers made from soy. We serve Boca Burgers at the clinic, and the patients love them.

Egg Salad Sandwich

12 hard-boiled eggs
2 stalks finely chopped celery
¼ cup chopped scallions
¼ cup chopped green pepper
¼ teaspoon cayenne pepper
1 tablespoon chopped parsley
¼ teaspoon mustard powder
1 teaspoon vegetable seasoning or salt substitute
½ cup mayonnaise (fat-free or homemade)

Remove yolks from six eggs and discard. Chop egg whites with remaining whole hard-boiled eggs. Combine all ingredients and stir until the desired moistness is reached.

Serves 4

Hummus Sandwich

1 can garbanzo beans, rinsed and drained
½ cup sesame tahini
2 cloves minced garlic
¼ teaspoon salt (or salt substitute to taste)
2 sprouted-grain or whole wheat pita bread rounds
1 tomato, chopped
½ cup lettuce, chopped

In a blender or food processor, mix garbanzo beans, tahini, garlic, and salt or salt substitute. If necessary, add a tablespoon or two of water to thin. Slice pita in half, open each half, and spread with hummus. Fill each half with tomatoes and lettuce.

Serves 2

Open-Faced Goat Cheese Sandwich

2 teaspoons Dijon mustard
2 slices sprouted-grain bread
½ avocado
2 ounces goat cheese, thinly sliced
½ cup alfalfa sprouts
1 small tomato, thinly sliced

Spread mustard on the bread slices, then layer as following: avocado, thin slices of goat cheese, sprouts, and tomato slices.

Serves 2

Tuna Melt

1 6-ounce can water-packed tuna
¼ cup mayonnaise (fat-free or homemade)
1 tablespoon chopped green onion
1 tablespoon pickle, chopped
1 tablespoon finely chopped celery
2 slices sprouted-grain bread, lightly toasted
2 thin slices of cheese (low-fat preferred)
2 tomato slices

Mix tuna with next four ingredients. Spread on toast and top with cheese. Place under broiler until cheese is melted and bubbly. Top with a fresh tomato slice.

Serves 2

Falafel

½ cup bulghur
1 cup boiling water
2 cups canned garbanzo beans, rinsed and drained
3 cloves garlic, minced
¼ cup lemon juice
½ teaspoon salt (or salt substitute to taste)
¼ teaspoon Tabasco
3 egg whites
½ cup dry bread crumbs
1 teaspoon olive oil
6 sprouted- or whole-grain pita bread rounds
2 tomatoes, thinly sliced
1 cucumber, thinly sliced
1½ cups lettuce, chopped
Tahini Sauce

Soak the bulghur in the boiling water for 20 minutes, then drain well in a colander. In a blender or food processor combine the garbanzo beans, garlic, lemon juice, salt or salt substitute, and Tabasco. In a large bowl beat the egg whites, then mix in the bread crumbs, pureed garbanzo mixture, the drained bulghur, and olive oil. Shape mixture into 6 thin patties. On a nonstick medium-hot griddle sprayed with olive-oil cooking spray, brown the patties for 3 to 5 minutes on each side. Serve immediately in pita pockets with vegetables and tahini sauce (1 tablespoon for each pita, recipe on next page). Falafel makes a great snack and also freezes well.

Serves 6

Tahini Sauce

3 tablespoons sesame tahini
½ teaspoon olive oil
2 tablespoons water (or more)
1 clove garlic, minced
2 teaspoons lemon juice
Dash of cayenne pepper

In a small bowl, stir all ingredients until thoroughly mixed, adding a little extra water if needed. Serve with falafel.

Makes 6 tablespoons

Veggie Salad Spread

2 grated carrots
3 grated zucchini
½ cup finely chopped parsley
½ cup finely chopped pecans or other nuts
½ cup finely chopped sunflower seeds
½ cup plain nonfat yogurt
1 teaspoon vegetable seasoning or salt substitute to taste

Mix all ingredients together to moisten well. Serve on whole grain bread or crackers, in pita bread, or on a bed of crisp greens.

Serves 4 to 6

BREADS AND MUFFINS

If there's one comfort food that just about everyone longs for, it is bread. Just thinking about the smell of freshly baked bread or muffins makes my mouth water. Most recipes, however, call for white flour and/or unhealthy sweeteners. We hope you enjoy these healthful recipes.

Blueberry Muffins

1 cup water
2–3 drops stevia
1 orange, peeled and sectioned
1 small apple, chopped
1 teaspoon vanilla
½ cup xylitol
1 teaspoon cinnamon
1 tablespoon olive oil
1 tablespoon baking powder
1 cup whole wheat flour
¾ cup ground almonds
1 cup blueberries (fresh or frozen)
2 egg whites, stiffly beaten

In a blender or food processor, puree the orange and apple together with the water. Add the vanilla, xylitol, cinnamon, and olive oil and continue to blend. Pour mixture into a large bowl and, with a hand mixer, beat in the baking powder, flour, and almonds. Fold in the berries, then the beaten egg whites. Pour into a nonstick muffin pan, sprayed with olive-oil pan spray, and bake in preheated 350-degree oven for 20 to 30 minutes, until centers spring back when touched.

Makes 1 dozen

Whole Wheat Bread

1 tablespoon dry yeast
2 cups lukewarm water
½ teaspoon brown rice syrup
4½ cups stone-ground whole wheat flour

Add the yeast and brown rice syrup to the water. Cover with a cloth and let sit about 15 minutes, until mixture begins to bubble. Add flour and knead in large bowl for about 10 minutes. Set the bowl in a warm place, cover it, and let it rise for 45 minutes. Punch down. Place dough in warmed olive oil-sprayed nonstick loaf pan. After loaf has doubled in size, bake for 40 minutes in a preheated 350-degree oven. Crust should sound hollow when tapped.

Makes 1 loaf

Garlic Bread

1 clove garlic, peeled and sliced
4 slices whole grain bread
4 teaspoons olive oil
4 teaspoons Parmesan cheese

Rub garlic halves over each piece of bread. Brush olive oil on bread. Sprinkle 1 teaspoon parmesan cheese on each slice. Broil until toasty.

Serves 4

Cinnamon Cheese Toast

1 cup nonfat cottage cheese
2 tablespoons plain nonfat yogurt
4 slices whole grain bread
1 tablespoon cinnamon
2 tablespoons xylitol or another granulated sweetener

Cream together the cheese and the yogurt. Spread thickly on the bread slices. Sprinkle with a mixture of the cinnamon and xylitol or another sweetener. Broil until bubbly. Serve immediately.

Serves 4

Bread Sticks

2 tablespoons Butter Buds liquid
3 tablespoons brown rice syrup
8 slices sprouted-grain or whole wheat bread
¼ cup sesame seeds

Mix the Butter Buds with the brown rice syrup. Cut bread into 4 strips per slice. Spread the Butter Buds mixture on the bread and sprinkle with the sesame seeds. Bake in a preheated 400-degree oven 8 to 10 minutes or until crisp.

Makes 32 sticks

FISH AND POULTRY MAIN DISHES

- As you know, cold-water fish are among the heart-healthiest of all foods because of their omega-3 fatty acid content. Try to eat two or three servings a week of salmon, trout, tuna, sardines, or mackerel. Broiling or sautéing fish steaks or fillets takes only a few minutes (baking takes a little longer), and all they require is a light garnish with lemon, olive oil, and a little salt and pepper. Once you realize how easy it is to prepare fish, you'll probably make it a mainstay of your diet.
- Purchase skinless poultry. We like to keep individually frozen skinless, boneless chicken breasts in the freezer and pull them out as needed. A chicken breast lightly sautéed in olive oil, flavored with a light sauce and served with a side dish of vegetables and a big salad make a tasty, quick, and easy dinner.
- Use ground turkey or chicken breast in place of ground beef. It is better than regular ground turkey or chicken because no skin has been added to increase the saturated fat content.

Broiled Salmon Steaks

2 4-ounce salmon steaks (or other favorite fish)
¼ teaspoon salt (or a salt substitute to taste)
2 teaspoons olive oil (divided use)
Parsley
Lemon wedges

Preheat broiler to high and set oven rack so the top of the fish will be two inches from the heating element. Dry fish with paper towels. Season by rubbing with salt or salt substitute and one teaspoon of olive oil. Broil for about two minutes, turn; brush with additional oil, and broil for another five minutes or so. It will be ready when it lightly springs to the touch yet is still moist. (When in doubt, cut into the fish to see if it is done.) Garnish with parsley and lemon before serving.

Serves 2

Fish and Salsa Bake

2 4-ounce tuna fillets (or other cold-water fish)
1 teaspoon olive oil
¼ teaspoon each onion and garlic powder
½ cup mild salsa

Brush fish with olive oil. Sprinkle with onion and garlic powder. Place fish in baking dish sprayed with olive-oil pan spray and cover with salsa. Bake for 15 to 20 minutes just until fish is flaky.

Serves 2

Rolled Fillet of Sole

4 6-ounce sole fillets
Juice of 1 lemon
¼ teaspoon garlic powder
¼ teaspoon dry mustard
¼ teaspoon pepper
¼ teaspoon curry powder
¼ cup chopped chives
1 cup fat-free sour cream

Rub both sides of the fish with lemon juice and sprinkle with garlic powder, dry mustard, pepper, and curry powder. Mix the chives with the sour cream and spread one-fourth of the mixture on each fillet. Roll up the fillets and fasten each with a toothpick. Bake in a preheated 350-degree oven for 20 minutes or until fish is flaky.

Serves 4

Tasty Trout

1 teaspoon olive oil
1 chopped onion
3 stalks chopped celery
4 4-ounce trout fillets
Juice of 1 lemon
1 cup whole-grain bread crumbs
1 tablespoon parsley
Lemon Sauce (recipe on next page)

Heat olive oil in nonstick skillet over medium heat, add onions and celery, and cook until tender. Rub both sides of the fish with lemon juice. Place in a baking dish oiled with olive-oil pan spray and cover with onion and celery mixture. Mix the bread crumbs with the parsley and sprinkle over the fish. Bake in a preheated 350-degree oven for 20 to 30 minutes. Serve with Lemon Sauce.

Serves 4

Lemon Sauce

2 tablespoons arrowroot or cornstarch
½ teaspoon salt (or salt substitute to taste)
1 cup water
3 tablespoons lemon juice
1 teaspoon grated lemon rind

Combine the arrowroot or cornstarch, salt or salt substitute, and water together in saucepan over medium heat. Stir constantly until thick. Simmer covered on low heat for 10 minutes. Remove from heat and blend in lemon juice and lemon rind. Beat well with wire whisk. Serve hot on fish or vegetables.

Makes about 1 cup

Shrimp Pasta

2 medium tomatoes
½ cup fresh basil
½ cup fresh parsley
Vegetable seasoning
Dash red pepper
1 pound shrimp, fresh or frozen
8 ounces fettuccine, linguine, or other pasta
1 tablespoon olive oil
2–3 cloves garlic (or more if you really like garlic)
¼ cup Parmesan cheese

Chop tomatoes, basil, and parsley. Mix with vegetable seasoning and a dash of red pepper and set aside. Shell and devein shrimp, leaving tails on if desired. Cook pasta until just tender (al dente), per package instructions. While pasta is cooking, heat olive oil in skillet over medium heat. Add shrimp and sauté until pink and firm, turning and stirring frequently, about five minutes. Add minced garlic and continue cooking until garlic is golden brown. Remove from heat. Drain pasta, and toss together with shrimp, parsley, basil, chopped tomatoes, and ¼ cup Parmesan cheese. Serve immediately.

Serves 4

Marinated Chicken Breasts

Juice of 1 lemon
¼ teaspoon salt (or salt substitute to taste)
1 clove garlic, minced
2 small or 1 large, halved chicken breast (4 ounces each; ½ pound total)
2 tablespoons parsley, chopped

Mix the lemon juice with salt or salt substitute and garlic. Marinate chicken breasts several hours or overnight in mixture. Bake in an uncovered casserole, sprayed first with olive-oil spray, at 350 degrees for 45 minutes. Garnish with parsley.

Serves 2

Teriyaki Chicken

2 chicken breasts, 4 ounces each
¾ cup water (divided use)
2 tablespoons low-sodium soy sauce (divided use)
½ teaspoon vinegar (rice vinegar preferred)
1 clove garlic, minced

Brown chicken breasts in medium skillet over medium heat for 3 to 4 minutes on each side. Add 2 tablespoons of water plus 1 teaspoon of the soy sauce, cover, reduce heat, and continue cooking for about 10 minutes, until cooked through. Meanwhile, cook remaining ingredients in a small saucepan over low heat for 10 minutes. Pour sauce over chicken before serving.

Serves 2

Turkey Enchiladas

1 pound ground turkey breast
2 teaspoons olive oil
1 teaspoon garlic powder
1 teaspoon onion powder
3 cups cooked navy, kidney, or pinto beans
1 cup frozen corn, thawed
1 6-ounce can tomato paste
3 cups water
1 teaspoon cumin
1 teaspoon salt (or salt substitute to taste)
1 dozen corn tortillas
4 ounces low-fat cheese, grated

Sauté turkey breast in nonstick skillet in olive oil, adding garlic and onion powders. Turn off heat and add beans and corn. Mix the tomato paste with water, cumin, and salt or salt substitute and stir well. Soften each tortilla in an ungreased, nonstick frying pan over medium heat, about 1 minute on each side. Dip the tortillas in the tomato sauce, lay flat, then fill with bean/turkey/corn mixture. Fold over and place in 9-inch by 13-inch baking pan coated with olive-oil spray. Pour any extra tomato sauce over enchiladas and sprinkle cheese over top. Cover and bake in a preheated 350-degree oven for 25 minutes.

Serves 6

Asparagus Chicken

1 onion, chopped
2 cloves garlic, minced
1 teaspoon olive oil
3 cups asparagus spears, cut into 1-inch pieces
1 cup sliced mushrooms
1 pound skinless, boneless chicken breasts, sliced into 2-inch strips
Juice and peel of 1 lemon
½ cup water
½ teaspoon salt (or salt substitute to taste)
¼ teaspoon pepper
3 tablespoons parsley, chopped

Sauté onion and garlic in oil for about 3 minutes. Add asparagus and mushrooms and cook for 3 more minutes. Remove from pan and set aside. Add chicken to the pan and cook until lightly browned, about 3 minutes. Return vegetables to the pan along with the chicken, and add the lemon juice and peel, salt or salt substitute, and pepper. Add water, stir and let simmer for ten minutes, or until heated and chicken is cooked through. Sprinkle with parsley before serving.

Serves 4

Chicken-Broccoli Pasta

1 large head broccoli (2 cups), cut into 1-inch pieces
1 pound boneless chicken breasts, cut into ½-inch-thick slices
1 teaspoon olive oil
1 clove minced garlic or ½ teaspoon garlic powder
½ teaspoon onion powder
½ teaspoon salt (or salt substitute to taste)
8 oz. spaghetti or other pasta
1 tablespoon olive oil
2 tablespoons parsley, chopped
4 tablespoons Parmesan cheese

Lightly steam broccoli until tender-crisp and set aside. Brown chicken in 1 teaspoon olive oil in large skillet until cooked through, 5–10 minutes, adding seasonings during the last minute. Add steamed broccoli to chicken. Meanwhile cook spaghetti until just tender (al dente), following package directions. Toss cooked pasta with chicken and broccoli mixture, and 1 tablespoon olive oil. Stir over low heat until heated through. Add parsley and cheese, stir well, and serve.

Serves 4

Mexican Supper

1 tablespoon olive oil (divided use)
1 pound ground turkey breast
1 zucchini, sliced and quartered
1 onion, chopped
1 green pepper, chopped
1 16-ounce can tomatoes, drained and chopped
4 tablespoons salsa (or more to taste) (recipe below)
½ teaspoon salt (or salt substitute to taste)
2 cups cooked brown rice or barley

Cook brown rice or barley as directed. Meanwhile, brown ground turkey in half of the olive oil. Drain and remove. Sauté vegetables in the remaining olive oil until tender-crisp. Add the turkey, tomatoes, salsa, and salt or salt substitute and cook for 3 minutes. Serve over ½ cup brown rice or barley per serving and top with extra salsa. For salsa recipe, see below.

Serves 4

Salsa

1 small chopped green pepper
1 large chopped onion
1 small can chopped green chili peppers
1 can tomatoes, drained and chopped
½ teaspoon salt (or salt substitute to taste)
Red pepper flakes or Tabasco sauce, to taste

Combine all ingredients. Modify amount of pepper or Tabasco to obtain desired hotness. Refrigerate for at least an hour to blend flavors.

Makes about 3 cups

Sesame Ginger Chicken

2 small chicken breasts (4 ounces each)
1 tablespoon olive oil
1 cup plain nonfat yogurt
1 tablespoon brown rice syrup
¼ cup toasted whole-grain bread crumbs
1 teaspoon freshly grated ginger (or to taste)

Brown the chicken in olive oil in a skillet. Do not cook completely. Mix the yogurt, brown rice syrup, bread crumbs, and grated ginger. Arrange the chicken in a single layer in an oven-safe dish, and spread the yogurt mixture over the surface of each piece of chicken. Place uncovered in a 325-degree oven and bake ½ hour or until chicken is tender.

Serves 2

Chicken Stir Fry

2 chicken breasts (4 ounces each), sliced into 1-inch strips
2 teaspoons olive oil (divided use)
2 cups snow peas
1 small can water chestnuts
1 cup sliced fresh mushrooms
2 stalks sliced celery
2 tablespoons arrowroot or cornstarch
1 cup low-sodium fat-free chicken broth
1 tablespoon low-sodium soy sauce

Sauté chicken pieces in 1 teaspoon olive oil until cooked through, about five minutes. Remove from skillet. Add second teaspoon of olive oil and stir-fry snow peas, water chestnuts, mushrooms, and celery until tender-crisp. Return chicken to pan with vegetables, combine arrowroot or cornstarch with the chicken broth and soy sauce, add, and cook, stirring constantly, until thickened. Serve over brown rice.

Serves 4

VEGETARIAN MAIN DISHES

- We have included a few main dish vegetarian dishes, since this may be the category you are least familiar with. You can also eat these dishes in smaller servings as a side to fish or poultry.
- You may find yourself resorting to pasta for quick and easy dinners. Consider making a pot of Spaghetti Sauce (recipe below). It may be stored in the refrigerator or frozen in 1- or 2-cup portions. You may also purchase fat-free, low-sodium spaghetti sauce and spice it up a bit by adding your favorite sautéed vegetables.

Spaghetti Sauce

6 cups chopped canned tomatoes (two 28-ounce cans)
½ cup tomato paste
2 cups minced green pepper
2 cups fresh minced onion (approximately 1 medium onion)
4 teaspoons oregano
2 tablespoons vegetable seasoning (or salt substitute to taste)
8 cloves garlic, minced or pressed in garlic press (or less, to taste)

Combine all the ingredients in a large pot and simmer slowly for 1 hour. You may add more tomato puree for thickness or more water if you desire your sauce less thick. The amount of vegetable seasoning may be increased to taste.

Variations: You may add 1 to 2 cups chopped mushrooms, 1 to 2 cups browned lean ground turkey, and/or 1 cup low-salt soy protein substitute. Increase the seasoning to 4 tablespoons of vegetable seasoning.

Makes 8½ cups

Pasta Putanesca

12 ounces penne pasta
1 teaspoon olive oil
1 onion, coarsely chopped
1–2 cloves minced or pressed garlic (to taste)
½ cup black olives, preferably strong, fresh olives from deli section
2 cups spaghetti sauce (recipe on page 397 or bottled)
¼–½ teaspoon red pepper flakes, to taste
¼ cup Parmesan cheese

Cook pasta al dente, according to package directions. Meanwhile, heat olive oil in a nonstick skillet, add onion and garlic, and sauté over medium heat until tender. Add remaining ingredients to the skillet and cook until hot. Serve over hot pasta and top with Parmesan cheese.

Serves 4

Stuffed Peppers

4 large green or red bell peppers
2 cups cooked barley
½ cup chopped parsley
1 medium carrot, grated
1 can tomatoes, chopped
¾ pound mushrooms, chopped

Cook the bell peppers by removing the caps and seeds and standing on end in a pot filled with 1 inch of water. Steam 10 to 15 minutes or until tender. Combine remaining ingredients and stuff into peppers. Bake in a covered baking dish in a preheated 350-degree oven for 20 minutes.

Serves 4

Tofu Steaks

1 pound extra-firm tofu
4 teaspoons low-sodium soy sauce

Slice tofu lengthwise into four slices. Sprinkle each slice with 1 teaspoon soy sauce. Heat a large nonstick skillet over medium heat. Spray with olive oil and add tofu steaks, two at a time. Cook for 3 to 5 minutes on each side, until brown.

Serves 4

Ratatouille

1 tablespoon olive oil
1 onion, cut in chunks
1 green pepper, cut in chunks
2 zucchini, cut in chunks
1 eggplant, peeled and cut in chunks
1 cup mushrooms
½ teaspoon salt (or salt substitute to taste)
1 16-ounce can tomatoes, chopped and drained

In a large skillet, heat the olive oil, then add the vegetables in the following order, cooking and stirring for about three minutes between each addition: onion, green pepper, zucchini, eggplant, and mushrooms. Add salt or salt substitute and tomatoes, stir until hot and mixture begins to dry. Serve ratatouille over hot pasta or quinoa.

Serves 4

Spinach Lasagna

12 lasagna noodles
½ pound ground turkey breast
½ teaspoon minced garlic or garlic powder
½ teaspoon onion powder
1½ cups fat-free ricotta cheese
1 small eggplant, sliced into paper-thin slices
4 tablespoons Parmesan cheese
1 large bunch fresh spinach, washed and stems removed
1 teaspoon oregano
12 ounces fresh mushrooms, sliced
2½ cups spaghetti sauce

Precook the lasagna noodles until just tender. When cooked, drain immediately and separate. Brown ground turkey with garlic and onion powders in olive-oil-sprayed pan. Add to spaghetti sauce. Spray a 9-inch by 13-inch baking dish with olive oil. Layer in this order: ½ cup of the spaghetti sauce, one layer of the noodles (4 noodles), ½ cup ricotta cheese, eggplant. Spread this with ½ cup of the spaghetti sauce and sprinkle with 1 tablespoon Parmesan cheese. Now layer a second layer of lasagna noodles. Spread another ½ cup of ricotta over the noodles. Heap the spinach over this second layer, about 4 leaves thick. Add another ½ cup sauce, then sprinkle with the oregano. Add a third layer of four lasagna noodles, followed by the last ½ cup of ricotta and another tablespoon of Parmesan. Top with the mushrooms, 1 more cup of spaghetti sauce, and 2 tablespoons of Parmesan, being careful to sprinkle it lightly so that it will cover the top. Cover with foil and bake at 350 degrees for 45 minutes. Cut into squares to serve. You may layer 2 squares so it will be thicker.

Serves 4

Tamale Pie

Filling:

1 chopped onion
1 chopped bell pepper
1 stalk chopped celery
1 minced garlic clove
1 teaspoon olive oil
2 cups tomato sauce
3 cups cooked pinto beans
2 cups fresh or frozen corn
1½ teaspoons chili powder
1 4-ounce can sliced or chopped black olives
½ cup low-fat cheese, grated

Crust

1 cup stone-ground cornmeal
1 cup cold water
½ teaspoon salt (or salt substitute to taste)
2 tablespoons olive oil
1 cup boiling water

Sauté onion, pepper, celery, and garlic in olive oil. Blend tomato sauce, pinto beans, corn, chili powder, and olives with sautéed vegetables. Pour into baking dish. Top with cheese.

Blend cornmeal with cold water. Add salt or salt substitute and olive oil to boiling water, then pour in cornmeal mixture and stir until thickened. Spread cornmeal mixture evenly over casserole and bake uncovered in a preheated 350-degree oven for 40 to 50 minutes.

Serves 6

Noodle Casserole

8 ounce package egg noodles

Sauce:
1 teaspoon olive oil
½ cup chopped onion
½ cup chopped celery
1 cup sliced mushrooms
1 cup fresh or frozen peas
2 cups nonfat milk
1 tablespoon vegetable seasoning (or salt substitute to taste)
2 tablespoons arrowroot or cornstarch mixed to a smooth paste in ¼ cup cold water

Topping:
½ cup whole-grain bread crumbs
⅓ cup finely chopped almonds
½ cup low-fat cheese, grated
1 tomato, chopped
2 tablespoons fresh parsley, chopped

Cook noodles per package directions. Do not overcook. Drain and set aside. Heat olive oil in large nonstick skillet. Add onion and sauté for 3 or 4 minutes. Add celery, mushrooms, and peas and cook another five minutes. Pour in milk and vegetable seasoning or salt substitute and bring to a low boil over medium-low heat, stirring constantly. Meanwhile, mix cornstarch in water, then slowly add to sauce, stirring constantly for a few minutes until thick and creamy. Mix sauce and noodles, then place in a medium-size baking dish sprayed with olive oil. Top with bread crumbs, almonds, and cheese. Bake uncovered in a preheated 350-degree oven for 30 to 40 minutes. Garnish with tomato and parsley.

Serves 4

SIDE DISHES

- Choose a side dish that complements your main dish—think color, texture, taste, and type. If your main dish is red, choose a green side dish. If your main dish is creamy, choose a crunchy side dish. If your main dish is strongly flavored, choose a mild side dish. And if you are featuring grains in your main dish, choose a nonstarch side dish.
- The easiest side dishes are your favorite vegetables lightly steamed or quickly cooked in the microwave. You may season them with a little salt or salt substitute, pepper, low-sodium soy sauce, lemon juice, a drizzle of olive oil, or your favorite healthful sauce. We are not going to include recipes for simple steamed veggies. If you do not know how to fix them, consult any traditional cookbook—but omit excess salt and oil.
- Make a point to eat the vegetable superstars often, such as leafy greens, broccoli and other cruciferous vegetables, and, of course, beans.

Green Beans Provençale

1 pound green beans
1 onion, chopped
1 16-ounce can tomatoes, chopped but not drained
¼ teaspoon basil
½ teaspoon salt (or salt substitute to taste)
½ teaspoon pepper

Snap the ends off the beans and add them to a medium saucepan, along with the other ingredients. Cover and bring to a boil. Reduce heat and simmer for about 20 minutes, until tender.

Serves 4

German Cabbage

4 cups shredded red or green cabbage
2 onions, chopped fine
1 tablespoon caraway seeds
Juice of 2 lemons
2 apples, unpeeled and diced
⅛ teaspoon ground allspice
¼ cup apple juice or cider
3 tablespoons brown rice syrup

Place all ingredients in a covered saucepan. Bring to a boil and simmer until tender, 10 to 15 minutes.

Serves 6

Mock Mashed Potatoes

4 cups cauliflower, cooked until soft
2 cups nonfat cottage cheese
¾ cup plain nonfat yogurt
½ finely chopped onion
½ teaspoon salt (or salt substitute to taste)
2 tablespoons liquid Butter Buds
1 cup whole-grain bread crumbs

Mash cauliflower in blender, food processor, or with mixer. Stir in cottage cheese, yogurt, onion, and salt. Pour into nonstick baking dish oiled with olive-oil pan spray. Brush top with liquid Butter Buds. Top with bread crumbs. Bake in a preheated 350-degree oven 30 to 40 minutes. Serve with Mushroom Gravy (recipe on next page).

Serves 6

Mushroom Gravy

3 tablespoons arrowroot or cornstarch mixed into ¼ cup cold water
1 large onion, finely chopped
1 teaspoon olive oil
1 pound sliced mushrooms
4 cups water or fat-free, low-sodium chicken broth
2 tablespoons vegetable seasoning
2 tablespoons low-sodium soy sauce

Make a paste by stirring cold water into the arrowroot or cornstarch until a creamy consistency is reached. Sauté the onion in olive oil in a nonstick pan until tender. Add mushrooms and continue cooking for another five minutes. Add water or chicken broth, vegetable seasoning, and soy sauce and bring to a boil. When very hot, stir in the cornstarch mixture and continue to cook, stirring constantly, until thick and smooth. Serve with Mock Mashed Potatoes (recipe on page 404), rice, or other starchy dishes.

Makes about 6 cups

Greens and Spuds

2 bunches greens (mustard, kale, etc.)
Water
2 unpeeled, cubed small red potatoes
Salt (or salt substitute to taste)

Clean greens and remove stems. In a large pot, put 2 inches of water and add greens. Steam until they start to become tender, about 20 minutes. Add potatoes and continue cooking until the potatoes are tender, about 15 minutes. During the last 5 minutes of cooking, add salt or salt substitute.

Serves 2

Creamed Spinach

1 10-ounce package frozen spinach or 1 large bunch fresh
¼ cup nonfat yogurt
½ teaspoon onion powder
¼ teaspoon nutmeg

Cook spinach until wilted. Drain. Blend yogurt with onion powder and nutmeg. Stir seasoned yogurt into spinach and cook over medium heat to serving temperature. Serve immediately.

Serves 2

Mushroom Pilaf

1 teaspoon olive oil
1½ cups finely chopped mushrooms
1 cup bulghur
2 teaspoons vegetable seasoning
¼ teaspoon pepper
2 cups water
2 green onions, thinly sliced

Heat olive oil over medium-high heat in a medium saucepan. Add mushrooms and cook, stirring often, for 5 minutes. Add bulghur, seasonings, and water, bring to a boil, then reduce heat to a simmer, cover pan, and cook for 20 minutes. Pilaf is done when all the liquid is absorbed. Fluff with a fork, garnish with green onions, and serve.

Serves 4

Curried Quinoa

1 cup quinoa
2 cups water
1 teaspoon curry powder

Rinse quinoa in medium saucepan. Add 2 cups water and curry powder. Bring to a boil, reduce heat, and simmer for about 15 minutes, until water is absorbed and grains have turned from white to transparent.

Serves 4

Barley Pilaf

1 tablespoon olive oil
1 medium onion, chopped
½ pound mushrooms, sliced
1 cup pearl barley
2 cups water
½ teaspoon salt (or salt substitute to taste)

Preheat oven to 350 degrees. Heat olive oil in medium skillet with a lid. Add onion and mushrooms and cook for 5 minutes. Add the barley, stirring to coat. Meanwhile, bring the water to a boil. Add to skillet with vegetables and barley, along with salt or salt substitute. Cover and cook in 350-degree oven for 30 minutes. Add a little water if pilaf becomes too dry.

Serves 4

DESSERTS

- The sweet tooth. I don't know if it's genetic or not, but either you have it or you don't. If you dream of chocolate and wax poetic about your mom's apple pie, you've got it bad, and we do not want to deny you.
- You'll notice that many of our dessert recipes are fruit-based. Plain whole or sliced fruit is also a great, healthful dessert.
- We hope you'll enjoy these recipes. Eat one serving—too much of even a good thing is not healthy.

Baked Apples

2 tart cooking apples (not delicious apples)
Water
2 teaspoons brown rice syrup
2 tablespoons chopped almonds
¼ teaspoon cinnamon

Core apples, leaving a little flesh at bottom to hold sauce. Place apples in an ovenproof dish with 1 inch of water in the bottom. Mix last three ingredients and spoon half into each apple. Cover and bake in a preheated 400-degree oven for about 45 minutes or until apples are soft.

Serves 2

Yogurt "Ice Cream"

1 cup plain nonfat yogurt
⅓ cup brown rice syrup
2 cups fresh fruit (strawberries, peaches, blueberries)
1 tablespoon lemon juice

Mix all together in a blender or food processor and freeze in a shallow pan. Can take out after several hours, stir or blend again, and return to freezer till firm.

Serves 3 to 4

Fresh Fruit "Ice Cream"

1 banana
1 pint strawberries
8 ounces nonfat yogurt
Stevia to taste

Combine the ingredients in a blender or food processor until smooth. Freeze in a loaf pan until firm. Scrape with an ice cream scoop to serve.

Serves 6 to 8

Apple Crisp

4 cups peeled, sliced apples (tart apples are best—anything but delicious)
1 tablespoon lemon juice
1 teaspoon cinnamon
1½ cups oatmeal (not instant)
½ cup whole wheat flour
¼ cup xylitol
⅓ cup chopped almonds
2 tablespoons Butter Buds liquid

Fill an olive-oil-sprayed pie plate with the apples. Sprinkle with lemon juice and cinnamon. Crush the oatmeal with a rolling pin and mix with flour, xylitol, almonds, and Butter Buds liquid. Sprinkle over the apples. Bake in a preheated 350-degree oven for 30 minutes.

Serves 8

Nutty Piecrust

1 cup Grape Nuts cereal
1–2 tablespoons frozen apple juice concentrate

Spray a 9-inch pie plate with olive-oil pan spray. Sprinkle Grape Nuts into pan and moisten with apple juice concentrate. Press against sides and bottom of pie plate—¼ to ½ inch thick. When filled and baked it tastes like a graham-cracker piecrust. This will be used in several of the pie recipes that follow.

Cheesy Lemon Pie

16 ounces nonfat cottage cheese
1 cup nonfat milk
6 ounces frozen orange juice concentrate
1 teaspoon vanilla extract
1 teaspoon lemon extract
4 stiffly beaten egg whites
Nutty Piecrust (recipe on page 410)

Blend first 5 ingredients. Fold the mixture into the egg whites. Pour into pie plate with Nutty Piecrust and bake in a preheated 350-degree oven for 1 hour. Serve warm or chilled.

Serves 8

Pumpkin Pie

1 16-ounce can unsweetened pumpkin
⅛ teaspoon cloves
⅛ teaspoon nutmeg
1 6-ounce can thawed frozen apple juice concentrate
1 teaspoon vanilla extract
1 teaspoon cinnamon
¼ teaspoon allspice
¼ teaspoon ginger
6 stiffly beaten egg whites
Nutty Piecrust (recipe on page 410)

Blend all ingredients except for the egg whites. In mixing bowl fold beaten egg whites into the pumpkin mixture. Pour into Nutty Piecrust in pie pan. Bake in a preheated 350-degree oven for 1 hour or until toothpick inserted into center shows it is firm but still moist.

Serves 8

Cherry Pie

2½ tablespoons tapioca granules
⅓ teaspoon nutmeg
3–4 drops of stevia mixed into ½ cup water
3 cups unsweetened cherries (not in thick syrup) frozen, canned, or fresh and pitted
¼ teaspoon almond extract
½ cup Grape Nuts cereal, soaked in 2 tablespoons water for 30 minutes
Nutty Piecrust (recipe on page 410)

Blend together the tapioca, nutmeg, sweetened water, and let stand for 15 minutes. Then stir in the cherries and almond extract. Pour into prepared Nutty Piecrust and top with soaked Grape Nuts. Bake in a preheated 425-degree oven for about 50 minutes.

Serves 8

Berry Delicious

3 tablespoons tapioca granules
1½ cups berries, unsweetened (boysenberries, blackberries, or raspberries) pureed and sweetened with stevia or xylitol, to taste
1 teaspoon vanilla
2 apples or pears, peeled and sliced
1 cup whole berries
¾ cup oatmeal (not instant)
¼ cup raw, unhulled sesame seeds
1 teaspoon cinnamon

Mix tapioca with the pureed berries and vanilla. Spread over the bottom of a pie plate sprayed with olive-oil pan spray. Place the apple or pear slices in a layer on top of the pureed berries. Next layer the whole berries. Blend the oatmeal, sesame seeds, and cinnamon in a bowl, then sprinkle on top. Bake in a preheated 350-degree oven for 30 minutes. Serve warm.

Serves 8

Dessert Fruit Salad

4 cups of your favorite fruit, cut (berries; peeled and sliced oranges; cored, peeled, and cubed apples; seedless grapes; peach slices; or bananas)

Combine fruits as desired. Refrigerate to combine flavors. Top with Fruit Salad Dressing (recipe below).

Serves 4

Fruit Salad Dressing

2 cups plain nonfat yogurt
½ cup berries
½ cup water
Stevia, xylitol, or brown rice syrup to taste

Blend all ingredients until smooth. Serve over fruit.

Makes 3 cups

Sesame Balls

1 cup oatmeal, ground coarsely in a grinder or blender
½ cup raw sesame seeds
½ cup brown rice syrup

Form the oats and seeds into 1-inch balls by mixing with the brown rice syrup, adding more syrup if necessary.

Serves 3 to 4

Rice Pudding

1½ cups nonfat milk
4 egg whites
2 tablespoons brown rice syrup
½ teaspoon nutmeg
1 teaspoon cinnamon
1 tablespoon tapioca granules
2 cups cooked brown rice
1 cup peeled, chopped apple

In a double boiler, heat the milk. In a bowl, beat egg whites lightly. Add the brown rice syrup, nutmeg, cinnamon, and tapioca to the egg whites. Slowly add the egg white mixture to the hot milk, stirring constantly about 10 minutes or until mixture starts to thicken. Remove from heat and add the rice. Mix well. Add the apple. Mix well. Pour into a buttered nonstick 2-quart baking dish. Bake in a preheated 350-degree oven for 15 minutes or until set. Serve warm or cold.

Serves 5 to 6

Poached Fruit

Water
2–4 fresh apples, pears, peaches, or nectarines, chopped
½ teaspoon cinnamon
¼ teaspoon stevia

Put one inch of water in a saucepan. Add chopped fruit, cinnamon, and stevia and simmer for 5 to 10 minutes. This is good eaten alone as a dessert, mixed with plain yogurt, or spooned over hot cereal or French toast.

Serves 2

BEVERAGES

- Your beverage of choice should be water, preferably filtered or purified. Drink at least eight 8-ounce glasses every day.
- One or two cups (not giant mugs) of regular coffee per day are acceptable for most people. If you have very high blood pressure, arrhythmias, elevated homocysteine, or if you are pregnant or nursing, go easy on coffee. A better choice for everyone is heart-healthy green and black tea. (For more on coffee and tea, see Chapter 12.)
- A little alcohol is also an approved part of the diet for reversing heart disease. One to two drinks per day for women and two to three for men are the limit. Do not start drinking for your health or use this as an excuse to drink if you have a problem with alcohol.
- We do not recommend unbridled consumption of fruit juice. It is just too high in sugar. A little on occasion is fine, especially if you dilute it with water.
- Vegetable juices, because they contain less sugar, are fine. Drinking 12 ounces of *low-sodium* V-8 or tomato juice every day will provide you with a hefty dose of potassium and other nutrients for the heart. (Do not drink regular V-8 or tomato juice. It has too much sodium.)
- Also see the Smoothie recipe on page 359. It makes a great between-meal snack.

Perrier Surprise

Orange juice
Perrier, seltzer, or club soda

Freeze orange juice in ice cube tray. Add a cube or two to chilled Perrier, seltzer, or club soda. Good for entertaining.

Hot Carob Cocoa

1 tablespoon carob powder
1 teaspoon brown rice syrup
¼ teaspoon vanilla
⅛ teaspoon cinnamon
1 cup heated nonfat milk

Stir all ingredients into heated milk. Serve hot.

Serves 1

Fruity Tea Punch

6 cups fruity herbal tea (your favorite)
1 pint club soda or Perrier
Stevia, xylitol, or another sweetener to taste
½ cup lemon juice
1 orange, lemon, and/or lime, thinly sliced

Mix the tea, club soda or Perrier, and lemon juice together and sweeten to taste. Decorate with the citrus fruit slices. Serve cold.

Serves 6

Hot Apple Cider

4 cups unsweetened apple cider or apple juice
½ teaspoon whole cloves
3 cinnamon sticks
½ teaspoon whole allspice

Bring apple cider or juice to a boil. Add the spices and cook an additional 10 minutes. Strain out spices and serve hot.

Serves 4

Cranberry Cooler

4 tablespoons cranberry juice concentrate, unsweetened
1 cup Perrier or club soda
Stevia, xylitol, or another sweetener, to taste

Stir or shake all ingredients together. Serve with frozen fruit juice ice cubes.

Serves 1

Creamy Orange Drink

8 ounces plain nonfat yogurt
¼ cup orange juice or 2 tablespoons thawed orange juice concentrate

Stir together. Add more juice to thin, if needed. Serve cold.

Serves 1

Strawberry Shake

1 cup water
½ cup frozen whole unsweetened strawberries
⅛ teaspoon almond extract (optional)
Stevia, xylitol, or other sweetener, to taste

Combine all ingredients in blender, blend, and serve cold.

Serves 1

Apple/Pear Shake

½ cup water
¼ cup apple juice
1 ripe peeled and cored pear
4 ice cubes
Stevia to taste

Combine all ingredients in blender and blend until smooth. Serve ice cold.

Serves 1

Lemonade

3 cups water
Juice of 2 lemons
Stevia, xylitol, or other sweetener to taste

Mix water and lemon juice. Sweeten to taste with stevia, xylitol, or other sweetener. Add ice and serve.

Serves 3

Part V

The Program in Action

CHAPTER 22

Getting Started, Staying on Track

An illness is not an abstraction. It happens to a human being. In this age of high-tech medicine and managed care, it is easy for doctors to forget the humanity of their patients. This is particularly unfortunate in dealing with heart disease, for the only real cure for the condition must be effected by the patients themselves. Atheroscleorsis, as I hope I have made clear in this book, is a multifaceted, progressive problem. A comprehensive program of diet, exercise, nutritional supplementation, and stress management is the only approach that systematically attacks the underlying causes of heart disease. With or without drugs and surgery, it is absolutely essential for successful management of the disease. To ignore this, particularly in light of all the supporting research and scientific studies, is just plain foolish.

Despite the rush of some cardiologists to go in and "do" something to their patients, what patients with heart disease really need is a guide, a monitor, and, most important, a teacher. We need to remember that the word doctor means "one who teaches." "Curing" people with sick arteries is not done by simply running tests, performing bypass surgery or angioplasty, or handing the patient a prescription to be filled at the pharmacy. For real healing to take place, doctors must talk to their patients, answer their questions, and take a very personal interest in getting them to change their unhealthy habits. This means helping patients understand the mechanisms underlying their illness, showing them how to implement lifestyle changes, and building enthusiasm for the process.

When I opened the Whitaker Wellness Institute in 1979, I wanted to create a comfortable environment where patients could learn the basics of lifestyle changes alongside others with similar health challenges, and by experiencing the short-term benefits of good nutrition and exercise become motivated to continue the program at home. My intention was to take patients with cardiovascular disease, diabetes, and high blood pressure, get them started in the right direction, and send them back to their own physicians for continued care.

I never envisioned my clinic as a substitute for hospitals or medical centers. Without question, your best place to be if a heart attack occurs is the hospital. But I did want to fill the void that our current approach to the treatment of heart disease has created so that patients could get the education and motivation necessary to successfully implement lifestyle changes. The physicians at the clinic are much more than astute examiners and skilled interpreters of tests. They are also educators, leaders, and motivators.

More than 60 million Americans suffer from cardiovascular diseases, and thousands of hospitals display the latest technology in the management of heart attacks and other acute coronary events. Yet there is a severe shortage of institutions designed to help people understand their condition, modify their underlying risk factors, and actually reverse the progression of atherosclerosis. What is needed is a dramatic shift of priorities. For the majority of patients who have symptoms of heart disease or have already had a heart attack, angioplasty or bypass surgery should not be considered until vigorous treatment with lifestyle changes and appropriate medications has first been tried.

The purpose of this book has been to share with you the

Whitaker Wellness Institute program for reversing heart disease. I sincerely hope that you have a physician who understands and respects the power of the therapies we have discussed and will help you implement them. Please understand the importance of working with a healthcare professional. Under no circumstances should you decide on your own to discontinue medications or begin training for a marathon. On the other hand, if your doctor is less than supportive, don't let that hold you back. I have provided you with all the information you need to institute your own program for reversing heart disease: meal plans and recipes, the specifics of an exercise program, recommendations for a nutritional supplement regimen, and suggestions for getting stress under control. All that remains is for you to take that first step and get started.

I want to conclude by first taking you through a week at the clinic in hope that you can use some of the same techniques we use with our patients to motivate yourself to begin and stick with your own program of lifestyle changes. Then, I will share with you stories of some of the patients who have been through our program. Patients such as these have been my greatest teachers. They help me understand what works and what changes people are willing to make. Their successes motivate me to continue sharing with others this very effective program for reversing heart disease.

A TYPICAL DAY AT THE INSTITUTE

8:00 A.M. The day starts early. Patients weigh in, have their blood pressure and pulse recorded, and give a history of the day before—how far they walked, the pulse rate attained during exercise, and a rundown of any symptoms experienced. These daily reports help us to evaluate progress and alter medication dosage.

8:30 A.M. Breakfast: anything from oatmeal to French toast to scrambled eggs with fresh fruit. This is also when patients take their morning nutritional supplements.

9:00–11:00 A.M. Most mornings are devoted to education. Every day a different speaker from the Whitaker Wellness Institute professional staff instructs patients in the nuts and bolts of the program. Our research director explains the basics of nutritional supplementation, which is an important and for many patients confusing aspect of the program, making sure that each patient understands every item on his or her personalized supplement "action plan." Our exercise physiologist explains the mechanics of safe exercise. Our certified nutritionist outlines the diet and food plan, explaining the roles fat, protein, and carbohydrates play in optimal health. We spend several sessions discussing food from every angle conceivable: shopping, storage, preparation, cooking, even dining out. One of the sessions is a hands-on cooking demonstration by our professional chef, so that in addition to receiving printed recipes and menus, patients clearly understand the mechanics of following this program at home.

11:00–11:45 A.M. Scheduled exercise. Patients have already received an individualized exercise program based on the results of their stress test, and most exercise throughout the day, swimming or walking in the usually beautiful southern California weather. However, each morning the group also exercises together, led by our personal trainer. During this time we can determine if patients are taking their pulse accurately, exercising at an appropriate level, and warming up and cooling down properly. Symptoms are also monitored during exercise, which gives the staff a good sense of how each patient is doing.

Noon–1:00 P.M. Lunch. It could be spinach lasagna, stir-fried chicken and vegetables with noodles, soup and salad, or another of the many pleasing and healthful dishes prepared by our chef.

1:00–4:00 P.M. We try to leave some time open every afternoon for follow-up physician visits, specialized therapies such as EECP, chelation, or hyperbaric oxygen therapy—or just enjoy some downtime.

4:00–4:30 P.M. Several days a week patients gather for guided relaxation, to learn techniques for combatting stress. We also teach them "health visualization": seeing themselves as healthy, active, thin, and pain-free. We realize that stress plays a role in disease and learning to manage it takes some training and practice. Patients enjoy this peaceful interlude toward the end of the day.

4:30–5:30 P.M. Each day, one of the Whitaker Wellness Institute physicians presents a lecture on a specific subject, such as heart disease, bypass surgery, diabetes, arthritis, and other areas of interest to patients. These lectures, as well as the morning sessions, are the backbone of the educational program, for it is during these seminars that patients begin to understand their medical condition as well as the role lifestyle changes play in their improvement. Each session has been recorded on tape and every patient is given the complete series to provide reinforcement and motivation after they return home.

5:30–6:30 P.M. Dinner. This is a time to enjoy the end of a day of accomplishment. Delicious, healthful meals are enjoyed with good fellowship and leisurely conversation. Salmon, chicken, or low-fat quiche may appear on the menu. We even have a celebratory glass of heart-healthy wine at our final meal.

Obviously, the days are full and active. Patients, often for the first time in their lives, spend the whole day doing things to improve their health. Many accomplished and disciplined people, expert in their own fields, limp into the clinic riddled with heart disease, diabetes, high blood pressure, and other serious problems. For many, this is their first experience in prioritizing and seriously concentrating on their health needs.

GETTING THE MOST OUT OF YOUR PROGRAM

After observing thousands of patients start and complete this program—and hearing from hundreds more who have followed it on their own—I have noticed some general trends I would like to share with you to help you get the most out of it.

Almost everyone is a little skeptical at first. The program for reversing heart disease outlined in this book is quite different from any other you may have been offered before. Despite the abundance of scientific data underscoring the efficacy of nutrition and exercise presented in this book (and the downside of conventional therapies), you may still have a few doubts. However, like the patients who have come to the clinic, you believe that this approach makes a lot of sense, and you want to give it a try.

At the clinic we begin with a thorough physical examination, blood tests (including cholesterol, LDL, HDL, triglycerides, homocysteine, C-reactive protein, and DHEA-sulfate), exercise stress test, echocardiogram, and other tests as indicated. I suggest you do the same. When the results are back, ask your physician to spend time explaining them to you. This would be the ideal time to talk about your medications: potential adverse effects, alternatives, and the possibility of reducing or discontinuing some of them. Ask questions, and insist on details. Also tell your doctor about the nutritional supplements you are taking or planning to take—but don't be surprised if he or she dismisses them. (Keep taking them anyway, unless your doctor can give you a valid reason not to.) Finally, it is always prudent to get a physician's clearance before beginning an exercise program.

We place a lot of emphasis at the clinic on education. Read and reread this and other books on heart disease, go online and visit health Web sites, attend lectures offered in your area, and talk to people who have heart disease or have made similar changes in their lifestyle. If you can hook up with others who are in the same boat, going in the same direction with the same goals, so much the better. One of the best things about the clinic program is the group support. Even though everyone comes from a different walk of life, they're all learning the same thing: how to alter their lives in key areas to regain and maintain their health. This is fertile ground for camaraderie. You'll likely find the same sense of kinship with the friend you walk with every morning, or the coworker who helps you pass up the doughnuts and stay on your diet.

Beginning an exercise program and making dietary changes are not easy, whether you're doing it on your own or at the clinic (although having someone prepare your meals and lead you in exercise for a week helps). As I suggested earlier, you need to put some thought into this. Wanting to do it isn't enough. Sit down with your calendar and schedule your exercise sessions. Actually write the time you're going to walk or when you'll be going to the gym. Tell your friends and family what you're doing, and above all, make a commitment to yourself to follow through.

Likewise with diet changes. Decide how you're going to approach the diet (gradually or cold turkey) and enlist the support of others to keep you on track. For the most part, you will be surprised at how delicious the food is—and delighted that you are encouraged to eat many of the things you might have worried would be considered taboo, such as pasta, eggs, chicken, and olive oil.

As your efforts begin to pay off, the drudgery eases up as true motivation begins—and this will be sooner than you might expect. Sometimes dramatic improvements are noticed after only one week at the Whitaker Wellness Institute. Angina eases. Many patients who were unable to walk a block without pain are taking daily strolls without difficulty. Blood pressures are down. Extra pounds start coming off, and there are changes in cholesterol, triglycerides, and other markers of heart disease. As you begin to feel better, expect to experience a sense of enthusiasm and a marked change in attitude.

First, fear, which often immobilizes heart patients, is replaced with a resolve to lick the problem. Heart patients who choose a lifestyle program such as this are not deluded about the gravity of their problem. Quite the contrary. You understand how serious it is even more clearly than most. However, you now have a plan of action, a way of addressing these dangers head on.

Second, the lifestyle changes are no longer viewed as arduous or impossible. You come to view the program as an opportunity, even a challenge, to overcome your health problems, and as you do, you develop an increased respect for your body and ultimately for yourself. Health now becomes a high priority, and this program gives you the tools to achieve it.

Third, and most important, you are no longer a passive recipient of medications prescribed by a physician, left in the dark about your condition or what you can do about it. You are now an active partner in your health care. You understand the causes of heart disease and the importance of the various markers of heart health. You realize the integral role nutrition plays in your recovery, and you are determined to receive the benefits of exercise.

In the final analysis, these changes in attitude are essential for long-term success, and the information provided in this book is designed to effect them. My hope is that you take this information and utilize it to regain and maintain your health. My best to you for a long and healthy life.

SUCCESS STORIES: PEOPLE WHO REVERSED THEIR HEART DISEASE

Joann Lang, California

Because of "suspicious" chest pains, I had an angiogram followed by bypass surgery. I was frightened, and from that time on

I had considered myself a cardiac cripple. Seven years later I had a heart attack and a repeat angiogram, which showed that both the graft and the artery were completely closed.

I entered Dr. Whitaker's program to do something positive about this problem. Now I have no chest pain. I joyously walk two to three miles a day, feel fantastic, and no longer consider myself a cardiac cripple. I wish I had done this before surgery.

Donna Monroe, Idaho

I have been a patient of Dr. Julian Whitaker's and would like to express my gratitude and thanks. I had open heart surgery. However, after three or four months I again experienced angina and never felt like the surgery did me much good. I continued to go downhill and experienced the same symptoms as before surgery. Finally, my cardiologist suggested that I have surgery again. I refused, and with the help of my daughter in California and friends who had heard of Dr. Whitaker, I decided I had nothing to lose by attending the institute.

Within one week of entering the Whitaker Wellness Institute, my blood pressure dropped considerably. I experienced less angina and my cholesterol drop was amazing. At the time of my surgery, I weighed 130 pounds at five feet one inch tall. At present I weigh exactly 100 pounds, and my blood pressure has stabilized to a safe and unbelievable level. As a mother of three children and a grandmother of seven, I now feel that life is once again worthwhile. I am no longer taking the high blood pressure medication that I had taken for thirty-two years. I exercise and try to keep on my diet. I feel that Dr. Whitaker and his methods are much more helpful and encouraging than surgery. At least I now know that I never would go through that surgery again. If I do have problems, I know what I am doing wrong and can correct them.

William Wolf, New York

I had a heart attack and went through the University of Washington Hospital, where I was diagnosed as having approximately 20 percent damage to my left ventricle and two blocked arteries. My left anterior descending artery was 100 percent blocked, and the doctors were very forceful in advising that I have bypass surgery. Instead, I elected to follow a medical program. The statistics I was able to find indicated that bypass surgery would reduce pain but would not increase longevity. In addition, I was aware that there were a number of hazards or risks in bypass surgery. Consequently, I was very disturbed by the prescription of bypass surgery.

I had a negative reaction to the angiogram and was placed in intensive care at the University of Washington Hospital. While in intensive care, one of the nurses advised me against rushing into an operation and suggested that I first try the Pritikin program of a very low-fat diet and exercise. She was so positive about the program that when I got out of the hospital, I immediately bought Dr. Pritikin's book and tried to follow the program on my own. I must say that although I read the book about seven times, I did not seem to make complete progress. I was still having pain. When I tried to exercise or walk, I frequently just had to stop to sit down and rest. I could not keep going. Thus, I was distraught and thought that I would have to go in for bypass surgery.

By chance, I met a man, Don Kennedy, on the beach. He had been fighting the same problem and had given up and was planning to go in for a bypass. When I saw him again several weeks later, he looked great. I asked him about his bypass operation. He informed me that rather than a bypass, he had been at the Whitaker Wellness Institute. Thus, I called and immediately tried to get into the institute.

At the time I entered the institute, I was doing fairly well, but my blood pressure was still a little high. My triglycerides were way up, around 238. My cholesterol was high at 261. My HDL was also very low, about 30. I began to improve immediately. By the end of two weeks I was able to walk and jog slowly for seven or eight miles without undue fatigue. I was having only very minor pains, occurring usually when I was warming up. My cholesterol level was down to 154, my triglycerides were down to 90, and my HDL was now up to 94. In short, all the measures of risk for heart attack had improved significantly.

I was amazed at the results. I have returned to work and have been doing relatively well. I find prolonged walking and jogging difficult in this climate in New York, but I am able to swim approximately thirty-five to forty lengths of the swimming pool, and usually I walk and jog two to five miles every other day. In short, I find that I am able to function effectively.

Carlo Teodori, Pennsylvania

I started looking for alternatives when my doctor of nine years told me I should increase my medication for high blood pressure. Since I was already taking three pills a day, I didn't want to increase that dosage. I read in *Prevention* magazine that Dr. Whitaker was having success in lowering blood pressure by proper diet and exercise, and I decided to enroll in the institute and try the program. My wife and I arrived and started right in on the food prepared especially for the patients at the institute. The very next morning we were up and walking with the other patients. Within a few days Dr. Whitaker suggested that I reduce my medication under his careful supervision. By the end of our two-week stay, I was off all medication and walking eight to ten miles a day and feeling great.

Since leaving the institute, I have taken medication only twice, when my pressure started to go back up. This program is really working for me and I am grateful for Dr. Whitaker and the approach he used to eliminate my high blood pressure problem.

Homer G. Ray, Georgia

The time my wife and I spent at the Whitaker Wellness Institute was undoubtedly one of the finest things we have done for our health and well-being in many years. The time and energy consumed and the expense of travel from Atlanta to California were worthwhile. We have unhesitatingly recommended the institute to friends here in Georgia. That time brought about changes in our lifestyles and eating habits that are continuing and benefiting us.

The good attention that Dr. Whitaker gave us, and the fellowship with others in attendance, made it a most stimulating and enjoyable two weeks. I am now considering making it an annual event in our lives because of the benefits and enrichment that it brought to us. Some of us are careless in our eating and our day-to-day habits, and what Dr. Whitaker offers is direction and supervision in making changes. I think we would all be far better off if we would take time every year and, in the spirit of Dr. Whitaker's program, give our health needs top priority.

Otto Lauf, Arizona

I would like to take this opportunity to join the thousands of others who have shared the experience of attending Dr. Julian Whitaker's institute. I suffered a total collapse and was told that I would be facing bypass surgery. My cholesterol level was so high, it seemed like the only solution if I wanted to live a normal life. It was not a prospect that I looked forward to, and I immediately began looking for an alternative solution. It was then that I heard about Dr. Whitaker's program.

I attended a session and found the only thing I had in my favor was my weight. I had never had a weight problem. But my eating habits and way of life were decreasing my longevity. Through Dr. Whitaker's program of diet and exercise, a whole new life has opened up to me. I've learned to eat properly and, though I sometimes yearn for a thick, juicy steak, I find that following his diet can be an enjoyable experience.

My cholesterol level has dropped drastically. Each checkup has shown very marked improvement. I walk three miles every morning, have played thirty-six holes of golf in one day, and have not been sick in over a year. I have a whole new attitude toward my health and life, feel years younger, and I am enjoying things that I never thought were possible. My thanks to Dr. Whitaker and his staff, who, through their care and guidance, have given me a new lease on life.

Joseph Moriconi, Connecticut

I spent twelve days at Dr. Whitaker's institute with my wife. It was the best money I have ever spent for my health. My cholesterol level dropped from 223 to 184. I stopped using Inderal (a beta-blocker), and my blood pressure stays steady at 120/80. I have 90 percent heart blockage of my two main arteries. The blockage is in a place where bypass surgery is risky. I know that if I continue to follow the program I went through at Dr. Whitaker's—which I will—I will be able to live a good, normal life.

Mildred Jessup, California

I think of Dr. Whitaker with appreciation for the way he changed my life. I went to him because I was sick. I had always had a weight problem and arthritis. I felt I had to do something to give my body all the help I could so I could feel good at my age. I also wanted to do what I could to avoid other degenerative problems, such as heart attack, stroke, diabetes, etc.

In going through his program, I learned the relationship of foods to the different organs of the body and also the damage that the wrong things can do. I lost fifteen pounds, but what is most important is that the weight has stayed off for over a year now. My arthritis has improved and I expect it to keep improving. My cholesterol and blood pressure both dropped. I have grown to love the taste of foods in their natural forms and do not find the fatty foods, red meat, and sweet junk palatable anymore.

Grace Mohler, California

I am willing to tell everyone the excellent results I have had since I attended Dr. Whitaker's program at the Whitaker Wellness Institute. My cholesterol dropped from 325 to 216 in two weeks and has stayed low since, without medication. My blood pressure has also maintained a healthy level with less medication. I had never eaten so much, yet I still lost 20 pounds. This all sums up to a better attitude and a happier life. I still walk two to five miles a day. Indigestion, which I frequently had, is no more. I feel just great.

Robert Clifford, California

After having an abnormal treadmill test I underwent an angiogram. Even though I did not have chest pain or angina, I was advised to have bypass surgery. I enrolled in the Whitaker Wellness Institute the day before I was to have surgery. Now my cholesterol and triglycerides are very low. I've lost 27 pounds in eight weeks, and I am walking two miles a day with no pain. I feel great and plan to stay on this program and avoid surgery.

Dale Harris, Missouri

If I had known about this program earlier, I could have avoided a lot of grief and surgery. By the time I was fifty-four, I had already had the large artery in my stomach replaced with a plastic graft as well as bypass surgery on my heart for clogged arteries. In spite of this surgery, I still could not walk because of severe pain in my calves, due to the blockages in the other arteries as well as blockages coming on in the graft. It was time I did something, so I went to the Whitaker Wellness Institute. I learned how to eat, how to exercise, the role of vitamins and minerals, and just, in general, how to take care of myself.

I was amazed at how rapidly changes occur on this program. I had always had a cholesterol problem and was taking a cholesterol-lowering drug without success. On the program for reversing heart disease, my cholesterol fell from 324 to 130, my triglycerides went from 413 to 123, and my blood pressure from 130/78 to 108/66. Other studies improved dramatically as well.

Exactly three years after leaving the institute, I am happy to report that I am completely pain-free in my legs and have been so for the last two-and-one-half years. I am walking two miles every day without any pain at all, feeling great and doing anything that I want to do. What a joy it is to be pain-free and getting healthy.

Howard B., New York

I had an angiogram after an abnormality showed up on a stress test. My cardiologist convinced me that I needed an angioplasty—even though I had no symptoms of chest pain or other signs of heart disease (except for an arrhythmia). During surgery, a blood vessel was punctured. My right leg swelled up and I had to stay in the hospital for some time. I eventually recovered, although later I developed high blood pressure and had to take another drug, in addition to one for my arrhythmia.

About eighteen months later, after another abnormal stress test, my doctor recommended a repeat angioplasty and stent placement. I wasn't too happy about the idea and when I balked, he told me that if I didn't have this procedure, I could drop dead at any moment. That didn't sound right, so I came to the Whitaker Wellness Institute for a second opinion.

After running a lot of tests, my doctor at the institute thought I was a good candidate for a more conservative course. I started on nutritional supplements and a good diet. I was already exercising thirty minutes a day and was encouraged by him to keep up the good work. I also did a course of EECP, and when I finished I felt better than ever. My blood pressure, which had stayed high while I was taking a beta blocker, went down, and I was able to get off that drug.

Terry Scott, California

I had triple bypass surgery in February of 1985, and over the years, each of these grafts closed up. Finally, in August 1997 the largest graft closed and I suffered a heart attack. After recovery I returned to work, but by March 1998, I was placed on disability from work. I was no longer able to do much—no flying, skiing, running, or anything strenuous and was told to stay below 2,000 feet in altitude. As the months passed my angina increased to the point where I was having pain going up and down my stairs at home. On January 4, 2000, an angiogram was performed and it was determined that I should undergo a quadruple heart bypass. Surgery was scheduled for March 8, 2000.

Thanks to a suggestion from a neighbor, I visited the Whitaker Wellness Institute and had a conference with a doctor there. Although dubious, I began the treatments suggested.

What a difference a year makes! In the last twelve months I have undergone a real transformation—*without surgery*. My doctor at the Whitaker Wellness Institute changed my diet and exercise, added supplements, adjusted my prescription drugs, and most important restored my health. The EECP, chelation, hyperbaric oxygen therapy, and acupuncture have now allowed me to return to the life I had before.

By October 2000, I was well enough to enjoy a week-long bike ride with Dr. Whitaker and some *Health & Healing* subscribers. I flew, for the first time in years, to and from Virginia for the trip. This year I have returned to snow skiing and running—all without pain!

What is particularly interesting is that my cardiologist thinks

I am wasting my time and money at the Whitaker Wellness Institute.

Barney M., Missouri

My cardiologist suggested that I have a test that may have necessitated bypass surgery. Having read Dr. Whitaker's *Health & Healing* newsletter for many years, I decided to check into the Whitaker Wellness Institute before submitting to the examination. After a complete physical checkup, it was determined that I could avoid surgery by diet, exercise, and the use of supplements. I was given a regimen to follow and for two years I have followed it as closely as possible.

At the age of eighty-six I work in the garden, mow most of an area of several acres, and am otherwise quite active. I look forward to the future with a positive attitude and am certainly thankful that I did not submit to invasive procedures.

It is my hope that Dr. Whitaker can influence other members of the medical profession to follow his type of medicine. I have recently been made aware of a cardiologist who advocates a similar program, so perhaps Dr. Whitaker is no longer a voice crying out alone.

Charles White, Alabama

I believe the reason I am alive today is because I attended Dr. Whitaker's program. Most all my family deceased before age sixty-five, many in their fifties. Father, mother, brother, aunt, uncles—and most of them had heart disease. I knew I had to do something different but did not know what to do.

I first went through Dr. Whitaker's program in the mid-1980s. It changed my lifestyle, eating habits, and exercise. I have kept my weight down, and my health is good. Dr. Whitaker took me off all my medications, and to this day I take no prescription drugs. I have returned to the clinic several times over the years, and I continue to feel great.

Bob D., California

Six and a half years ago I developed rather severe chest pain and had an angiogram at a prestigious medical center. I was told I needed immediate bypass surgery, as two of my arteries were significantly blocked. I went to Dr. Whitaker who said we could try conservative therapy, including lifestyle change. It worked like a charm. I lost thirty pounds, started an exercise regimen which I have maintained and, in short, was probably the healthiest I've been in my life.

Eighteen months ago, however, the chest pain started coming back, likely due to my high-stress lifestyle. I went on virtually a worldwide search for an option to surgery and found EECP. I discussed this with Dr. Whitaker, who enthusiastically encouraged me to pursue it.

Remarkably, in only three weeks the pain went away. I'm taking less medication, and I can now do my exercise routine without any pain at all.

I'm now convinced that Dr. Whitaker's diet, nutritional supplement program, and EECP can eliminate the need for the overwhelming majority of bypass operations. It certainly did for me.

RESOURCES

Medical Clinics and Physician Referrals

Whitaker Wellness Institute
4321 Birch Street
Newport Beach, CA 92660
800-488-1500
www.whitakerwellness.com

Dr. Whitaker's institute is a full-service medical clinic that specializes in outpatient care, as well as a weeklong residence program of medical evaluation and examination, patient education, and instruction in implementing lifestyle changes. Areas of specialty include heart disease, hypertension, diabetes, arthritis, and other degenerative diseases.

American College for Advancement in Medicine
P.O. Box 3427
Laguna Hills, CA 92654
800-532-3688
www.acam.org

This is a professional organization of alternative health medical doctors and osteopathic physicians, many of whom utilize many of the therapies discussed in this book. A majority of them administer chelation therapy. To receive a list of such physicians in your area, visit the Web site or send a self-addressed, stamped envelope (two stamps).

American Association of Naturopathic Physicians
8201 Greensboro Drive, Suite 300
McLean, VA 22102
703-610-9037
www.naturopathic.org

Naturopathic physicians are licensed professionals who have attended four-year graduate level naturopathic medical school. Their education covers the same basic sciences as an M.D. but they are also schooled in nutritional and other natural approaches. This organization publishes a national referral directory.

American Association for Health Freedom
P.O. Box 458
Great Falls, VA 22066
800-230-2762

This political action group is involved in lobbying for legislation that allows medical freedom. It offers a directory of practitioners, books, and other resources on alternative medicine.

RESOURCES FOR SPECIFIC THERAPIES

Nutritional Supplements

Healthy Directions, Inc.
P.O. Box 6000
Kearneysville, WV 25430
800-722-8008
www.drwhitaker.com

Dr. Whitaker's line of high-quality nutritional supplements is distributed by Healthy Directions. It includes many of the supplements discussed in this book for reversing heart disease.

Enhanced External Counterpulsation (EECP)
Vasomedical, Inc.
180 Linden Avenue
Westbury, NY 11590
800-455-3327
www.naturalbypass.com

Vasomedical, Inc., provides information on EECP and a list of clinics offering the therapy. If you would like to consider EECP treatment at the Whitaker Wellness Institute, call 800-488-1500.

Hyperbaric Medicine Education and Research Institute
P.O. Box 9653
Newport Beach, CA 92658
909-883-0821
www.whitakerwellness.com

The Hyperbaric Medicine Education and Research Institute organization provides information on hyperbaric oxygen therapy and offers education programs for physicians. It also has a listing of chamber locations throughout the country. To contact the Whitaker Wellness Institute's hyperbaric department, call 800-488-1500.

MAIL-ORDER SOURCES OF FOOD ITEMS

Healthful Sweeteners

STEVIA

Wisdom of the Ancients
2546 West Birchwood Avenue, Suite 104
Mesa, AZ 85202
800-899-9908
www.wisdomherbs.com
www.steviaplus.com

Body Ecology
1266 West Paces Ferry Road, Suite 505
Atlanta, GA 30327
800-4-STEVIA
www.bodyecologydiet.com

XYLITOL

Advantage International
61 West 74 Street, Suite 6B
New York, NY 10023
917-441-1038
www.advantageintl.qupg.com
www.xerix.com/cavityfree

BROWN RICE SYRUP

Mother's Market
225 East 17 Street
Costa Mesa, CA 92627
800-595-MOMS or 949-631-4741

Healthy Salt Substitutes

VEGETABLE SEASONING

Bernard Jensen's Vegetable Seasoning
P.O. Box 8
Solana Beach, CA 92075
800-755-4027

CARDIA SALT

Whitaker Wellness Institute Vitamin and Book Store
4301 Birch Street
Newport Beach, CA 92660
800-810-6655

WHITAKER WELLNESS HEALTH AND NUTRITION BAR

Whitaker Wellness Institute Vitamin and Book Store
4301 Birch Street
Newport Beach, CA 92660
800-810-6655

ADDITIONAL INFORMATION AND SUGGESTED READING

Hypertension

Reversing Hypertension by Julian Whitaker (New York, N.Y.: Warner Books, 2000)

Diabetes

Reversing Diabetes by Julian Whitaker (New York, N.Y.: Warner Books, 2001)

General Health

Health & Healing, Dr. Whitaker's monthly newsletter, informs 500,000 readers every month about a variety of aspects of health and cutting-edge alternative therapies. Subscriptions are available from Phillips Publishing Company, 800-539-8219 or www.drwhitaker.com

Dr. Whitaker's Guide to Natural Healing by Julian Whitaker (Rocklin, Ca.: Prima Publishing, 1995)

Encyclopedia of Natural Medicine by Michael Murray, N.D., and Joseph Pizzorno, N.D. (Rocklin, Ca.: Prima Publishing, 1998)

Encyclopedia of Nutritional Supplements by Michael Murray, N.D. (Rocklin, Ca.: Prima Publishing, 1996)

The Healing Power of Herbs by Michael Murray, N.D. (Rocklin, Ca.: Prima Publishing, 1995)

Glycemic Index of Foods

www.mendosa.com

Medical writer Rick Mendosa's Web site contains extensive lists of the glycemic indexes of specific foods. He also has links to many excellent articles explaining the glycemic index.

NOTES

EPIGRAPHS

1. Thomas, L. *Lives of a Cell*. New York, N.Y.: Viking Press, 1974.
2. Carrel, A. London: *Man the Unknown*. 1935.
3. Thomas Edison quotes. http://www.thomasedison.com/edquote.html.
4. Works by Hippocrates. http://classics.mit.edu/Browse/browse-Hippocrates.html.

CHAPTER 1

5. American Heart Association, *2001 Heart and stroke statistical update*. http://www.americanheart.org/statistics/coronary.html.
6. Ibid.
7. Enos, W. F. et al. Coronary disease among United States soldiers killed in action in Korea. *Journal of the American Medical Association*, 1953;152: 1090–3.
8. Strong, J. P. et al. The natural history of coronary atherosclerosis. *American Journal of Pathology*, 1958;34: 209–35.
9. Rich-Edwards, J. W. et al. The primary prevention of coro-

nary heart disease in women. *New England Journal of Medicine*, June 29, 1995;332(26): 1758–66.
10. Bales, A. C. In search of lipid balance in older women. *Postgraduate Medicine*, 2000 Dec;108(7): 57–72.
11. American Heart Association, *2001 Women, heart disease and stroke statistics*. http://www.americanheart.org/statistics/.
12. Legato, M. J. and Colman, C. *The Female Heart*. New York, N.Y.: Simon & Schuster, 1991.
13. Hu, F. B. et al. Trends in the incidence of coronary artery disease and changes in diet and lifestyle in women. *New England Journal of Medicine*, August 24, 2000;343(8): 530–37.
14. Tunstall-Pedoe, H. et al. for the WHO MONICA Project. Contribution of trends in survival and coronary event rates to changes in coronary heart disease mortality: 10-year results from 37 WHO MONICA Project populations. *The Lancet*, 1999;353: 1547–57.
15. Kuulasmaa, K. et al. Estimation of contribution of changes in classic risk factors to trends in coronary-event rates across the WHO MONICA Project. *The Lancet*, Feb. 26, 2000;355: 675–87.

CHAPTER 2

1. Gibbons, G. H. Endothelial function as a determinant of vascular function and structure: a new therapeutic target. *American Journal of Cardiology*, 1997;79(5A): 3–8.
2. Luscher, T. F. The endothelium and cardiovascular disease—a complex relation. *New England Journal of Medicine*, April 14, 1994;330(15): 1081–2.
3. Imai, Hideshige. Angiotoxicity of oxygenated sterols and possible precursors. *Science*, 1980; 207: 651–653.
4. Shah, P. K. Role of inflammation and metalloproteinases in

plaque disruption and thrombosis. *Vascular Medicine*, 1998;3(3): 199–206.

5. Falk, E. et al. Coronary plaque disruption. *Circulation*, 1995;92: 657–71.
6. Canto, J. G. et al. Prevalence, clinical characteristics, and mortality among patients with myocardial infarction presenting without chest pain. *Journal of the American Medical Association*, 2000 June 28;283(24): 3223–9.
7. Luepker, R. V. et al. Effect of a community intervention on patient delay and emergency medical service use in acute coronary heart disease: the Rapid Early Action for Coronary Treatment (REACT) Trial. *Journal of the American Medical Association*, July 5, 2000;284(1): 60–7.
8. American Heart Association, *2001 Heart and stroke statistical update*. http://www.americanheart.org/statistics/coronary.html.
9. Williams, D. R. *Dead by Now*. San Diego, Ca.: ProMotion Publishing, 1995.

CHAPTER 3

1. Kannell, W. B. et al. Serum cholesterol lipoproteins and risk of coronary heart disease, The Framingham study. *Annals of Internal Medicine*, Jan. 1971;24(1): 1–12.
2. Levy, R. I. Report on the Lipid Research Clinic Trials. *European Heart Journal*, August 1987;8 Suppl E: 45–53.
3. Kwiterovich, P. O. Jr. The antiatherogenic role of high-density lipoprotein cholesterol. *American Journal of Cardiology*, 1998;82(9A): 13Q–21Q.
4. Castelli, W. P. et al. Incidence of coronary heart disease and lipoprotein cholesterol levels: the Framingham Study. *Journal of the American Medical Association*, 1986;256(20): 2835–8.
5. Executive Summary of the Third Report of the National

Cholesterol Education Program (NCEP), Expert Panel on Detection, Evaluation, and Treatment of High Blood Cholesterol in Adults (Adult Treatment Panel III). *Journal of the American Medical Association*, May 16, 2001;285(19): 2486–97.

6. Safeer, R. S. et al. The emerging role of HDL cholesterol. *Postgraduate Medicine*, 2000 Dec.;108(7): 87–98.
7. Reaven, G. M. *Syndrome X: Overcoming the Silent Killer That Can Give You a Heart Attack*. New York, N.Y.: Simon & Schuster, 2000.
8. Austin, M. A. Epidemiology of hypertriglycidemia and cardiovascular disease. *American Journal of Cardiology*, 1999 May 13;83(9B): 13F–16F.
9. Chanu, B. Hypertriglyceridemia: danger for the arteries. *Presse Med*, 1999 Nov. 20;28(36): 2011–17.
10. Danesh, J. et al. Lipoprotein(a) and coronary heart disease. Meta-analysis of prospective studies. *Circulation*, September 2000;102(10): 1082–5.
11. Rath, M. and Pauling, L. Hypothesis: lipoprotein(a) is a surrogate for ascorbate. *Proceedings of the National Academy of Science, USA*, 1990;87: 6204–6207.
12. Graham, I. M. et al. Plasma homocysteine as a risk factor for vascular disease. *Journal of the American Medical Association*, June 11, 1997;277(22): 1775–1786.
13. McCully, K. S. *The Homocysteine Revolution*, New Canaan, Conn.: Keats Publishing, 1997.
14. Marieb, E. N. *Human Anatomy & Physiology*, Menlo Park, Ca.: Benjamin/Cummings Science Publishing, 1998.
15. Robinson, K. et al. Other risk factors for coronary artery disease. *Comprehensive Cardiovascular Medicine*, Topol, E. J., ed. Philadelphia, Pa.: Lippincott-Raven Publishers, 1998.
16. Gey, K. F. et al. Inverse correlation between plasma vitamin E and mortality from ischemic heart disease in cross-cultural

epidemiology. *American Journal of Clinical Nutrition*, 1991;53: 326S–334S.

17. Ridker, P. M. et al. Inflammation, aspirin, and the risk of cardiovascular disease in apparently healthy men. *New England Journal of Medicine*, April 3, 1997; 336(14): 973–9.
18. Ridker, P. M. et al. C-reactive protein and other markers of inflammation in the prediction of cardiovascular disease in women. *New England Journal of Medicine*, 2000 Mar. 23;342: 836–43.
19. Ridker, P. M. Evaluating novel cardiovascular risk factors: Can we better predict heart attacks? *Annals of Internal Medicine*, 1999 June;130(11): 933–7.
20. Siscovick, D. S. et al. Chlamydia pneumoniae, herpes simplex virus type 1, and cytomegalovirus and incident myocardial infarction and coronary heart disease death in older adults: the Cardiovascular Health Study. *Circulation*, Nov. 7, 2000;102(19): 2335–40.
21. Zhu, J. et al. Host response to cytomegalovirus infection as a determinant of susceptibility to coronary artery disease: sex-based differences in inflammation and type of immune response. *Circulation*, 2000 Nov. 14;102(20): 2491–6.
22. Genco, R. et al. Periodontal disease and risk for myocardial infarction and cardiovascular disease. *Cardiovascular Reviews & Reports*, March 1998: 34–40.
23. Wu, T. et al. Examination of the relation between periodontal health status and cardiovascular risk factors: serum total and high density lipoprotein cholesterol, C-reactive protein, and plasma fibrinogen. *American Journal of Epidemiology*, Feb. 1, 2000;151(3): 273–82.

CHAPTER 4

1. Fifth Report of the Joint National Committee on the Prevention, Detection, Evaluation, and Treatment of High

Blood Pressure. *Archives of Internal Medicine*, 1993; 153, 154–83.

2. Kwah, K. T. et al. Glycated haemoglobin, diabetes, and mortality in men in Norfolk cohort of European prospective investigation of cancer and nutrition (EPIC-Norfolk). *British Medical Journal*, 2001 Jan. 6;322(7277): 15–8.
3. Sobal, G. et al. Why is glycated LDL more sensitive to oxidation than native LDL? A comparative study. *Prostaglandins Leukot Essent Fatty Acids*, 2000 Oct.;63(4): 177–86.
4. Vlassara, H. Intervening in atherogenesis: lessons from diabetes. *Hospital Practice*, 2000 Nov. 15: 25–39.
5. Reaven, G. M. et al. *Syndrome X, Overcoming the Silent Killer That Can Give You a Heart Attack*, New York, N.Y.: Simon & Schuster, 2000.
6. Bryant, M. Obesity eating away at American health, dollars. 2000 Oct. 17. www.reutershealth.com/2000/10/17.
7. Visser, J. et al. Elevated C-reactive protein levels in overweight and obese adults. *Journal of the American Medical Association*, 1999 Dec. 8;282(22): 2131–5.
8. Rexrode, K. M. et al. Abdominal adiposity and coronary heart disease in women. *Journal of the American Medical Association*, 1998 Dec. 2;280(21): 1843–8.
9. Baik, I. Adiposity and mortality in men. *American Journal of Epidemiology*, 2000 Aug. 1;152(3): 264–71.
10. Spake, A. How McNuggets changed the world. *U.S. News & World Report*. Jan. 2001, 22:54.

CHAPTER 5

1. Progress in the war against heart attacks. *Harvard Heart Letter*. 1994 April;4(8): 1–5.
2. Hillman, D. et al. The direct-to-consumer advertising dilemma. *Patient Care*, 2001 Mar. 30: 22–33.

3. Starfield, B. Is US health really the best in the world? *Journal of the American Medical Association*, 2000 July 26;284(4): 483–5.
4. New hope for heart patients. (from *The PDR Family Guide to Prescription Drugs*, chapter 1). http://www.healthsquare.com/fgpd/fg4ch01.htm#1.
5. Levy, R. I. Declining mortality in coronary heart disease. *Arteriosclerosis*. 1981 Sept./Oct.; 1(5): 312–325.
6. McGovern, P. G. et al. Recent trends in acute coronary heart disease. *New England Journal of Medicine*. April 4, 1996;334: 884–90.
7. Kuulasmaa, K. et al. Estimation of contribution of changes in classic risk factors to trends in coronary-event rates across the WHO MONICA Project populations. *The Lancet*, Feb. 26, 2000;355: 675–77.
8. Ibid.
9. Tunstall-Pedoe, H. et al. for the WHO MONICA Project. Contribution of trends in survival and coronary-event rates to changes in coronary heart disease mortality: 10-year results from 37 WHO MONICA Project populations. *The Lancet*, 1999;353: 1547–57.

CHAPTER 6

1. Van Vlaanderen, E. A new view on heart disease. *Cortland Forum*, 2000 Mar.;150–6.
2. Bates, B. Angiograms miss most atheromas. *Family Practice News*. July 2001; 31(19): 1–4.
3. Arnett, E. N. et al. Coronary artery narrowing in coronary heart disease: comparison of cineangiographic and necropsy findings, *Annals of Internal Medicine*, 1979;91: 350–356.
4. Optimal approaches to diagnosis and treatment of chest pain topic of core curriculum session. *Medical Meeting Highlights*,

American College of Cardiology, 45th Annual Scientific Sessions, 1996: 3–4, 8.

5. Zir, L. M. et al. Interobserver variability in coronary angiography. *Circulation*, April 1976;53(4): 627–632.
6. White, C. W. et al. Does visual interpretation of the coronary arterio-gram predict the physiologic importance of a coronary stenosis? *New England Journal of Medicine*, 1984;310: 819–824.
7. Graboys, T. B., et al. Results of a second-opinion trial among patients recommended for coronary angiography. *Journal of the American Medical Association*, 1992;268: 2537–40.
8. CASS principle investigators and their associates. Coronary Artery Surgery Study (CASS): a randomized trial of coronary artery bypass surgery. Survival data. *Circulation*, 1983; 68(5): 939–950.
9. Detrano, R. C. et al. Coronary calcium does not accurately predict near-term future coronary events in high-risk adults. *Circulation*, 1999 May 25;99: 2633–8.
10. Detrano, R. C. Pro & con: Is screening for coronary calcium by electron beam CT a valuable adjunct for risk stratification? *Family Practice News*, 2001 Jan. 1: 9.
11. Taylor, A. J. et al. Self-referral of patients for electron-beam computed tomography to screen for coronary artery disease. *New England Journal of Medicine*, 1998 Dec. 31;339(27): 2018–9.
12. Ashley, E. A. et al. Exercise testing in clinical medicine. *The Lancet*, 2000 Nov. 4;356: 1592–7.
13. Thomas, J. D. et al. Cardiac imaging techniques: which, when, and why. *Cleveland Clinic Journal of Medicine*, 1996 July/Aug.;63: 213–20.
14. Squires, S. Promising technologies augur a new era for cardiac medicine. *Los Angeles Times*, Sept. 11 2000:S5.

CHAPTER 7

1. Van Vlaanderen, E. A new view on heart disease. *Cortland Forum*, 2000 March: 150–6.
2. Hultgren, H. N. et al. Aortocoronary-artery-bypass assessment after 13 years. *Journal of the American Medical Association*, 1978 Sept. 22;240(13): 1353–4.
3. Murphy, M. L. et al. Treatment of chronic stable angina; a preliminary report of survival data of the randomized Veterans Administration Cooperative study. *New England Journal of Medicine*, 1977 Sept. 22; 297(12): 621–7.
4. Braunwald, E. Coronary-artery surgery at the crossroads (editorial). *New England Journal of Medicine*, 1977 Sept. 22;297(12): 661–3.
5. Kroncke, G. M. et al. Five-year changes in coronary arteries of medical and surgical patietns in the Veterans Administration randomized study of bypass surgery. *Circulation, Supplement I*, 1988 Sept.;78(3): I–44—I–50.
6. Sharma, G. V. et al. Identification of unstable angina patients who have favorable outcome with medical or surgical therapy. *American Journal of Cardiology*, 1994 Sept. 1;74: 454–8.
7. CASS principal investigators and their associates. Coronary artery surgery study (CASS): A randomized trial of coronary artery bypass surgery, survival data. *Circulation*, 1983 Nov.; 68(5): 939–50.
8. CASS principle investigators and their associates. Myocardial infarction and mortality in the coronary artery surgery study (CASS) randomized trial. *New England Journal of Medicine*, 1984 Mar. 22;310(12): 750–8.
9. Rogers, W. J. et al. Ten-year follow-up of quality of life in patients randomized to receive medical therapy or coronary artery bypass graft surgery. *Circulation*, 1990 Nov.;82(5): 1647–58.

10. Caracciolo, E. A. et al. Comparison of surgical and medical group survival in patients with left main equivalent coronary artery disease. *Circulation*, 1995 May 1;91(9): 2335–44.
11. Yusuf, S. et al. Effect of coronary artery bypass graft surgery on survival: overview of 10-year results from randomized trials by the Coronary Artery Bypass Graft Trialists Collaboration. *The Lancet*, 1994 Aug. 27;344: 563–70.
12. Boden, W. E. et al. Outcomes in patients with acute non-Q-wave myocardial infarction randomly assigned to an invasive as compared with a conservative management strategy. *New England Journal of Medicine*, June 18, 1998;338(25): 1785–1792.
13. Wexler, L. F. et al. Non-Q-wave myocardial infarction following thrombolytic therapy: a comparison of outcomes in patients randomized to invasive or conservative post-infarct assessment strategies in the Veterans Affairs non-Q-wave Infarction Strategies In-Hospital (VANQWISH) Trial. *Journal of the American College of Cardiology*, 2001 Jan.;37(1): 19–25.
14. Mundth, E. D. Surgical measures for coronary heart disease. *New England Journal of Medicine*, July 17, 1975;293(3): 124–130.
15. Preston, T. *The Clay Pedestal*. Madrona Publishers, Seattle, WA, 1981.
16. Coronary artery surgery study (CASS). A randomized trial of coronary artery bypass surgery, quality of life in patients randomly assigned to treatment groups. *Circulation*, 1983;68: 951–960.
17. Rogers, W. J. et al. Ten-year follow-up of quality of life in patients randomized to receive medical therapy or coronary artery bypass graft surgery. *Circulation*, 1990 Nov.;82(5): 1647–58.
18. Seides, S. F. Coronary problems after bypass surgery. *New England Journal of Medicine*, 1978;298: 1213–17.

19. Maurer, B. J. Changes in grafted and non-grafted coronary arteries following saphenous vein bypass grafting. *Circulation*, 1974;50: 293.
20. Griffith, L. S., Changes in intrinsic coronary circulation and segmental ventricular motion after saphenous vein coronary bypass graft surgery. *New England Journal of Medicine*, 1973;288: 589.
21. Cashin, L. W. et al. Accelerated progression of atherosclerosis in coronary vessels with minimal lesions that are bypassed. *New England Journal of Medicine*, 311: 824428, 1984.
22. Chenoweth, D. E. Complement activation during cardiopulmonary bypass. *New England Journal of Medicine*, 1981;304: 497–503.
23. Top 100 in cardiac care perform 4.7% to 31% better than others. *Clinical Resource Management*, 2000 June;1(6): 92–4, 81.
24. Selnes, O. A. et al. Coronary artery bypass surgery and the brain. *New England Journal of Medicine*, 2001 Feb. 8;44(6): 451–2.
25. Newman, M. F. et al. Longitudinal assessment of neurocognitive function after coronary-artery bypass surgery. *New England Journal of Medicine*, 2001 Feb. 8;344(6): 395–402.
26. Henriksen, L., Evidence suggestive of diffuse brain damage following cardiac operations. *The Lancet*, 1984 April 14; 816–820.
27. Price, D. L. Cholesterol emboli and cerebral arteries as a complication of retrograde aortic profusion during cardiac surgery. *Neurology*, 1970;20: 1209–1214.
28. Buccino, R. A. Aorto-coronary bypass grafting in patients with coronary artery disease. *Primary Cardiologym*, 1981 Jan.; 91–95.
29. Lown, B. *The Lost Art of Healing*. New York, N.Y.: Houghton Mifflin, 1996.

30. Bates, M. S. A critical perspective on coronary artery disease and coronary bypass surgery. *Social Science & Medicine*, 1990;30: 249–60.
31. Podrid, P. J. et al. Prognosis of medically treated patients with coronary artery disease with profound ST segment depression during exercise testing. *New England Journal of Medicine*, 1981;305: 1111–1116.
32. Graboys, T. B. et al. Results of a Second-Opinion Program for Coronary Artery Bypass Graft Surgery, *Journal of the American Medical Association*, 1987; 258: 1611–1616.

CHAPTER 8

1. Greuntzig, A. Transluminal dilatation of coronary-artery stenosis. *The Lancet*, 1978;1: 263.
2. Greuntzig, A. R. et al. Non-operative dilation of coronary artery stenosis: percutaneous transluminal coronary angioplasty. *New England Journal of Medicine*, 1979 July 12;301(2): 61–8.
3. Sapirstein, W. et al. FDA approval of coronary-artery brachytherapy. *New England Journal of Medicine*, 2001 Jan. 25;344(4): 297–8.
4. Topol, E. J. Coronary-artery stents—gauging, gorging, and gouging, *New England Journal of Medicine*, 1998 Dec. 3;339(23): 1702–4.
5. Sheppard, R. et al. Intracoronary radiotherapy for restenosis. *New England Journal of Medicine*, 2001 Jan. 25;344(4): 295–6.
6. Versaci, F. et al. A comparison of coronary-artery stenting with angioplasty for isolated stenosis of the proximal left anterior descending coronary artery. *New England Journal of Medicine*, 1997 Mar. 20;336(12): 817–22.
7. Jacobs, A. K. Coronary stents—have they fulfilled their

promise? *New England Journal of Medicine*, 1999 Dec. 23;341(26): 2005–6.

8. Pocock, S. J. et al. Quality of life after coronary angioplasty or continued medical treatment for angina: three-year follow-up in the RITA-2 trial. Randomized Intervention Treatment of Angina. *Journal of the American College of Cardiology*, 2000 Mar. 15;35(4): 907–14.
9. RITA-2 trial participants. Coronary angioplasty versus medical therapy for angina: the second Randomized Intervention Treatment of Angina (RITA-2) trial. *The Lancet*, 1997;350: 461–8.
10. Pitt, B. et al. Aggressive lipid-lowering therapy compared with angioplasty in stable coronary artery disease. *New England Journal of Medicine*, 1999 June 8;341(2): 70–6.
11. Holmboe, E. S. Perceptions of benefit and risk of patients undergoing first-time elective percutaneous coronary revascularization. *Journal of General Internal Medicine*, 2000;15(9): 632–7.
12. Hannan, E. L. et al. Coronary angioplasty volume-outcome relationships for hospitals and cardiologists. *Journal of the American Medical Association*, 1997 Mar. 19;277(11): 892–8.
13. Verin, V. et al. Endoluminal beta-radiation therapy for the prevention of coronary restenosis after balloon angioplasty. *New England Journal of Medicine*, 2001 Jan. 25;344(4): 243–9.
14. Leon, M. B. et al. Localized intracoronary gamma-radiation therapy to inhibit the recurrence of restenosis after stenting. *New England Journal of Medicine*, 2001 Jan. 25;344(4): 250–6.
15. Moscucci, M. et al. Today's approach to PTCA: how it is performed, who might benefit. *Journal of Critical Illness*, 1993 Feb.;8(2): 185–208.
16. Koster, R. et al. Nickel and molybdenum contact allergies in

patients with coronary in-stent restenosis. *The Lancet*, Dec. 2000;356(2945): 1895–7.

17. Barton, S., ed. *Clinical Evidence*. London: BMJ Publishing Group, 2000.
18. CASS principle investigators and their associates. Myocardial infarction and mortality in the coronary artery surgery study (CASS) randomized trial. *New England Journal of Medicine*, 1984 Mar. 22;310(12): 750–8.

CHAPTER 9

1. Pinkowish, M. D. Prescribing for older patients: 5 points to remember. *Patient Care*, August 2000;15: 45–52.
2. Kohn L., ed., et al. *To Err Is Human: Building a Safer Health System*. Washington, D.C.: National Academy Press, 1999.
3. The Lipid Research Clinics Coronary Primary Prevention Trial results. I. Reduction in incidence of coronary heart disease. *Journal of the American Medical Association*, Jan. 20, 1984;251(3): 351–64.
4. Committee of Principal Investigators. World Health Organization Clofibrate Trial: A co-operative trial in the primary prevention of ischemic heart disease using clofibrate. *British Heart Journal*, 1978; 40: 1069–1118.
5. *Physicians' Desk Reference, 54th Edition*, Montvale, N.J.: Medical Economics, 2001.
6. Zoler, M. Statins may help a wider range of coronary risks. *Family Practice News*, 2000 Sept. 1: 5.
7. Streja, D. If LDL lowering is the answer, why conduct more trials? *Cardiology Review*, 2000 June: 1056.
8. LaRosa, J. C. et al. Effect of statins on risk of coronary disease, a meta-analysis of randomized controlled trials. *Journal of the American Medical Association*, 1999 Dec. 22/29;282(24): 2340–6.

9. FDA approves Mevacor in people with average cholesterol levels. *Doctor's Guide*, Mar 16; http://www.palgroup.com
10. Goldstein, S. Over-the-counter statins? *Family Practice News*, 2000 Sept. 1: 9.
11. Brown, D. Cholesterol drug taken off market. *Washington Post*, Aug. 9, 2001; www.washingtonpost.com.
12. Associated Press. Anti-cholesterol drugs taken by millions are said to kill 81. *Baltimore Sun*, Aug. 21, 2001. www.baltimoresun.com.
13. Ghirlanda, G. et al. Evidence of plasma CoQ10-lowering effect by HMG-CoA reductase inhibitors: a double-blind, placebo-controlled study. *Journal of Clinical Pharmacology*, 1993;33: 226–229.
14. Langsjoen, P. H. et al. Coenzyme Q10 in cardiovascular disease with emphasis on heart failure and myocardial ischaemia. *Asia Pacific Heart Journal*, 1998;7(3): 160–168.
15. Turpeinen, O. Dietary prevention of coronary heart disease: the Finnish Mental Hospital Study. *International Journal of Epidemiology*, June 1979;8(2): 99–118.
16. Saunders, C. S. Navigating the nitrate maze. *Patient Care*, 1998 Oct. 30: 23–51.
17. Krasuski, R. A. et al. Nitrates: still an essential weapon against heart disease. *Emergency Medicine*, 2000 Nov.: 56–65.
18. *Physicians' Desk Reference*, 54th Edition, Montvale, N.J.: Medical Economics Data, 2001.
19. Psaty, B. M. et al. The risk of myocardial infarction associated with antihypertensive drug therapies. *Journal of the American Medical Association*, 1995;274, 620–625.
20. Stelfox, H. T. et al. Conflict of interest in the debate over calcium-channel antagonists. *New England Journal of Medicine*, 1998 Jan. 8;338(2): 101–6.
21. Pahor, M. et al. Health outcomes associated with calcium antagonists compared with other first-line antihhyperten-

sive therapies: a meta-analysis of randomized controlled trials. *The Lancet*, 2000 Dec. 9;356: 1949–54.

22. Pahor, M., et al., Calcium-channel blockade and incidence of cancer in aged populations. *The Lancet*, 1996;348 (9026): 493–7.
23. Fitzpatrick, A. L. et al. Use of calcium channel blockers and breast carcinoma risk in postmenopausal women. *Cancer*, 1997;80: 1438–47.
24. Heart Outcomes Prevention Evaluation Study Investigators, Effects of an angiotensin-converting-enzyme inhibitor, ramipril, on death from cardiovascular causes, myocardial infarction, and stroke in high-risk patients. *New England Journal of Medicine*, 2000 Jan. 20;342(3): 145–53.
25. Ridker, P. M. et al. Inflammation, aspirin, and the risk of cardiovascular disease in apparently healthy men. *New England Journal of Medicine*, 1997;336: 973–9.
26. Steering Committee of the Physicians' Health Study Research Group: Final report on the aspirin component of the ongoing Physicians' Health Study. *New England Journal of Medicine*, 1989; 321: 129–135.
27. ISIS-2 Collaborative Group: Randomized trial of intravenous streptokinase, oral aspirin, or both, or neither among 17,187 cases of suspected acute myocardial infarction: ISIS-2. *The Lancet*, 1988;318: 349–360.
28. Prescott, L. Aspirin recommended for primary and secondary prevention of cardiovascular disease. *Internal Medicine World Report*, 1995 Jan. 1–14;36.
29. Stafford, R. S. Aspirin use is low among United States outpatients with coronary artery disease. *Circulation*, March 14, 2000;101(10): 1097–101.
30. Multiple Risk Factor Intervention Trial Research Group. Multiple risk factor intervention trial. Risk factor changes and mortality results. *Journal of the American Medical Association*, 1982;248(12): 1465–77.

31. Grimm, R. H. Effects of thiazide diuretics on plasma lipids and lipoproteins in mildly hypertensive patients. *Annals of Internal Medicine*, 1981;94: 7–11.

CHAPTER 10

1. Ignatowski, A. Ober die Wirkung des tierischen Eiweisses auf die Aorta und die parkenchromatsen Organe der Kaninchen. *Virchos Arch*, 1909;198: 248.
2. Anitschkow, N. Ober experimentelle Cholesterin Steatose und ihre Bedeutung fur die Entstehung einiger pathologischer. *Prozesse: Zbl. Path*, 1913;26: 1.
3. Vesselinovitch, D. Regression of atherosclerosis in rabbits, treatment with low fat diet, hyperoxia, and hypolipidemic agents. *Atherosclerosis*, 1974, 19: 259–275.
4. Vesselinovitch, D., Studies of reversal of advanced atherosclerosis in rhesus monkeys. *American Joumal of Pathology*, 1973;70: 41A.
5. *Taber's Cyclopedic Medical Dictionary*, Philadelphia, Pa.: F. A. Davis Company, 1977.
6. Ashoff, T. *Lectures in Pathology*. New York: Hoeber, 1924.
7. Vartiainen, I. Wartime immortality of certain diseases in Finland. *Annals of Internal Medicine, Finland*, 1946;535: 234–240.
8. Strom, A. Examination of the diet of Norwegian families during the war years, 1942–1944. *Active Medicus Scandinavia*, 1948;Sup. 214: 47.
9. Vartiainen, I. et al. Arteriosclerosis in wartime. *Annals of Internal Medicine*, 1947;536: 748–758.
10. Strom, A. Mortality from circulatory diseases in Norway, 1940–1945. *The Lancet*, 1951;126–129.
11. Ibid.
12. Ibid.

13. Bassler, T. Regression of athroma. *Western Journal of Medicine*, 1980;132: 474–75.
14. Roth, D. Non-invasive and invasive demonstration of spontaneous regression of coronary artery disease. *Circulation*, 1980; 62, 888–896.
15. Ornish, D. et al. Effects of stress management training and dietary changes in treating ischemic heart disease. *Journal of the American Medical Association*, 1983;249: 54–59.
16. Ornish, D. et al. Can lifestyle changes reverse coronary heart disease? *The Lancet*, 1990 July 21;336: 129–133.
17. Ornish, D. et al. Intensive lifestyle changes for reversal of coronary heart disease. *Journal of the American Medical Association*, 1998 Dec. 16;280(23): 2001–7.
18. Khaw, K. T. et al. Relation between plasma ascorbic acid and mortality in men and women in EPIC-Norfolk prospective study: a prospective population study. Euroean Prospective Investigation into Cancer and Nutrition. *The Lancet*, 2001 March 3; 357 (9257): 657–63.
19. Stampfer, M. H. et al. Vitamin E consumption and the risk of coronary disease in women. *New England Journal of Medicine*, 1993 May 20;328(20): 1444–9.
20. Steffen-Batey, L. Change in level of physical activity and risk of all-cause mortality or reinfarction: The Corpus Christi Heart Project. *Circulation*, 2000 Oct. 31;102(18): 2204–9.
21. Smith, S. S. et al. The epidemiology of tobacco use, dependence, and cessation in the United States. *Primary Care*, Sept. 1999;26(3): 433–61.
22. The dangers of smoking. http://www.redcross.org/services/hss/tips/healthtips/smoking.html.

CHAPTER 12

1. Regan, T. Myocardial blood flow and oxygen consumption during postprandial lipernia and heparin-induced lipolyse. *Circulation*, 1961;23: 55–63.

2. Kuo, P. T. Angina pectoris induced by fat ingestion in patients with coronary artery disease. *Journal of the American Medical Association*, 1955 July 23;1008–1013.
3. Plotnick, D. G. et al. Effect of antioxidant vitamins on the transient impairment of endothelium-dependent brachial artery vasoactivity following a single high-fat meal. *Journal of the American Medical Association*, November 26, 1997;278: 1682–1686.
4. Jee, S. H. et al. The effect of chronic coffee drinking on blood pressure; a meta-analysis of controlled clinical trials. *Hypertension*, 1999 Feb.;33(2): 647–52.
5. Mercola, J. Coffee may damage blood vessels. 2000 Sept. 17; www.mercola.com.
6. Sesso, H. D. et al. Coffee and tea intake and the risk of myocardial infarction. *American Journal of Epidemiology*, 1999;149: 162–7.
7. Ishikawa, T. et al. Effect of tea flavonoid supplementation on the susceptibility of low-density lipoprotein to oxidative modification. *American Journal of Clinical Nutrition*, 1997;66: 261–6.
8. Vogel, R. A. et al. Effect of a single high-fat meal on endothelial function in healthy subjects. *American Journal of Cardiology*, 1997 Feb. 1;79(3): 350–4.
9. Howell, W. H. et al. Plasma lipid and lipoprotein responses to dietary fat and cholesterol: a meta-analysis. *American Journal of Clinical Nutrition*, 1997;65(5): 1747–64.
10. Beveridge, J. M. R. The response of man to dietary cholesterol. *Journal of Nutrition*, 1960;71: 61.
11. Hu, F. B. et al. A prospective study of egg consumption and risk of cardiovascular disease in men and women. *Journal of the American Medical Association*, 1999 Apr. 21;281(15): 1387–94.
12. Ascherio, A. and W. C. Willett. Health effects of trans fatty acids. *American Journal of Clinical Nutrition*, 1997 Oct.;66(4 Suppl): 1006S–1010S.

13. Vigilante, K. et al. *Low-Fat Lies*. Washington, D.C.: Lifeline Press, 1999.
14. Ferrara, L. A. et al. Olive oil and reduced need for antihypertensive medications. *Archives of Internal Medicine*, 2000 Mar. 27;160(6): 837–42.
15. De Lorgeril, M. et al. Mediterranean diet, traditional risk factors, and the rate of cardiovascular complications after myocardial infarction. Final report of the Lyon Diet Heart Study. *Circulation*, 1999 Feb. 16; 99(6): 779–785.
16. Highlights of the International Workshop on omega-3 fatty acids, diabetes and cardiovascular risk. *Holistic Primary Care*, 2001 Feb. 14: 13.
17. How much protein is enough? *Consumer Reports on Health*, 2001 Feb.; 13(2): 8–10.
18. Ibid.
19. World Health Organization Technical Report. Series No. 522. Energy and protein requirements. Geneva, 1973.
20. Mazess, R. B. Bone mineral content of North Alaskan Eskimos. *American Journal of Clinical Nutrition*, 1974;27: 916–925.
21. How much protein is enough? *Consumer Reports on Health*, 2001 Feb.;13(2): 8–10.
22. Walker, R. M. Calcium retention in the adult human male, as effective by protein intake. *Journal of Nutrition*, 1972;102: 1297–1302.
23. Grant, W. B. Milk and other dietary influences on coronary heart disease. *Alternative Medicine Review*, 1998;3(4): 281–294.
24. Cohen, R. *Milk, the Deadly Poison*, Englewood Cliffs, N.J.: Argus Publishing, Inc., 1997.
25. Brody, J. Eat your fruits, veggies, but choose wisely. *Orange County Register*, December 31, 2000.
26. Chandalia, M. et al. Beneficial effects of high dietary fiber intake in patients with type 2 diabetes mellitus. *New England Journal of Medicine*, 2000;342 (19): 1392–1398.

27. Meyer, K. A. et al. Carbohydrates, dietary fiber, and incident type 2 diabetes in older women. *American Journal of Clinical Nutrition*, 2000 Apr.;71(4): 921–30.
28. Rimm, E. B. et al. Vegetable, fruit, and cereal fiber intake and risk of coronary heart disease among men. *Journal of the American Medical Association*, February 14, 1996;275(6): 447–451.
29. Wolk, A. et al. Long-term intake of dietary fiber and decreased risk of coronary heart disease among women. *Journal of the American Medical Association*, 1999 June 2;281(21): 1998–2004.
30. He, J. et al. Dietary sodium intake and subsequent risk of cardiovascular disease in overweight adults. *Journal of the American Medical Association*, 1999 Dec. 1;282(21): 2027–35.
31. Kaplan, N. Current controversy: salt in hypertension. *Dateline Hypertension*, Jan. 1984, 2: 1.
32. MacGregor, Graham A. Moderate potassium supplementation in essential hypertension. *The Lancet*, Sept. 11, 1982; 567–570.
33. Mozes, A. FDA allows foods to claim heart benefits of potassium. *Reuters Health Information*, 2000 Oct. 30; www.reuthershealth.com/archi...0.
34. Grant, W. B. Milk and other dietary influences on coronary heart disease. *Alternative Medicine Review*, 1998 Aug.;3(4): 281–94.
35. Jarvi, A. E. et al. Improved glycemic control and lipid profile and normalized fibrinolytic activity on a low-glycemic index diet in type 2 diabetic patients. *Diabetes Care*, 1999; 22(1): 10–18.
36. Bierenbaum, M. L. Reducing atherogenic risk in hyperlipidemic humans with flaxseed supplementation: a preliminary report. *Journal of the American College of Nutrition*, Oct. 1993;12(5): 501–504.
37. Anderson, J. W. et al. Meta-analysis of the effects of soy pro-

tein intake on serum lipids. *New England Journal of Medicine*, Aug. 3, 1995; 333(5): 276–282.

38. Upritchard, J. E. et al. Effect of supplementation with tomato juice, vitamin E, and vitamin C on LDL oxidation and products of inflammatory activity in type 2 diabetes. *Diabetes Care*, 2000 June;23(6): 733–8.
39. Arab, L. et al. Lycopene and cardiovascular disease. *American Journal of Clinical Nutrition*, 2000 June;71(6 Suppl): 1691S–7S.
40. Goodnight, Scott, H., M.D. and Dr. W. E. Connor, M.D. The effects of dietary omega-3 fatty acids on platelet composition and function in man: A perspective control study. *Blood*, 1981 Nov.; 58(5): 880–885.
41. Ibid.
42. Hu, F. B. et al. Frequent nut consumption and risk of coronary heart disease in women. *British Medical Journal*, 1998 Nov. 14;317: 1341–5.
43. Warshafsky, S. et al. Effect of garlic on total serum cholesterol. *Annals of Internal Medicine*, 1993;119: 599–605.
44. DeMott, K. Oatmeal, vitamin E ease endothelial dysfunction. *Family Practice News*, 1999 Nov. 15: 26.

CHAPTER 13

1. Herbert, V. The vitamin craze. *Archives of Internal Medicine*, 1980;148: 173.
2. National Institutes of Health, Office of Dietary Supplements, IBIDS Database, http://odp.od.nih.gov/ods/databases/ibids. html.
3. Murray, M. T. *Encyclopedia of Nutritional Supplements*, Rocklin, Ca.: Prima Publishing, 1996.
4. Bayourni, R. A. et al. Evaluation of methods of coenzyme activation of erythrocyten enzymes of detection of defi-

ciency of Vitamins B1, B2, B6. *Clinical Chemistry*, 1976;22: 327.

5. Enstrom, J. E. et al. Vitamin C intake and mortality among a sample of the United States population. *Epidemiology*, 1992 May; 3(3): 194–202.
6. Williams, Roger J., Concept of genetotrophic disease. *Nutrition Review*, 1950;8: 257–260, 1950.
7. Lonsdale, D. and R. J. Shamberger. Red cell transketolase as an indicator of nutritional deficiency. *American Journal of Clinical Nutrition*, 1980 33(2): 205–211.
8. Graci, S. *The Power of Superfoods*, Scarborough, Ontario: Prentice Hall Canada, Inc., 1997.
9. Lazarou, J. et al. Incidence of adverse drug reactions in hospitalized patients. *Journal of the American Medical Association*, 1998;279(15): 1200–1205.

CHAPTER 14

1. Khaw, K. T. et al. Relation between plasma ascorbic acid and mortality in men and women in EPIC-Norfolk prospective study: a prospective population study. European Prospective Investigation into Cancer and Nutrition. *The Lancet*, 2001 Mar. 3;357(9257): 657–63.
2. Kontush, A. et al. Lipophilic antioxidants in blood plasma as markers of atherosclerosis: the role of beta-carotene and gamma tocopherol. *Atherosclerosis*, 1999;144: 117–22.
3. Watkins, M. L. et al. Multivitamin use and mortality in a large prospective study. *American Journal of Epidemiology*, 2000 July 15;152(2): 149–62.
4. Vitamins reduce risk of death from heart disease, stroke. *Reuters Health Information*, 2000 July 21; www.reuters-health.com.
5. Plotnick, D. G. et al. Effect of antioxidant vitamins on the

transient impairment of endothelium-dependent brachial artery vasoactivity following a single high-fat meal. *Journal of the American Medical Association*, Nov. 26, 1997;278: 1682–1686.

6. Stampfer, M. J. et al. Vitamin E consumption and the risk of coronary disease in women. *New England Journal of Medicine*, May 20, 1993;328: 1444–1449.
7. Rimm, E. B. et al. Vitamin E consumption and the risk of coronary disease in men. *New England Journal of Medicine*, May 20, 1993;328: 1450–1456.
8. Stephens, N. G. et al. Randomized controlled trial of vitamin E in patients with coronary disease: Cambridge Heart Antioxidant Study (CHAOS). *The Lancet*, Mar. 23, 1996;347: 781–786.
9. Motoyama, T. Vitamin E administration improves impairment of endothelium-dependent vasodilation in patients with coronary spastic angina. *Journal of the American College of Cardiology*, 1998 Nov. 15;32(6): 1672–9.
10. Haeger, K. Long-term treatment of intermittent claudication with vitamin E. *The American Journal of Clinical Nutrition*, 1974;27: 1179–1181.
11. Willis, G. C. The reversibility of atherosclerosis. *Canadian Medical Association Journal*, 1957, 77: 106.
12. Enstrom, J. E. et al. Vitamin C intake and mortality among a sample of the United States population. *Epidemiology*, 1992;3: 194–202.
13. Beaglehold, R. et al. Decreased blood selenium and risk of myocardial infarction. *International Journal of Epidemiology*, 1990;19: 918–22.
14. Nester, P. J. Fish oil and cardiovascular disease: lipids and arterial function. *American Journal of Clinical Nutrition*, 2000;71(suppl): 228S–31S.
15. Murray, M. T. *Encyclopedia of Nutritional Supplements*. Rocklin, Ca.: Prima Publishing, 1996.

16. Montori, V. et al. Fish oil supplements in type 2 diabetes. *Diabetes Care*, 2000 Sept.;23(9): 1407–15.
17. Illingworth, D. R. et al. Comparative effects of lovastatin and niacin in primary hypercholesterolemia. *Annals of Internal Medicine*, 1994;154: 1586–95.
18. Dorner, V. G. et al. The influence of m-inositol hexanicotinate ester on the serum lipids and lipoproteins. *Arzneim Forsch*, 1961;11: 110–113.
19. Kiff, R. S. et al. Does inositol nicotinate (Hexopal) influence intermittent claudication? A controlled trial. *British Journal of Clinical Practice*, 1988;42: 141–145.
20. Patrick, L. et al. Cardiovascular disease: C-reactive protein and the inflammatory disease paradigm: HMG-CoA reductase inhibitors, alpha-tocopherol, red yeast rice, and olive oil polyphenols. A review of the literature. *Alternative Medicine Review*. 2001 June;6(3): 248–71.
21. Mas, R. et al. Effects of policosanol in patients with type II hypercholesterolemia and additional coronary risk factors. *Clinical Pharmacology and Therapeutics*. 1999 Apr.; 65(4): 439–47.
22. Stampfer, M. J. et al. A prospective study of plasma homocysteine and risk of myocardial infarction in US physicians. *Journal of the American Medical Association*, August 19, 1992;268(7): 877–881.
23. McCully, K. *The Homocysteine Revolution*, New Canaan, Conn.: Keats Publishing, Inc., 1997.
24. Ridker, P. M. Evaluating novel cardiovascular risk factors: Can we better predict heart attacks? *Annals of Internal Medicine*, 1999 June;130(11): 933–7.
25. Simopoulos, A. P. Essential fatty acids in health and chronic disease. *American Journal of Clinical Nutrition*, 1999;700(suppl): 560–9S.
26. Devaraj, S. et al. Alpha tocopherol supplementation decreases serum C-reactive protein and monocyte interleukin-

6 levels in normal volunteers and type 2 diabetic patients. *Free Radical Biology & Medicine*, 2000 October 15;29(8): 790–2.

27. Mabile, L. et al. Moderate supplementation with natural alpha-tocopherol decreases platelet aggregation and low-density lipoprotein oxidation. *Atherosclerosis*, 1999 November 1;147(1): 177–85.
28. Pryor, W. A. Vitamin E and heart disease: basic science to clinical intervention trials. *Free Radical Biology Medicine*, 2000 January 1;28(1): 141–64
29. Kim, J. M. et al. Effect of vitamin E on the anticoagulant response to warfarin. *American Journal of Cardiology*, 1996 March 1;77(7): 545–6
30. Folkers, K. et al. Biochemical rationale and myocardioal tissue data on the effective therapy of cardiomyopathy with coenzyme Q10. *Proceedings of the National Academy of Science*, 1985 February;62: 901–4.
31. Langsjoen, P. H. et al. Long-term efficacy and safety of coenzyme Q10 therapy for idiopathic dilated cardiomyopathy. *American Journal of Cardiology*, 1990;65: 521–523.
32. Ghirlanda, G. et al. Evidence of plasma CoQ10-lowering effect by HMG-CoA reductase inhibitors: a double-blind, placebo-controlled study. *Journal of Clinical Pharmacology*, 1993;33: 226–229.
33. Cacciatore, L. et al. The therapeutic effect of l-carnitine in patients with exercise-induced stable angina: a controlled study. *Drugs Under Experimental and Clinical Research*, 1991;17: 225–35.
34. Kawano, Y. et al. Effects of magnesium supplementation in hypertensive patients: assessment by office, home, and ambulatory blood pressures. *Hypertension*, August 1998;32(2): 260–265.
35. Shechter, M. et al. Magnesium therapy in acute myocardial infarction when patients are not candidates for thrombolytic

therapy. *American Journal of Cardiology*, February 15, 1995;75(5): 321–323.

36. Fried, R. and Merrell, W. C. *The Arginine Solution*. New York: Warner Books, 1999.
37. Cooke, J. P. Is atherosclerosis an arginine deficiency disease? *Journal of Investigative Medicine*, October 1998;46(8): 377–80.
38. Casino, P. R. The role of nitric oxide in endothelium-dependent vasodilation of hypercholesterolemic patients. *Circulation*, December 1993; 88(6): 2541–47.
39. Salonen, Jukka T. et al. High stored iron levels are associated with excess risk of myocardial infarction in Eastern Finnish men. *Circulation*, 1992; 86(3): 803–11.
40. Elwood, J. C., Effect of high chromium brewers yeast on human serum lipids. *Journal of American College of Nutrition*, 1982;1: 263–274.
41. Newman, H. A. Serum chromium and angiographically determined coronary artery disease. 1978; *Clinical Chemistries*, 24: 541.
42. Borden, G. et al. Effects of vanadyl sulfate on carbohydrate and lipid metabolism in patients with non-insulin-dependent diabetes mellitus. *Metabolism*, September 1996;45(9): 1130–1135.
43. Jacob, S. et al. Oral adminisration of RAC-a-lipoic acid modulates insulin sensitivity in patients with type-2 diabetes mellitus: a placebo-controlled pilot trial. *Free Radical Biology Medicine*, 1999, 27(3/4): 309–314.

CHAPTER 15

1. Speed, C. A. et al. Exercise prescription in cardiac disease. *The Lancet*, 2000 October 7;356: 1208–9.

2. Morris, J. N. Coronary heart disease and physical activity of work. November 21 and 28, 1953; *The Lancet*. 2: 1053, 111.
3. Morris, J. N. Vigorous exercise in leisure time in the incidence of coronary heart-disease. *The Lancet*, 1973;1: 333–339.
4. Paffenbarger, R. S. Work energy level: Personal characteristics and fatal heart attack, a birth cohort effect. *American Journal of Epidemiology*, 1977;105: 200–213.
5. Steffen-Batey, L. et al. Change in level of physical activity and risk of all-cause mortality or reinfarction: The Corpus Christi Heart Project. *Circulation*, 2000 October 31;102(18): 2204–9.
6. Lee, I. M. et al. Exercise intensity and longevity in men. The Harvard Alumni Health Study. *Journal of the American Medical Association*, 1995 April 19;273(15): 1179–84.
7. Mann, G. G. Cardiovascular disease in the Masai. *Journal of Atherosclerosis Research*, 1964;4: 239.
8. Mann, G. G. Atherosclerosis in the Masai. 1972; *American Journal of Epidemiology*, 95: 26–37.
9. Halbert, J. A. et al. The effectiveness of exercise training in lowering blood pressure: a meta-analysis of randomized controlled trials of 4 weeks or longer. *Journal of Hypertension*, 1997;11(10): 641–9.
10. Wolfe, M. M. et al. Gastrointestinal toxicity of nonsteroidal anti-inflammatory drugs. Glucose transporters and insulin activity. *New England Journal of Medicine*, 1999;340(24); 342(4).
11. Pratley, R. E. et al. Aerobic exercise training-induced reductions in abdominal fat and glucose-stimulated insulin responses in middle-aged and older men. *Journal of the American Geriatrics Society*, 2000 September;48(9): 1055–61.

12. Greist, J. H. Antidepressant running, running as a treatment for non-psychotic depression. *Behavioral Medicine*, July 19,1979.
13. Bortz, W. M. II et al. Catecholamines, dopamine, and endorphin levels during extreme exercise. *New England Journal of Medicine*, 1981 August 20;305(8): 466–7.
14. Exercise could help beat depression. *Reuters Health Information*, 2000 September 25, http://www.reutershealth.com.
15. Dustman, R. E. et al. Aerobic exercise training and improved neuropsychological function of older individuals. *Neurobiological Aging*, spring 1984;5(1): 35–42.
16. Caspersen, C. J. et al. Changes in physical activity patterns in the United States, by sex and cross-sectional age. *Medicine and Science in Sports and Exercise*, 2000 September;32(9): 1601–9.
17. Lee, I. M. et al. Physical activity and coronary heart disease risk in men: does the duration of exercise episodes predict risk? *Circulation*, 2000 August 29;102(9): 981–6.
18. Gibbons, L. W. et al. The acute cardiac risk of strenuous exercise. *Journal of the American Medical Association*, 1980 October 17;244(16): 1799–801.
19. Albert, C. M. et al. Triggering of sudden death from cardiac causes by vigorous exercise. *New England Journal of Medicine*, 2000 November 9;343(19): 1355–61.

CHAPTER 16

1. Meisel, S. et al. Effect of Iraqi missile war on incidence of acute myocardial infarction and sudden death in Israeli civilians. *The Lancet*, 1991;338: 660.
2. Tofler, G. H. Analysis of possible triggers of acute myocardial infarction (the MILIS study). *American Journal of Cardiology*, 1990 July 1;66(1): 22–7.

3. Bosma, H. et al. Low job control and risk of coronary heart disease in Whitehall II (prospective cohort) study. *British Medical Journal*, 1997 February 22;314(7080): 558–65.
4. Orth-Gomer, K. et al. Marital stress worsens prognosis in women with coronary heart disease: The Stockholm Female Coronary Risk Study. *Journal of the American Medical Association*, 2000 December 20;284(23): 3008–14.
5. Rosenman, R. et al. Coronary heart disease in the Western Collaborative Group Study: final follow-up experience of 812 years. *Journal of the American Medical Association*, 1975;233: 872.
6. Mittleman, M. A. et al. Triggering of acute myocardial infarction onset by episodes of anger. Determinants of Myocardial Infarction Onset Study Investigators. *Circulation*, 1995 October 1;92(7): 1720–5.
7. Leor, J. et al. Sudden cardiac death triggered by an earthquake. *New England Journal of Medicine*, 1996;334: 413.
8. Haines, A. et al. Psychological characteristics and fatal ischaemic heart disease. *Heart*, 2001 April;85(4): 385–9.
9. Anda, R. et al. Depressed affect, hopelessness, and the risk of ischemic heart disease in a cohort of U.S. adults. *Epidemiology*, 1993 July;4(4): 285–94.
10. Penninx, B. W. et al. Depression and cardiac mortality: results from a community-based longitudinal study. *Archives of General Psychiatry*, 2001 March;58(3): 221–7.
11. Frasure-Smith, N. et al. Depression following myocardial infarction. Impact on 6-month survival. *Journal of the American Medical Association*, 1993 October 20;270(15): 1819–25.
12. Frasure-Smith, N. et al. Depression and 18-month prognosis after myocardial infarction. *Circulation*, 1995 February 15;91(4): 999–1005.
13. Williams, R. B. et al. Prognostic importance of social and economic resources among medically treated patients with angiographically documented coronary artery disease. *Journal of the American Medical Association*, 1992;267: 520–524.

14. White, J. M. Effects of relaxing music on cardiac autonomic balance and anxiety after acute myocardial infarction. *American Journal of Critical Care*, 1999 July;8(4): 220–30.
15. Volz, H. P. et al. Kava-kava extract WS 1490 versus placebo in anxiety disorders—a randomized placebo-controlled 25-week outpatient trial. *Pharmacopsychiatry*, 1997;30(1): 1–5.
16. Cohen, H. W. et al. Excess risk of myocardial infarction treated with antidepressant medications: association with use of tricyclic agents. *American Journal of Medicine*, 2000 January;108(1): 2–8.

CHAPTER 17

1. Mitchell, L. E. et al. Evidence for an association between dehydroepiandrosterone sulfate and nonfatal, premature myocardial infarction in males. *Circulation*, January 1994;89: 89–93.
2. Feldman, H. A. et al. Low dehydroepiandrosterone and ischemic heart disease in middle-aged men: prospective results from the Massachusetts Male Aging Study. *American Journal of Epidemiology*, 2001 January 1;153(1): 79–89.
3. Porsova-Dutoit, I. et al. Do DHEA/DHEAS play a protective role in coronary heart disease? *Physiological Research*, 2000;49 Suppl 1: S43–56.
4. Kreze, A. Jr. et al. Dehydrdoepiandrosterone, dehydroepiandrosteron-sulfate and insulin in acute myocardial infarct. *Vnitrÿni Lekarÿstvi*, 2000 December;46(12): 835–8.
5. Kahaly, G. J. Cardiovascular and atherogenic aspects of subclinical hypothyroidism. *Thyroid*, 2000 August;10(8): 665–79.
6. Phillips, G. B. et al. The association of hypotestosteronemia with coronary artery disease in man. *Arteriosclerosis Thrombosis*, 1994 May;14(5): 701–6.

7. Zhao, S. et al. Plasma levels of lipids, lipoproteins and apolipoproteins affected by endogenous testosterone. *Hunan Yi Ke Da Xue Xue Bao* 1998;23(3): 299–301.
8. Webb, C. M. et al. Effects of testosterone on coronary vasomotor regulation in men with coronary heart disease. *Circulation*, 1999 October;100(16): 1690–6.
9. Stellato, R. K. et al. Testosterone, sex hormone-binding globulin, and the development of type 2 diabetes in middle-aged men: prospective results from the Massachusetts male aging study. *Diabetes Care*, 2000 April;23(4): 490–4.
10. English, K. M. et al. Low-dose transdermal testosterone therapy improves angina threshold in men with chronic stable angina: A randomized, double-blind, placebo-controlled study. *Circulation*, 2000 October 17;102(16): 1906–11.
11. Stampfer, M. J. et al. Estrogen replacement therapy and coronary heart disease: a quantitative assessment of epidemologic evidence. *Preventive Medicine*, 1991;20: 47–63.
12. Effects of estrogen or estrogen/progestin regimens on heart disease risk factors in postmenopausal women. The Postmenopausal Estrogen/Progestin Intervention (PEPI) Trial. *Journal of the American Medical Association*, 1995 January 18;273(3): 199–208.
13. Hemminki, E. et al. Impact of postmenopausal hormone therapy on cardiovascular events and cancer: pooled data from clinic trials. *British Medical Journal*, 1997;315: 149–53.
14. Hulley, S. et al for the H Heart and Estrogen Replacement Study (HERS) Research Group. Randomized trial of estrogen plus progestin for secondary prevention of coronary heart disease in postmenopausal women. *Journal of the American Medical Association*, 1998;280: 605–13.
15. Herrington, D. M. et al. Effects of estrogen replacement on the progression of coronary-artery atherosclerosis. *New England Journal of Medicine*, 2000;343: 522–9.
16. Wenger, N. K. HRT and CHD: Balancing risk and suggested benefit. *Patient Care*, 2000 October 30; 32–55.

17. Wolfe, S. M. Postmenopausal estrogen replacement therapy: is its value exaggerated and its role vanishing? *Worst Pills, Best Pills News*, 2001 February;7(2): 9–11.
18. Ibid.
19. Westendorp, I. C. et al. Hormone replacement therapy and peripheral arterial disease: the Rotterdam study. *Archives of Internal Medicine*, 2000 September 11;160(16): 2498–502.
20. Reis, S. E. et al. Estrogen is associated with improved survival in aging women with congestive heart failure: analysis of the vesnarinone studies. *Journal of the American College of Cardiology*, 2000 August;36(2): 529–33.
21. Sitruk-Ware, R. Progestins and cardiovascular risk markers. *Steroids*, 2000 October–November;65(10–11): 651–8
22. Rosano, G. M. et al. Natural progesterone, but not medroxyprogesterone acetate, enhances the beneficial effect of estrogen on exercise-induced myocardial ischemia in postmenopausal women. *Journal of the American College of Cardiology*, 2000 December;36(7): 2154–9
23. Rudman, D. et al. Effects of human growth hormone in men over 60 years of age. *New England Journal of Medicine*, 1990 July 5;323(1): 1–6.
24. Bocchi, E. A. et al. Growth hormone for optimization of refractory heart failure treatment. *Arquivos Brasileiros de Cardiologia*, 1999 October;73(4): 391–8.

CHAPTER 18

1. Lawson, W. E. et al. Efficacy of enhanced external counterpulsation in the treatment of angina pectoris. *American Journal of Cardiology*, October 1, 1992;70: 859–862.
2. Fricchione, G. L. et al. Psychosocial effects of enhanced external counterpulsation in the angina patient. *Psychosomatics*, September–October 1995;36(5): 494–49.

3. Aurora, R. R. et al. The Multicenter Study of Enhanced External Counterpulsation. *Journal of the American College of Cardiology*, 1999;33(7): 1833–40.
4. Arora, R. R. et al. Results of the multicenter study of Enhanced External Counterpulsation (MUST-EECP): clinical benefits are sustained at a mean follow-up time of one year. *Supplement, Journal of the American College of Cardiology*, (abstracts, 47th annual scientific session), February 1998;31(2, suppl. A): abstract 859–62.
5. Meltzer, L. E. Report on therapy, the treatment of coronary artery disease with disodium EDTA, a reappraisal. *American Journal of Cardiology*, 1963 April;0: 501.
6. Chappel, L. T. et al. The correlation between EDTA chelation therapy and improvement in cardiovascular function: a meta-analysis. *Journal of Advancement in Medicine*, 1993 fall;6(3): 139–60.
7. Chappel, T. *Questions from the Heart*. Charlottesville, Cal: Hampton Roads Publishing Company, Inc., 1995.
8. Walker, M. Cardiac therapy: hyperbaric oxygen and your heart. *Explore*, 1998;9(1).

INDEX

more . . .

REVERSING ASTHMA

Breathe Easier with This Revolutionary New Program

by Richard N. Firshein, D.O.

Here is a guide that not only helps relieve the symptoms of asthma but gets to the root of your problem. From a nationally renowned asthma specialist who is also a lifelong asthma sufferer, this acclaimed book gives you the program Dr. Firshein developed for himself and his patients. This groundbreaking new program will help you cut down on wheezing, allergic reactions, and asthma drugs. You'll learn to change your lifestyle and breathe easier—in a way that boosts your vitality and improves your general health.